Y0-BCO-682

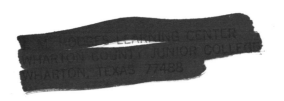

HOSPITAL QUALITY ASSURANCE

Risk Management and Program Evaluation

Edited by

Jesus J. Peña, M.P.A., J.D.
Senior Vice President
St. Michael's Medical Center
Newark, New Jersey

Bernard Rosen, Ph.D.
Director—Program Evaluation
Kingsboro Psychiatric Center
Brooklyn, New York

Alden N. Haffner, O.D., Ph.D.
Associate Chancellor for Health
  Sciences
State University of New York
Albany, New York

Donald W. Light, Ph.D.
Professor of Community Medicine
  and Medical Sociology
University of Medicine and
  Dentistry of New Jersey/
  NJSOM
Camden, New Jersey

68874

AN ASPEN PUBLICATION®
Aspen Systems Corporation
Rockville, Maryland
Royal Tunbridge Wells
1984

Library of Congress Cataloging in Publication Data
Main entry under title:

Hospital quality assurance.

"An Aspen publication."
1. Hospital care — Quality control. 2. Hospital care — Evaluation.
3. Quality assurance. I. Peña, Jesus J. [DNLM: 1. Quality
assurance, Health care. 2. Financial management. 3. Evaluation
studies. 4. Hospital administration — Economics. WX 153 H8255]
RA972.H683   1984   362.1'1'0685   83-21486
ISBN: 0-89443-942-1

Publisher: John R. Marozsan
Associate Publisher: Jack W. Knowles, Jr.
Editor-in-Chief: Michael Brown
Executive Managing Editor: Margot G. Raphael
Managing Editor: M. Eileen Higgins
Printing and Manufacturing: Debbie Collins

Library of Congress Catalog Card Number: 83-21486
ISBN: 0-89443-942-1

Printed in the United States of America

2   3   4   5

Table of Contents

Editors

Jesus J. Peña, M.P.A., J.D.
Senior Vice President
St. Michael's Medical Center
Newark, New Jersey

Bernard Rosen, Ph.D.
Director—Program Evaluation
Kingsboro Psychiatric Center
Brooklyn, New York

Alden N. Haffner, O.D., Ph.D.
Associate Chancellor for Health
   Sciences
State University of New York
Albany, New York

Donald W. Light, Ph.D.
Professor of Community Medicine
   and Medical Sociology
University of Medicine and
   Dentistry of New Jersey/
   NJSOM
Camden, New Jersey

Contributors

John E. Affeldt, M.D.
President, Joint Commission on
   Accreditation of Hospitals
Chicago, Illinois

*Marianne D. Araujo, R.N.,
M.S.N.*
Vice President, Nursing and
   General Administration
Mercy Hospital and Medical
   Center
Chicago, Illinois

Joseph N. Cintron, M.H.A.
Executive Director
Lincoln Hospital
Bronx, New York

*Avedis Donabedian, M.D.,
M.P.H.*
Nathan Sinai Distinguished
   Professor of Public Health
The University of Michigan
Ann Arbor, Michigan

B. Abbott Goldberg, LL.B.
Judge of the Superior Court
   (Retired)
Scholar in Residence, McGeorge
   School of Law University of
   the Pacific
Sacramento, California

Alden N. Haffner, O.D., Ph.D.
Vice Chancellor for Research,
   Graduate Studies, and
   Professional Programs
State University of New York
Albany, New York

*James W. Holsinger, Jr.
M.D., Ph.D.*
Professor of Medicine and
   Health Administration
Virginia Commonwealth
   University
Richmond, Virginia, and,
Medical Director, V.A. Hospital
Richmond, Virginia

ix

Steven Jonas, M.D., M.P.H.
Associate Professor of
    Community and Preventive
    Medicine
State University at Stony Brook
Stony Brook, New York

*Joanne T. Jurkovic, R.N.,
M.S.*
Director, Quality Assurance
    Program
Mercy Hospital and Medical
    Center
Chicago, Illinois

Patricia M. Kearns, M.S.
Assistant Administrator
Malcolm Grow Medical Center
Andrews Air Force Base,
    Maryland

*Christine T. Kovner, R.N.,
M.S.N.*
New York University
New York, New York

Alan M. Leiken, Ph.D.
Assistant Professor, Department
    of Allied Health Resources
State University of New York at
    Stony Brook
Stony Brook, New York

Donald W. Light, Ph.D.
Professor and Director of
    Behavioral and Social
    Medicine
Department of Psychiatry
U.M.D.-New Jersey Medical
    School of Osteopathic
    Medicine
Camden, New Jersey

William E. McAuliffe, Ph.D.
Associate Professor of Sociology
Department of Behavioral
    Sciences
Harvard University School of
    Public Health
Boston, Massachusetts

*Edmund J. McTernan, M.P.H.,
Ed.D.*
Professor of Allied Health
    Sciences
School of Allied Health
    Professions
State University of New York at
    Stony Brook
Stony Brook, New York

Gregory Parston, Ph.D.
Assistant Professor
Graduate School of Public
    Administration
New York University
New York, New York

Beatriz M. Peña, M.P.H.
Manager, Occupational Health
    Information System
Merck & Company, Incorporated
Rahway, New Jersey

Jesus J. Peña, M.P.A., J.D.
Senior Vice President
Saint Michael's Medical Center
Newark, New Jersey

*Burton Pollack, M.P.H.,
D.D.S., J.D.*
Professor of Dental Health
State University of New York at
    Stony Brook
Stony Brook, New York

James R. Posner, Ph.D.
Vice President and Director,
    Special Hospital Program
Marsh & McLennan,
    Incorporated
New York, New York

Richard Quan, M.B.A., J.D.
Hospital Litigation Specialist
Quan & Nodroff
New York, New York

Robert M. Refowitz, M.D., Ph.D.
Medical Director
United States Metal Refining
    Company
Carteret, New Jersey

Bernard Rosen, Ph.D.
Director of Program Evaluation
Kingsboro Psychiatric Center
Brooklyn, New York

David J. Slawkowski, J.D.
Malpractice Specialist
Lord, Bissell and Brook
Chicago, Illinois

Regina M. Walczak, M.P.H.
Director of Quality Assurance
Joint Commission on
    Accreditation of Hospitals
Chicago, Illinois

John R.C. Wheeler, Ph.D.
Assistant Professor
School of Public Health
The University of Michigan
Ann Arbor, Michigan

Sankey V. Williams, M.D.
Assistant Professor of Medicine
Henry J. Kaiser Family
    Foundation Faculty Scholar
Section of General Medicine
    and
Associate Director for Medical
    Affairs
Leonard Davis Institute of Health
    Economics
University of Pennsylvania
Philadelphia, Pennsylvania

Leon Wyszewianski, Ph.D.
Associate Professor
School of Public Health
The University of Michigan
Ann Arbor, Michigan

Preface

During the past 20 years, a number of important developments have had a profound impact on the delivery of health care in the United States. Perhaps the most important of these, to both administrators and patients, has been the change in society's attitudes toward the quality of care that a patient could expect a hospital to deliver. At one time, a hospital could be legally held only to that standard of care that was "customarily offered by hospitals generally in its community."[1] However, by 1979, this had changed drastically. The Pediatric Bill of Rights states expressly that patients are entitled to "competent health care,"[2] and the Joint Commission in its 1979 edition of the *Accreditation Manual for Hospitals* stated that "The hospital shall demonstrate that the quality of care provided to all patients is consistently optimal. . . ."[3] The Joint Commission modified this requirement in subsequent standards to "The hospital shall demonstrate a consistent endeavor to deliver patient care that is optimal within available resources and consistent with achievable goals."[4] However, in their statutory laws or in administrative regulations having the force of law, many states have mandated that hospitals, through their medical staffs, have responsibility for the quality of care given to their patients.

This increased emphasis on the provision of quality health care stems, in large part, from the greater involvement of governmental and insurance agencies in health care, through their role as third party payers. As the amount of money spent by these third party payers increased, their concern that their money was being used efficiently also increased. The care given by hospitals began to be scrutinized with increasing frequency, with the result that, in many instances, payment for services had been refused by third party payers because the patient's length of stay was unnecessarily long or aspects of the care were inconsistent with the diagnosis. Concomitantly, juries began increasingly to find for the plaintiff in malpractice and negligence suits against hospitals. The large monetary settlements in these suits caused the providers of negligence and malpractice liability insurance to put additional pressure on hospitals to monitor the quality of care provided.

Thus, while there is general agreement on the need to provide quality health care and to conform to the regulations requiring the monitoring of this care, there is little agreement as to what constitutes quality care or what form the monitoring should take. The definition of quality assurance in the health field is generally elusive, if not controversial. In manufacturing, *quality assurance* can be defined simply as a program to minimize the number of defective parts produced, but it is not as easy to define in the health field. *Quality of care* in the health field implies more than reducing the number of malpractice suits or the number of deaths from a given procedure. Rather, it implies that health care is provided in such a manner as to improve the health and functioning of the patient. As such, quality of care can be seen as an all-encompassing term, which can include anything that influences the health and functioning of the patient, from the environment, to staff morale and training, the evaluation of programs, and the efficiency of the various departments in the facility.

In our view one of the biggest obstacles to the provision of quality health care on a consistent basis is the complex nature of hospitals. There are enormous pressures on the administrator to deal with a large number of emergencies— political, financial, and medical. It is impossible, in this complex setting, for any administrator to keep abreast of all aspects of the operation of the institution, or even his or her section of it. In addition, since the existence of problems often can be ascertained only by examining trends, organized information must be available to the administrator so that he or she can assess the facility's performance against the standards it has set up.

Within the above framework, quality assurance can be defined as the process that sets the standards for performance, provides information about the achievement of those standards, and monitors whether improvement has taken place and whether the standards are being met. Because the delivery of quality care is dependent upon the availability of sufficient funds, cost containment and quality care may seem to be contradictory terms. However, as pointed out in this book, the two processes can be compatible. Thus, the authors approach quality assurance in practical terms with an emphasis on the relationship between quality assurance, program evaluation, and risk management. The joint aim of these components is to provide practical information for improving the efficiency of the facility, as well as reducing or eliminating risks to patients and employees.

The current emphasis on quality assurance programs may indicate a final attempt on the part of the regulatory agencies and third party payers to permit the industry to regulate itself. It is the authors' hope that this book will provide some help in the success of this attempt and in the overall improvement of health care in this country.

NOTES

1. In Darling 33 Ill.2d at 331, 211 N.E.2d at 257; 50 Ill. App.2d at 309, 200 N.E.2d at 277.

2. W. Curran & E. Shapiro, *Law Medicine and Forensic Science* (3rd edition), 1982, p. 757.

3. Joint Commission on Accreditation of Hospitals, *Accreditation Manual for Hospitals*, J.C.A.H., Chicago, 1975.

4. Joint Commssion on Accreditation of Hospitals, *Accreditation Manual for Hospitals*, J.C.A.H., Chicago, 1981.

Acknowledgments

Editing a book with such a large number of contributors requires a great deal of coordination with regard to peoples' differences and styles. The editors thank the contributors for their patience and their cooperation in responding to the demands made upon them.

In addition, we also thank Christine Baumgartner for her invaluable assistance in coordinating the work. Such coordination was necessary to ensure the successful completion of this book. Thanks also go to Susan Lulek for her work in verifying the references and retyping portions of the manuscripts.

Part I

Quality Assurance: Historical, Legal, and Social Perspectives

Chapter 1

Regulating the Quality of Patient Care*

Alden N. Haffner, O.D., Ph.D., Steven Jonas, M.D., M.P.H., and
Burton Pollack, D.D.S., M.P.H., J.D.

INTRODUCTION

According to Avedis Donabedian, professor of public health at the University of Michigan:

> We have granted the health professions access to the most secret and sensitive places in ourselves and entrusted to them matters that touch on our well-being, happiness, and survival. In return, we have expected the professions to govern themselves so strictly that we need have no fear of exploitation or incompetence. The object of quality assessment is to determine how successful they have been in doing so; and the purpose of quality monitoring is to exercise constant surveillance so that departure from standards can be detected early and corrected.[1] (p.11)

A number of measures show that health care delivered in the United States varies sharply in quality. In fact, quality health care is professed by many but achieved by few. Is it a concept that eludes achievement because it is not understood? Is quality care too costly and, therefore, difficult to secure? Or, is it a concept that is not sufficiently ingrained so that it is relatively easily obviated? The answers to the three questions, are, in our opinion, "yes." In the climate of today's public opinion and attitudes, it would be tragic to define quality health care as that which is delivered in the absence of malpractice suits. The lack of legal action does not, perforce, mean quality health services, and the presence (or the threat) of a legal action does not automatically mean poor health care.

---

*Sections of this chapter are taken from Steven Jonas, *Health Care Delivery in the United States*, (2nd edition). Copyright ©1981 by Springer Publishing Company, Inc., New York. Used by permission. Other sections are taken from "Essential Administrative Ingredients of Risk Management as a Preventive Against Malpractice" by Alden N. Haffner in *Public Health Reports*, 92, 462, 1977.

In a sense, quality care is like honesty. It must pervade the very fiber of the individual or the institution. It is particularly important that quality care be an ingrained philosophy in an institution where there is a complexity of behavior and performance patterns, secured by rules, and developed through some rational plan. To be effective and to reflect the character of the institution, quality care and the striving for it must be intrinsic in the myriad of decision-making processes that make up the totality of the institution's operations.

But why *must* quality pervade the very fiber of the individual or the institution? First, perhaps, is the principle *primum non nocere:* "Primarily, do no harm." The precept is at least as old as the Hippocratic Oath, of which it is a part. As the following discussion of the results of quality determinations will demonstrate, this consideration is important in a health care delivery system in which a substantial minority of care delivered is of less than good quality and could be harmful.

Second, our society devotes a significant and increasing portion of its economic resources to providing health services. Americans have a strong interest in obtaining a good product for the money spent. Further, there are social and humanitarian motivations to see that the large sums of money spent actually help those persons who are receiving the services.

Third, from the providers' point of view, a major motivation for doing good work in health care is professionalism. The concepts of "profession" and "professionalism" are related to quality. A profession is, in part at least, a field of human endeavor in which the practitioners themselves control entry and exit, in which a common body of knowledge exists, and in which the practitioners attempt to expand and develop that body of knowledge to improve the quality of human life and extend the understanding of human existence. This last aspect of professionalism, aside from personal pecuniary and self-protective interests, adds a strong impetus to the thrust of at least part of the medical profession to regulate and improve the quality of medical care.

Finally, there is a strong social ethic in our culture to value doing a good job in and of itself. This principle has deep historical roots in the Judeo-Christian tradition; its origins probably stem from the individual and species survival value of performing tasks well. In health care, of course, there is a direct link between both individual and species survival and doing a good job in personal and community health services.

If quality assurance in health care is a good thing, how can it be achieved?

CAN QUALITY BE EVALUATED?

But how is quality measured? Do procedures exist that permit a rational method or means by which to "stamp" one institution as being of a higher quality than another? The answers to both questions are elusive and given the rudimentary state of the art, undoubtedly controversial. In the words of McKillop:

Primitive is perhaps the best word to describe the present state of the art of quality assessment. The analysis of one chart by an individual member of a medical audit committee parallels the work of an individual artisan before the industrial revolution. The failure of this method to attain quality control is obvious. Many articulate spokesmen for the health care field acknowledge that hospital medical staff activities to ensure consistent quality and to maintain quality control have not been successful.

Nonsystematic is another descriptive term for the present state of the art. When medical care is evaluated, it is done on an individual, random, episodic basis. The results contribute little to continuing medical education, quality of patient care, and quality control of medical practice.

Episodic is another word that may be used to describe the present process of evaluating medical care in most hospitals. The episodic nature of the medical audit flows of necessity from the episodic nature of medical care. Physicians, sociologists, and representatives of many other disciplines have talked long and often about the nature of today's medical care, which is episodic, crisis-oriented, and disease-oriented. Those concerned with the nature of the evaluation of such care find themselves describing the review process in the same terms that those who describe the actual process of care use.[2] (pp.44–45)

Nevertheless, while the present system in practice, is primitive, nonsystematic, and episodic, its theory and techniques, at least for measurement if not assurance, are reasonably well developed. It is the implementation that is faulty.

The extent to which quality of care can be evaluated has been a subject of debate. A former president of the American Medical Association, Russell Roth, said in a presidential address that "good quality in medical care is not something which can be expressed in dollars of cost, hours of time, or for that matter, in decibels of political oratory. Quality of such medical care is not a tangible, qualifiable thing."[3] He added there are "immense difficulties" inherent in properly identifying high-quality care. On the other hand, many authorities in the field have thought it possible to measure and regulate the quality of discrete instances of care delivery. Codman has been recognized as the granddaddy of outcome studies.[4–7] Emphasizing his faith in their efficacy as measures of quality, he said, "While a layman could not authoritatively inquire into the details of the reasons why, he could insist that the end-result system should be used, that someone must see that it is used, and that an efficiency committee be appointed for the purpose."[6]

Lee and Jones wrote a landmark work on quality determination in 1933, which was built around the concept that "good medical care is the kind of medicine practiced and taught by the recognized leaders of the medical profession at a given time or period of social, cultural, and professional development in a community or population group."[8] Thus they felt that quality could be measured against the value judgments of recognized professional leaders. In 1951, Weinerman, reflecting the 1949 statement made by the Subcommittee on Medical Care of the American Public Health Association in "The Quality of Medical Care in a National Health Program,"[9] said: "The quality of medical care is a composite of all the technical, organizational, and financial aspects of any program for personal health service. Good quality can be defined, consciously planned, and evaluated."[10] Thus Weinerman introduced the concept of structural criteria (see below). The American Public Health Association's belief in the possibility of measuring quality was amply restated in the second volume of *A Guide to Medical Care Administration: Medical Care Appraisal—Quality and Utilization*.[11]

In their work describing the "tracer method" of quality measurement, Kessner and his co-authors said, "The question is no longer whether there will be intervention in health services to assure quality, but who will intervene and what methods they will use."[12] In a review article, Brook said, "Even though the perfect system for assessment and assurance of quality care may not yet exist, innumerable simple efforts can be made to improve quality of care. If applied in a systematic manner, many are likely to be successful."[13]

It happens, as it so often does, that there is nothing new about all of this. In 1732, Francis Clifton, an English physician, wrote: "Three of four persons should be employed in the hospitals to set down the cases of the patients from day to day candidly and judiciously without any regard to ɔrivate opinions and public systems, and at the year's end publish these facts just as they are—leaving everyone to make the best use he could for himself."[14]

HOW IS QUALITY OF HEALTH CARE PRESENTLY ASSESSED AND ASSURED?

The first problem in analyzing quality measurement in health care is to classify and understand the different methodologies. Many review articles[1,4,11,15,16,17,18,19] have established schemata for classifying the techniques or methodologies used for measuring the quality of medical care delivered by individuals or institutions. However, before examining the techniques for evaluating the quality of care, it is useful to understand the approaches to quality measurement and control that are actually in use in the United States. (See Exhibit 1-1.) In the early 1970s, Roemer,[20] Lewis,[6] and Ellwood et al.[21] began to take this necessary broader view.

The *approaches* are those various methods used to ensure quality in the health care delivery system, such as licensing, accreditation, and peer review through

Exhibit 1-1 Approaches, Techniques, and Criteria for Measuring the Quality of Health Care

1. Approaches
     General
        licensing
        accreditation
        certification
     Specific
        hospital medical staff review committees
        professional standards review organizations
        patient satisfaction
        malpractice litigation
2. Techniques
     Evaluation of structure; evaluation of physical facilities and administrative organization
     Evaluation of process: evaluation of activities of physicians and other health staff professionals in management of patients
     Evaluation of outcome: evaluation of effects of care on the end results in terms of health and satisfaction
3. Criteria
     Explicit—written down
     Implicit—exist only in the mind of the evaluator

hospital medical staff committees. *Techniques* are the ways quality is measured within the various approaches. Techniques are only tools; approaches use the tools to effect control or at least attempt to do so. Thus, techniques are scientific constructs, whereas approaches are political ones.

Approaches

The approaches may be divided into two groups—the general and the specific. The general approaches examine an individual's or an institution's ability to meet established evaluative criteria at a particular time. Individuals are evaluated in terms of experience, education, and knowledge (usually measured by examination). Institutions are evaluated on the basis of physical structure, administrative and staff organization, minimum capabilities and standards for the provision of service, and personnel qualifications. If the criteria are met at the time of evaluation, it is then predicted that the individual or institution will function well either indefinitely, as in the case of the medical license, or for a given period of time, as in the case of the hospital license. The general approaches used in the United States are licensing, accreditation, and certification.[22,23,24]

The specific approaches to quality measurement and control, on the other hand, look at discrete instances of provider-patient interaction and evaluate them using one of several available techniques. The major specific approaches in use in the United States are hospital medical staff review committees; Peer Review Organizations (formerly Professional Standards Review Organizations); patient satisfaction; and malpractice litigation, an extreme product of patient dissatisfaction.

Techniques

Donabedian has provided the generally accepted classification of the techniques of quality assessment:*

> Three major approaches to the evaluation of quality have been identified. These have been designated as the evaluation of structure, process, and outcome or end results.
>
> Appraisal of structure involves the evaluation of the settings and instrumentalities available and used for the provision of care. While including the physical aspects of facilities and equipment, structural appraisal goes far beyond to encompass the characteristics of the administrative organization and the qualifications of health professionals. . . . Two major assumptions are made when structure is taken as an indicator of quality: First, that better care is more likely to be provided when better qualified staff, improved physical facilities and sounder fiscal and administrative organization are employed. Second, that we know enough to identify what is good in terms of staff, physical structure and formal organization   . .
>
> Assessment of process is the evaluation of the activities of physicians and other health professionals in the management of patients. The criterion generally used is the degree to which management of patients conforms with the standards and expectations of the respective professions. These standards and expectations may be derived from what is considered to be ideal, good, or acceptable practice as formulated by recognized leaders in the profession. Such standards may also be inferred from patterns of care observed in actual practice. . . .
>
> When evaluation of process is the basis for judgments concerning quality, a major assumption is that health care is useful in maintaining or promoting health. Furthermore, there is the explicit or implicit assumption that particular elements and aspects of care are known to be specifically related to successful or unsuccessful health outcomes

---

*Donabedian uses the word *approaches* in the sense in which the word *techniques* is used in this chapter.

or end results. Assessment of outcomes is the evaluation of end results in terms of health and satisfaction. That this evaluation in many ways provides the final evidence of whether care has been good, bad or indifferent is so because of the broad fundamental social and professional agreement on what results are deemed desirable. Furthermore, it is assumed that good results are brought about, at least to a significant degree, by good care.[11] (pp.2–3)

Thus, the structural approach examines the setting of care; the process approach examines what goes on between the provider(s) and the patient; and the outcome approach examines the results of the encounter between the patient and the health care delivery system. In the main, the structural technique is used in the general approaches, while the process and outcome techniques are used in the specific approaches, sometimes in combination with the structural technique as well.

Criteria

Explicit Criteria

In all three techniques, criteria are used in the evaluation process. Explicit criteria are written down, and the work under study is checked against them. For example, in a process study of physician performance, an explicit criterion might be that, in the course of a good physical examination, a blood pressure measurement is taken. If a medical record is being used as the medium of evaluation, the evaluator would then check to see if a blood pressure measurement had been recorded. Actually, if the evaluation is being made solely on the basis of the medical record, a blood pressure notation can mean either that the pressure was taken and recorded or that it was not taken and a number was put down anyway. The absence of a blood pressure reading in the record can mean either that it was not taken or that it was taken and not recorded. Of the four possibilities, only the first represents good medical care.

Implicit Criteria

Implicit criteria, on the other hand, exist only in the mind of the evaluator. Nothing specific to look for is written down. Evaluators are picked on the basis of their own credentials and reputations. The assumption is made that since they are "good" physicians (or dentists, nurses, etc.), they will be able to distinguish between "good" and "bad" care and will be able to make valid and reliable assessments.

Thus, there are two groups of approaches, three sets of techniques, and two categories of criteria. They are organized in various combinations in practice in the United States.

HOW IS QUALITY ACTUALLY ACHIEVED BY INSTITUTIONS AND INDIVIDUALS?

As pointed out above, the techniques and methods are there. Over a long period of time, a variety of authorities have said that the job can be done. Yet there are serious gaps in the quality of the product provided by the U.S. health care delivery system. Over the years, a large number of research studies have been carried out in the problem area of measuring and controlling the quality of particular instances of medical care delivery using the process and/or outcome techniques. They have generally shown deficits in the quality of care, regardless of the methods used.

There have been a number of reviews of the literature. Sheps considered a large series of primarily clinical evaluations.[19] Her review included one of the earliest attempts to categorize the techniques of quality evaluation. Anderson and Altman produced an annotated bibliography covering the period 1955–1961.[25] Donabedian produced three major reviews in the late 1960s.[11,15,16] In the early 1970s, a large literature review was undertaken by Brook[4] and again by Brook and colleagues in 1977.[26] A major review of the state of the art in the early 1970s was held under the aegis of the Graduate Program in Hospital Administration of the University of Chicago in 1973.[27] Christoffel published a comprehensive bibliography in the mid-1970s,[28] as did the Institute of Medicine.[29] Christoffel and Lowenthal reviewed the literature on ambulatory care quality assessment in 1977.[30]

Certain studies can be considered landmarks. In 1953 to 1954, a study of general practice in North Carolina used both structural and process techniques and explicit criteria in a direct observation method. It was found that "Many physicians were performing at a high level of professional competence. Of greater importance is the fact that other physicians were performing at a lower level. . . ."[31] Of the various parameters measured, only the length of postgraduate hospital training in internal medicine was consistently related to the quality of a physician's clinical work. Academic performance, for example, was related to quality of clinical work only for physicians aged 35 and less.[31] Lembcke was one of the pioneers in developing the hospital medical audit, using analysis of clinical records.[32] As an example, he evaluated major female pelvic surgery in several hospitals and found that the introduction of auditing techniques reduced both the population hysterectomy rate and the proportion of unnecessary hysterectomies.

In the period 1957 to 1961, a review of medical records, process and outcome techniques, and implicit criteria[33] were used in a study of 406 admissions of members of the Teamsters Unions and their families to hospitals in New York City. The study found that 88 percent of admissions were justifiable. However, only 57 percent of the patients received "good or excellent medical care," while a fifth received fair care, and another fifth received poor care. A second study by the same researchers in 1962, using a slightly different evaluation technique, arrived at similar conclusions.[34] Some observers consider that implicit criteria have limited applicability since they rely entirely on the internal judgments of the evaluators.[35]

In the late 1960s and early 1970s, a series of studies on quality of medical care in neighborhood health centers, primarily using process techniques,[36,37,38] showed that such techniques could be widely applied; the quality of care in neighborhood health centers was found to be reasonably good compared to that found in other organized ambulatory care settings.

Applying the tracer method to two different pediatric population groups in Washington, D.C., Kessner and colleagues found that "inappropriate" or "ineffective" treatment for specific tracer conditions was documented in a large proportion of the children.[39,40]

At the same time that Kessner was breaking new ground in developing a quality measurement method combining the process and outcome techniques, Brook was carrying out another landmark study, comparing five different types of process and outcome evaluations of the same medical care episodes.[4,41] Brook and Appel summarized the work as follows:

> The care of 296 patients with urinary-tract infection, hypertension or ulcerated gastric or duodenal lesions was reviewed with the use of the five methods. Depending on the method, from 1.4 to 63.2 percent of patients were judged to have received adequate care. Judgment of process using explicit criteria yielded the fewest acceptable cases (1.4 percent). The largest differences found were between methods using different sources of data. Thus, medical care, judged with implicit criteria, was rated adequate for 23.3 percent of patients when process, and 63.2 percent when outcome was used.[41] (p.1,323)

In his major publication on his study, Brook[4] concluded that although serious methodological problems remain in assessment of the quality of care, it is still nevertheless true that as many as 25 percent of the patients would have had better outcomes if the medical processes had been better. Brook noted:

> It is, therefore, recommended that simple routine assessments of quality of care which employ carefully selected outcomes and processes should begin even while awaiting definitive methodologic research. Such studies using outcome measurements as a means to identify high priority areas could have a major impact on the health of the American people without dramatically increasing the cost of such care.

A number of other studies of the quality of medical care have been conducted. For example, in a national quiz of physician volunteers of their knowledge of the use of antibiotics, the average score was 68 percent.[42] In the New Mexico Medicaid program, a peer review program was designed to correct deficiencies. The use of injections, of which half were antibiotics, was considered by the peer reviewers to be inappropriate in 40 percent of cases. The peer review program did achieve a drop in the use of injections from 41 per 100 ambulatory visits to 16 per 100 ambulatory visits.[43]

In another study, fewer than 10 percent of patients admitted to a university hospital had a routine serologic test for syphilis performed, yet in those tested the response was positive in 6 percent of cases. Effective therapy was not given in one-third of them and in two-thirds of them, syphilis was not listed as a discharge diagnosis.[44] Whether or not any of the detected cases was reported to the local health department, a measure essential for control of the disease in the population, was not recorded in the study.

In an evaluation of burn care in Florida, it could not be shown that, even when adjusting for case severity, hospitals with burn units did better than those without, and "many records were poor, admissions were inappropriate, patients with minor burns stayed too long, and burn shock was too frequent."[45]

A study of the work of over 1,300 physicians in 22 Maryland and Pennsylvania hospitals used one of the classic process tools, the Physician Performance Index developed by Payne and colleagues at the University of Michigan. The average score was about 70 percent.[46]

In another study, 36 percent of 815 consecutive patients admitted to a general medical service showed evidence of an iatrogenic illness. For nine percent of these patients, iatrogenesis threatened life or produced considerable disability. In two percent of cases, it was considered to have contributed to the patient's death.[47]

Thus, there is plenty of evidence that the quality of care provided is not what it should or could be. However, changing the system and its results is another matter. What needs to be done?

Leadership for Quality

Adherence to principles of quality and the constant efforts needed to strive for them in a health care institution begin (and, indeed, may falter and end abruptly) with the element of leadership. Leadership is that aspect of administration that sets the tone of an institution. Clearly, as in any form of complex organization, the major function of the head of the institution, its chief administrative officer, is to exercise leadership to accomplish the stated and accepted goals and objectives. He or she enunciates them and interprets them to the staffs and to the community. He or she provides the inspiration for others to follow. It is that very leadership function that ingrains those desirable behavioral patterns that result in quality outcomes. As stated by Wilcox, "Their reasoning is that the hospital corporation is ultimately responsible for the quality of patient care provided in the hospital and may be named as a defendant and be held liable for any injury directly caused by a staff member's act that is performed within the hospital."[3] (p. 3)

Leadership that is goal and achievement oriented, with quality as a behavioral objective, is constant and never ending. Such leadership recognizes and rewards quality in all of its aspects and analyzes those areas and functions that are identified for their lack of quality in order to upgrade them.

Planning for Quality

If everything is done correctly, does that mean quality? The answer is "no," emphatically. Quality can be planned. Such planning is a deliberate and carefully thought out effort to identify omissions, delays, and inefficiencies in order to reduce time, conserve energies and resources, and allow for the achievement of objectives more directly, more successfully, and with a crispness of style. This is what patients feel and understand—an air of efficiency that comes about because a plan has been developed for the operation. The more effective the planning effort is as an administrative function, the clearer the element and process of accountability will be, particularly to the institution's clientele, the patients.

No plan achieves its goals—quality care and services—unless the plan is understood. There can be no commitment to carrying out the plan in the absence of that understanding. Commitment is total, not partial, and it is translated for all personnel of an institution, not just a few.

Molding Attitudes about Quality

Of course, everyone believes in quality care. But the reality frequently differs from the attitude, and it is the collective attitude of the institution's personnel that determines the relative degree of quality exhibited by the institution. An actively favorable attitude about all aspects of quality in the delivery of health care must be aggressively pursued. The lack of such an attitude, particularly on the part of administration, may result in a sense of passivity that leads to a "high verbal but low performance" environment. It becomes the ongoing role of the administrative leadership to analyze and to mold, in very lifelike situations, attitudes of staff members at all levels from the patients' viewpoints. A training program to foster positive attitudes toward patients should be continuous and unrelenting, and it should extend to all levels of the staff and to their performances. The key to molding staff members' attitudes is the fundamental understanding of their roles in patient care that, in totality, compose quality care.

Achievement of quality requires resources for implementing an administrative program. No program comes about by itself. It requires manpower, time, space, and money. Clearly, in any kind of administrative budget for which there are identifiable goals spelled out in terms of programs, one of the goals must be the achievement of excellence and quality. Such achievement requires funds, a trained staff, suitable space, and committed time during which professional and supporting staffs can develop administrative procedures and personal attitudes designed to promote the achievement of quality health care. The process requires continuing staff orientation and education as well as persistent patient orientation and education. If staff orientation and dedication proceed without an understanding of the patient orientation and dedication effort, a deficient program is promoted. It is just as much the responsibility of professional and supporting staffs to understand and to strive for the achievement of quality in the delivery of health care services as it is the responsibility of patients to understand the nature of the quality services that are being attempted. In order for patients to understand services a continuous program of patient education is required. An informed patient population is another mechanism to stimulate staff, both professional and supporting, to strive for and to achieve excellence in all phases of delivery of health care services.

The lack of budgetary support for achieving excellence, identifiable by specific program objectives, would constitute a serious deficiency in any administrative program that attempts to plan, mold, and evaluate a program effort to achieve quality. This is much more than an ombudsman effort or consciousness raising. Such a program must be total and pervasive and must be carried by the administration's dedication to quality and enunciated by the spirit of its leadership. This type of program undoubtedly is costly to an institution—but so is the settlement of grievances, malpractice claims, and lawsuits. Although no data base readily exists by which to make financial comparisons, an institution's risk management program, carefully planned and deliberately budgeted, will prove to be less costly. In terms of the sheer expenditure of time and aggravation, in attending to and pursuing grievances, malpractice claims, and legal suits, an institution's leadership-sponsored and administration-managed program of risk prevention and avoidance is less expensive. Such a program must lead to a more productive morale environment. Further research endeavors and demonstration programs are needed.

Nevertheless, it is apparent that some hospitals and some doctors are better than other doctors and hospitals. In some cases, patients can sense the differences. Some hospitals and doctors do have "good" reputations. Often the perception is objectively correct. How is it achieved? In the absence of some kind of grading system, reputation is the means by which some hospitals and clinics achieve the status of quality institutions. Rarely are the achievements of quality or of greatness in institutions obtained by accident. More often the achievement is by design, deliberate planning, and persistent hard work. Although quality depends greatly on the caliber of professional and support staffs and the administrative matrix, the caliber of personnel does not automatically mean quality care. The additional essential element is quality administration.

THE ROLE OF THE PATIENT

Whether or not useful quality assurance systems are in place (and in many institutions they are not) and whether or not those that are in place function to full effectiveness (and they do not always do so) how do patients determine if the health care delivery system in general and the medical profession in particular are meeting their responsibilities? Patient satisfaction is one specific approach to quality of care measurement and control that has received little attention. A review has pointed out that although little is known about patient satisfaction, patients generally appear to be less critical of the technical content of care than they are of attitudinal and situational components,[48] a conclusion confirmed in one of the largest-scale studies of patient satisfaction carried out by the mid-1970s.[49]

One gauge of patient satisfaction is the extent of medical malpractice litigation. By the mid-1970s, malpractice litigation had become a matter of major concern in the United States. In 1973, a major commission reported on the matter,[50] and its many findings and recommendations created a great deal of controversy.[51] During the 1970s, the volume of suits increased, the magnitude of settlements rose, and insurance premiums threatened to rise out of sight.[52] The problem is not entirely new. As Curran himself pointed out, in the 1940s there had been complaints about "a plague of malpractice suits."[52] Katz refers to physicians' "alarm at the increase in (malpractice) claims" in the 1840s![53] Nevertheless, by 1975 the situation had seriously worsened.[54] Insurance companies stopped writing malpractice policies in several states, often after requests for premium increases of 300 percent or more were denied by state insurance commissioners. In several states, medical societies set up their own insurance companies. Hospitals saw their rates skyrocket: the annual premium for the Massachusetts General Hospital increased 10 times between 1969 and 1975.[53] In California, physicians struck in the spring of 1975, seeking to force legislative changes[54a] as they did or threatened to do elsewhere.[55]

The wave of legislative remedies became a flood during that summer. Curran states, "The thrust of most of the enacted bills can be classified into three major categories: insurance coverage changes; legal-system reforms; and the strengthening of medical disciplinary mechanisms."[55] Most significant legislative changes, however, gored one ox or another, and, as well known, in the United States gored oxen often go to court seeking a remedy. Nevertheless, there were malpractice litigation system changes in a number of states that led to a leveling off in the number of suits, the average size of awards made in successful ones, and, as a result, the rate of premium increase. Nevertheless, in the early 1980s, the situation began to deteriorate again.

It is useful to examine some of the causes of the increase in malpractice litigation.[56] First of all, some care provided by physicians in this country is of poor or doubtful quality. Some, but not all, of this poor care involves negligence.

Second, physicians have not shown themselves to be particularly competent or capable of policing their own ranks.[57] This situation does not seem to have improved in recent years. Third, some observers think that an increasing supply of attorneys, particularly when it occurs in states with no-fault automobile insurance, may be a factor. Fourth, other observers think that the incidence of malpractice litigation is related to the deterioration of the doctor-patient relationship. A medical writer in the *Dallas Morning News* wrote a "Message to Doctors and Hospitals." In part she said: "Most of all, doctors and nurses . . . please listen to me. . . . You treat me like a human being, and I wouldn't sue you even if you sew up a scalpel in my stomach."[58] Finally, the rapidly rising cost of medical care may itself be a factor.

Thus, the principal role of the patient in the medical quality assurance/malpractice drama is as subject; respondent; victim; passive participant; angry, wronged adversary; and happy, better patient. Certain expectations are created for patients. They play little part in creating them. When things go well, or as well as they were led to believe they would, patients are happy. When things go poorly, or less well than the established level of expectation, patients are unhappy. Because their technical knowledge of and influence on the health care delivery system is limited, and because they can virtually never have impact upon the health care delivery system's own quality assurance mechanism, the only recourse is to sue. But how did this situation arise?

DETERMINATION OF PATIENT ATTITUDES AND PERCEPTIONS

Patient attitudes, perceptions, and responses to medical care problems when they arise are molded by a variety of factors. These include personal considerations, social influences, and the professional providers and institutions themselves. Taken together, these factors are powerful determinants of behavior.

Personal and Social Factors

Most people do not want to be ill. If they are ill, they want to get better. Furthermore, most people do not want to receive bad news about health and illness. However, in our medical/health culture, self-care and personal health promotion, while being given an increasing amount of lip service and even a certain amount of serious attention, are not strongly and widely held values. Therefore, most people when ill surrender most if not all control of the situation to the professional providers and institutions. Most people who use physicians thus consciously regard the physician as healer, a person with almost mystical powers. In many cases, the profession does nothing to alter this view.

The "he (or she) will fix it" attitude is reinforced by the intermittent nature of illness. Most people are well, or at least not ill, most of the time. Thus, since illness rather than wellness is stressed in our medical/health culture, most people have little inclination to learn much about health and medicine. The intermittent nature of illness further encourages the transfer of responsibility for getting better from the individual to the medical care provider. Once this rather complete transfer is accomplished, of course, the patient has to believe that his or her provider and institution are, if not the best, if not absolutely perfect, then very close to it. In this total social/personal context, less than perfect or close to perfect results can leave patients with little other recourse than to sue, even if negligence is not involved.

Many factors determine the social role and image of physicians. It is interesting to note how they are both reflected and molded by television. Prime time shows that do well generally show the physician as being in charge and coming out a winner even if problems are encountered along the way. Thus Drs. Kildare, Casey, Welby, Quincy, and Trapper John have had long lives, at least in television terms. Conversely, programs that show the medical profession and health care institutions as normal do not tend to have long runs. Normality in this context means that, while most of the time the person or institution does a good job, incompetence, negligence, ignorance, stupidity, cupidity, corruption, inefficiency, and ineffectiveness are not exactly uncommon.

In the mid-1970s, *Police Story*, a television program about the seamy side of police departments and police work, had a successful run of several years. Encouraged by this success, the producer, influenced in part by a family tragedy that resulted from negligent medical care, put together a show called *Medical Story*. A series of well done, critically acclaimed, one-hour dramas examined the seamy side of the medical profession. It lasted 13 weeks. In 1982, *St. Elsewhere*, a television program about a less-than-perfect hospital, with a good deal of humor in it, premiered to critical acclaim—and small audiences. Its survival was uncertain. Medical soap operas do well, of course, even though not all doctors and nurses on them are perfect. But the personal imperfections of the characters tend to outweigh (indeed, they overshadow their professional ones) and form the main focus of the stories. This principal focus probably accounts for the success of this category of medical program.

Professional Providers and Institutions

The successful T.V. image is the one that the providers and institutions tend to project and indeed get caught up in. It is the image of the "medical mystique," as Belsky has termed it.[59] The medical mystique covers both the content of medicine, which is so complex, and the process of medicine, which is so intricate and intense. It is accompanied by the aura of infallibility. In fact, mystery and infallibility are inextricably linked. If individuals own a mystery that they cannot share or is unsharable, then in performance of their public services, they must be infallible, otherwise there would be no reason to patronize them and to pay them good money. After all, if there is only a 50/50 chance of success, why should anyone try?

By projecting the mystique of infallibility, the profession promotes its image as healer, and the institution assumes its place as the focus of salvation. Central here once again is the issue of control. Physician and institution alike put themselves in control of the patient's illness, wellness, life, and destiny. Control is not shared. Physician and institution do not want to share control, and the patient is given no option to gain control. However, if total control is given to one side with total dependence on the other, look out. When something goes wrong, given the option, the controlled has a strong motivation to go after the controller.

A further influence on patient behavior is the medical profession's perception of its principal enemy. To the profession, death is the principal enemy of medicine. This accounts for the ever-increasing emphasis on high technology, acute care, an institutional focus, and late-stage medicine. In the U.S., five percent of nonpoor, nonelderly families have medical expenses of more than $5,000 in a given year, but these families account for one-half of the medical expenses incurred by all such families.[60]

If death is the principal enemy, illness that is unlikely to involve death is not considered interesting or worthy of serious attention. To most patients, however, illness is the principal enemy. Most people don't think about confronting death, most of the time. The individual is sick and simply wants to get better. This discordance of views can easily lead to conflict if, once again, the outcome is not what the patient bargained for.

To cap this all off, the medical profession has great difficulty in communicating its limitations to patients. First of all, some members of the profession truly believe that they have none. Second, the carefully constructed mystique allows little possibility for admitting possible fallibility. After all, how can an individual possibly be fallible and infallible at the same time?

Together, all of these factors and influences create the public expectations for medical care and its quality. There is limited recourse if a patient is let down. The patient may feel, "I trusted you, and look what you did to me." The letdown thus comes hard. As several studies have shown, if good doctor-patient communication exists (despite the above discussion, it sometimes does), the problem can be worked out short of litigation. Often, however, the only alternative is suit.[61]

RESPONSIBILITY OF THE MEDICAL PROFESSION AND THE HEALTH CARE INSTITUTIONS

The responsibility is so simple to state, but so hard to carry out. Two principal problems have been outlined. First, the quality of medical care is, in fact, not nearly as good as it could or should be. Second, the profession and the institutions have created for themselves an aura of infallibility, a state of control, and a projected expectation of near perfection. Both of these problems are largely created by the profession and the institutions. Thus it is their responsibility to solve them. But can they do so?

The technical means exist to solve the first problem. While perfection is no more achievable in medical care than it is in any other realm of human endeavor, quality could be significantly improved by using available means of audit and control, based upon well-developed, explicit, written criteria for both the process and substance of medical care. However, in this realm, the problem is not a lack of knowledge or skill but a lack of will. Over the past 20 years, the medical profession has clearly demonstrated that it is simply not interested in seriously doing anything about its own failures. Whether that will, that crucial change of attitude, can be created, remains to be seen.

The second problem is even more difficult to solve because it is almost completely ideological. (The first, in contrast, has both an ideological and a technical component.) There is no clear answer to the problem of transferring a significant part of the doctor-patient relationship to the patient. Attitudes, behaviors, and expectations are entrenched on both sides. However, if at least a start is not made toward the goal of breaking down the medical mystique, the overall problem will not be solved.

A measure of the difficulty of accomplishing this ideological and behavioral change is the impact that the medical graduates of the Vietnam War era have had on medical practice. This was a time of turmoil, of revolt, and of heightened social consciousness in medical schools. Many medical students and indeed some medical schools made statements that they were going to "do something" about medical inequity and social injustice. Certainly a major area of concern is quality of care. Many graduates of that era are now through their residency training and in practice, but their measurable impact upon the system is negligible to date.

Medicine is still a shortage profession. Work is still plentiful on a national scale, although certain areas are "full." Social consciousness does not always stand up well to the demands of families, the state requirements for professional development, and the allure of high incomes. It is easier to leave the status quo untouched when those demands are being met. Furthermore, medical education itself did not change in any significant ways during that era, any rhetoric to the contrary notwithstanding. With no technical equipment to make change and with no change in the ideology of the system as a whole, the young radicals of the late 1960s and early 1970s were ill equipped to become more than the next generation of conventional medical practitioners.

THE DUTY OF THE INSTITUTION TO REGULATE

What then, can be done? The medical profession as it is now constituted is unlikely to make the necessary changes discussed above. This puts the responsibility squarely on the shoulders of the institutions. But the policies of the institutions themselves are subject to the major influence of the profession. However, there is potential here, and it is starting to be felt. The nonmedical professional leadership, the administrators and the boards of trustees, as well as public officials in the case of public institutions, will have to move into the forefront of the change process. They will be assisted by a coming change in the nature of the medical profession, however.[62]

There is a coming oversupply of physicians. One likely outcome of this state of affairs is that an increasing number of young physicians will forsake the potential rewards but increasingly rigorous competition of private practice for the security of salaried service. This change will give the institutions more control over physician behavior than they have now. However, the struggle will not be an easy one to win. Even in the face of a salary structure, several hundred years of a medical tradition and an ingrained ideology continually reinforced by undergraduate, graduate, and continuing medical education will die hard.

Of course, there will be some external motivators for changes as well. With the continually rising costs of care, third party payers and behind them the ultimate payers of the bills are beginning to devote some attention to quality. The malpractice liability problem will not go away by itself. The situation cannot be significantly improved until both technical quality and control/communication are dealt with in a positive way.

The responsibility for change is there. The profession could take it on, but for historical and ideological reasons probably will not and cannot. That leaves the job to the institutions. Only history will tell if they are able to meet the challenge.

NOTES

1. A. Donabedian, "The Quality of Medical Care," in *Health: United States, 1978*, DHEW Pub. No. (PHS) 78-1232. (Hyattsville, Md.: DHEW, 1978), pp. 111–126.

2. W. McKillop, "Is High-quality Care Assessable?" *Hospitals*, (1975):43–47.

3. "Peers' Role Stressed by AMA President," *American Medical News*, (December 10, 1973):3.

4. R.H. Brook, *Quality of Care Assessment: A Comparison of Five Methods of Peer Review*, National Center for Health Services Research and Development (Washington, D.C.: USDHEW, 1973).

5. T. Christoffel, "Medical Care Evaluation: An Old New Idea," *Journal of Medical Education* 51 (1976):83–88.

6. C.E. Lewis, "The State of the Art of Quality Assessment—1973," *Medical Care* 12 (1974):799–806.

7. F.D. Moore, "Surgical Biology and Applied Sociology: Cannon and Codman Fifty Years Later," *Harvard Medical Alumni Bulletin* 53 (1975):12.

8. R.I. Lee and L.W. Jones, *The Fundamentals of Good Medical Care* (1933; reprint ed., Hamden, Conn.: Archon Books, 1962).

9. Subcommittee on Medical Care, American Public Health Association. "The Quality of Medical Care in National Health Program," *American Journal of Public Health* 39 (1949):898–905.

10. E.R. Weinerman, "The Quality of Medical Care." *The Annals of the American Academy of Political and Social Science* 13 (1951):185–191.

11. A. Donabedian, *A Guide to Medical Care Administration. II: Medical Care Appraisal—Quality and Utilization,* (Washington, D.C.: American Public Health Association, 1969), pp. 2–3.

12. D.M. Kessner et al., "Assessing Health Quality—The Case for Tracers," *New England Journal of Medicine* 288 (1973):189–194.

13. R.H. Brook, "Critical Issues in the Assessment of Quality of Care and Their Relationship to HMO's," *Journal of Medical Education* part 2, 48 (1973):114–134.

14. J. Lester, "By the London Post," *New England Journal of Medicine* 296 (1977):436–438.

15. A. Donabedian, "Evaluating the Quality of Medical Care," *Milbank Memorial Fund Quarterly* 44 (1966):166–171.

16. A. Donabedian, "Promoting Quality through Evaluating the Process of Patient Care," *Medical Care* 6 (1968):181–202.

17. H.L. Blum, "Evaluating Health Care," *Medical Care* 12 (1974):999–1011.

18. P.J. Sanazaro and J.W. Williamson, "End Results of Patient Care: A Provisional Classification Based on Reports by Internists," *Medical Care* 6 (1968):123–130.

19. M. Sheps, "Approaches to the Quality of Hospital Care," *Public Health Reports* 70 (1955):877–886.

20. M.I. Roemer, "Controlling and Promoting Quality in Medical Care," in *Health Care From the Library of Law and Contemporary Problems,* C.C. Havighurst and J.C Weistart, eds., (Dobbs Ferry, N.Y.: Oceania Publications, 1972):176–186.

21. P.M. Ellwood et al., "Assessing the Quality of Health Service," in *Assuring the Quality of Health Care* (Minneapolis, Minn.: Interstudy, 1973):193–207.

22. H.S. Cohen and L.H. Miike, *Developments in Health Manpower Licensure.* USDHEW, Pub. No. (HRA) 74-3101 (Washington, D.C., 1973).

23. USDHEW, *Secretary's Report on Licensure and Related Health Personnel Credentialing.* USGPO, Pub.N. (HSM) 72-11 (Washington, D.C., 1971).

24. USDHEW, *Credentialing Health Manpower,* Pub. No. (OS) 77-50057, USGPO (Washington, D.C., 1977).

25. A.J. Anderson and I. Altman. *Methodology in Evaluating the Quality of Medical Care* (Pittsburgh, Pa.: University of Pittsburgh Press, 1962).

26. R.H. Brook et al., "Assessing the Quality of Medical Care Using Outcome Measures: An Overview of the Method," *Medical Care* 15, (November 9 Supp., 1977):3.

27. E. Scheye, *The Hospital's Role in Assessing the Quality of Medical Care: Proceedings of the Fifteenth Annual Symposium on Hospital Affairs, May 1973,* (Chicago: Graduate Program in Hospital Administration and Center for Health Administration Studies, Graduate School of Business, University of Chicago, 1973).

28. T. Christoffel, "A Selected Bibliography of Literature of Quality Patient Care," *Quality Review Bulletin* 8 (Jan./Feb. 1976):30–33.

29. Institute of Medicine, *Assessing Quality in Health Care: An Evaluation* (Washington, D.C.: National Academy of Sciences, 1976).

30. T. Christoffel and M. Lowenthal, "Evaluating the Quality of Ambulatory Health Care: A Review of Emerging Methods," *Medical Care* 15 (1977):877–897.

31. O.L. Peterson et al., "An Analytical Study of North Carolina General Practice," *The Journal of Medical Education* 31, Dec. Part 2 Suppl. (1956):143.

32. P.A. Lembcke, "Medical Auditing by Scientific Methods," *Journal of the American Medical Association* 162 (1956):646–655.

33. R.E. Trussell et al., *The Quantity, Quality and Costs of Medical and Hospital Care Secured by a Sample of Teamster Families in the New York Area* (New York: Columbia University School of Public Health and Administrative Medicine, 1962).

34. M.A. Morehead et al., *A Study of the Quality of Hospital Care Secured by a Sample of Teamster Family Members in New York City* (New York: Columbia University School of Public Health and Administrative Medicine, 1964).

35. L.M. Koran, "The Reliability of Clinical Methods, Data and Judgments," *New England Journal of Medicine* 293 (1975):642–646 and 695–698.

36. M.A. Morehead, "Evaluating Quality of Medical Care in the Neighborhood Health Center Program of the Office of Economic Opportunity," *Medical Care* 8 (1970):118–131.

37. M.A. Morehead and R. Donaldson, "Quality of Clinical Management of Disease in Comprehensive Neighborhood Health Centers," *Medical Care* 12 (1974):301–315.

38. M.A. Morehead et al., "Comparisons between OEO Neighborhood Health Centers and Other Health Care Providers of Ratings of the Quality of Health Care," *American Journal of Public Health* 61 (1971):1294–1306.

39. D.M. Kessner and C.E. Kalk, *Contrasts in Health Status, 2: A Strategy for Evaluating Health Services* (Washington, D.C.: Institute of Medicine, 1973).

40. D.M. Kessner et al., *Contrasts in Health Status, 3: Assessment of Medical Care for Children* (Washington, D.C.: Institute of Medicine, 1974).

41. R.H. Brook and F.A. Appel, "Quality of Care Assessment: Choosing a Method for Peer Review," *New England Journal of Medicine* 288 (1973):1323–1329.

42. H.C. Neu and S.P. Howrey, "Testing the Physician's Knowledge of Antibiotic Use," *New England Journal of Medicine* 293 (1975):1291–1295.

43. R.H. Brook and K.N. Williams, "Effect of Medical Care Review on the Use of Injections," *Annals of Internal Medicine* 85 (1976):509–515.

44. S.J. Tomecki and M.E. Plaut, "Syphilis Surveillance," *Journal of the American Medical Association* 236 (1976):2641–2642.

45. B.S. Linn et al., "Evaluation of Burn Care in Florida," *New England Journal of Medicine* 296 (1977):311–315.

46. R.M. Saywell et al., "A Performance Comparison: USMC-FMG Physicians," *American Journal of Public Health* 69 (1979):57–62.

47. K. Steel et al., "Iatrogenic Illness on a General Medical Service at a University Hospital," *New England Journal of Medicine* 304 (1981):638–642.

48. J.L. Lebow, "Consumer Assessments of the Quality of Medical Care," *Medical Care* 12 (1979):328–337.

49. J.S. Birch and S. Wolfe, "Consumers Assess Alternative Kinds of Health Service," Delivered at annual meeting, American Public Health Association, Chicago, Ill., November 20, 1975.

50. USDHEW, *Report of the Secretary's Commission on Medical Malpractice* (Washington, D.C.: USGPO, 1973).

51. C.E. Welch, "Medical Malpractice," *New England Journal of Medicine* 292 (1975):1372–1376.

52. W.J. Curran, "Malpractice Crisis: The Flood of Legislation," *New England Journal of Medicine* 293 (1975):1182–1183.

53. B.F. Katz, "The Medical Malpractice Crisis—Its Causes and Effects," Presented at the annual meeting, American Public Health Association, Chicago, Ill., November 19, 1975.

54. J.K. Cooper and S.K. Stephens, "The Malpractice Crisis—What Was It All About?" *Inquiry* 14 (1977):240–253.

54a. D.F. Phillips, "The California's Physicians' Strike," *Hospitals* 49 (1975):49–52.

55. W.J. Curran, "Malpractice Insurance: A Genuine National Crisis," *New England Journal of Medicine* 292 (1975):1223–1224.

56. J.M. Vaccarino, "Malpractice: The Problem in Perspective," *Journal of the American Medical Association* 238 (1977):861–863.

57. "How Well Does Medicine Police Itself?" *Medical World News,* 15 March 1974, p. 62.

58. "In the Hospital, I Am a Bundle of Fears," *American Medical News,* 25 August 1974, p. 50.

59. M. Belsky and L. Gross, *Beyond the Medical Mystique: How to Choose and Use Your Doctor* (New York: Arbor House, 1975).

60. "How Catastrophic Are Medical Expenses?" *Washington Report on Medicine and Health/ Perspectives* 36 (December 10, 1982):50.

61. N.S. Blackman, "Professional Liability Insurance and Practice of Medicine," *New York State Journal of Medicine* 82 (1982):1387–1389.

62. S. Jonas, "Some Thoughts on the Future of Health Services in the United States," *Employee Benefits Journal* 6, no. 2 (1981):10–15.

Chapter 2

The Duty of Hospitals To Regulate the Quality of Patient Care: A Legal Perspective

B. Abbott Goldberg, LL.B. *

> *Greater than the tread of mighty armies is*
> *an idea whose hour has come.*
> *Victor Hugo (attributed)*

The idea whose hour has come is "Hospitals should, in short, shoulder the responsibilities borne by everyone else."[1] It is supported by two subsidiary ideas: (1) that hospitals, even charitable hospitals, are businesses; and (2) that hospitals treat patients. "This all seems so clear on principle that one wonders why there should ever have been any doubt about it."[2] The purpose here is to explain why there was doubt and why the application of ordinary legal principles to hospitals has produced so much concern and a small library of legal comment.

The explanation will focus on one topic—the potential liability of a hospital to a patient for the negligent appointment to or retention on its medical staff of the patient's private physician, that is, for its corporate negligence in the now common expression.[3] Eliminated from consideration is a hospital's liability for the negligence of its actual employees, ostensible or apparent employees, tenants such as radiologists or pathologists and emergency room contractors—persons for whose negligence the hospital may be held liable even though it was not negligent itself. In legal parlance what are omitted are cases explainable under the doctrine of *respondeat superior* ("let the master be responsible") except insofar as such cases are explanatory of the development of the concept of the hospital's corporate negligence.

---

*The author thanks Margaret E. Daily of Portland, Oregon, a graduating student at McGeorge School of Law, his research assistant during 1980–1982.

The leading case, although not the most illuminating one, is *Darling v. Charleston Community Memorial Hospital*,[4] an illustration of hospital inattention to the enforcement of obligations imposed by law and assumed by accreditation and its own bylaws. A young athlete broke a leg playing football. He was admitted as an emergency patient, and his leg was put in a cast by the private staff physician on emergency call pursuant to the hospital's medical staff bylaws.[5] The doctor applied no padding and put the cast on too tight. As a result of the constricture, the leg became necrotic, with obvious symptoms such as foul odor,[6] discoloration, and loss of sensation. No consultation was had despite the medical staff bylaw requiring one in "all major cases."[7] After 15 days of intense suffering, the lad was transferred to another hospital where, eventually, his leg was amputated.

The doctor settled in the ensuing litigation, but the hospital went to trial on the theories that its liability as a charity was limited and that it could be held to no higher standard of care than that "customarily offered by hospitals generally in its community."[8] It lost, but the grounds on which it lost are not particularly clear. Put narrowly, the grounds are that the nurses failed to call the patient's deteriorating condition to the attention of the hospital administration and that the hospital failed to review the doctor's work or require consultation as required by its own rules.[9] More broadly, they are that the hospital's duty of care was not defined by the customs of its community.

> The Standards for Hospital Accreditation, the state licensing regulations and the defendant's bylaws demonstrate that the medical profession and other responsible authorities regard it as both desirable and feasible that a hospital assume certain responsibilities for the care of the patient.[10]

Tested by conventional legal rules, the result of hospital liability is unremarkable. By 1965 charitable immunity, the proposition that a charity was not liable for the negligence of its agents, servants or employees, had been in process of judicial abandonment for more than two decades.[11]

> Institutions should shoulder the responsibilities all other citizens bear. They should minister as others do, within the obligation not to injure through carelessness. . . .
>
> The incorporated charity should respond as do private individuals, business corporations and others, when it does good in the wrong way.[12]

Adherence to community standards or even general standards for hospital conduct was obviously inappropriate for it could mean that hospitals could write their own tickets.[13] *Bing v. Thunig*,[14] relied on in *Darling*, had already abolished the special immunity enjoyed by hospitals but by no other employers and held a hospital liable for the negligence of its employed nurses. Under commonplace law, violation of a statute or regulation intended for the benefit of the public was either negligence or evidence of negligence.[15] The representation of particular competence or the voluntary assumption of a duty of care, as by seeking and obtaining accreditation, had long been a basis of liability.[16] The liability of a hospital for allowing the violation of its own rules, although a little more obscure, had been established generations before, and it is not a peculiarity of hospital law.[17]

Attributed to *Darling*,[18] although actually obscure in the case itself, a hospital may be liable for failing to review the work of a staff physician retained by a patient, it is, nevertheless, analytically simple. Although it had become conventional to refer to a staff physician as an independent contractor,[19] he or she was not an independent contractor employed by the hospital. The private staff physician who admits and cares for a private patient is not employed by the hospital in any sense, neither as an independent contractor, agent, or servant. The physician is actually a concessionaire or licensee of the hospital, a person allowed to do his or her own business in the hospital to help the hospital accomplish its function of treating the patient, very much as the proprietor of an amusement park may allow the operation of various attractions by third persons. If there is any consideration paid, it is not by the owner of the facility as an employer but rather by the concessionaire for the privilege of using the facility. Thus a staff physician may be required to pay dues,[20] to participate in staff activities,[21] and, as in *Darling*, to be available for emergencies, all as consideration for the privilege of remaining on the staff. Of course, the hospital, like any other possessor of land, is under a duty to use reasonable care to prevent harm by its concessionaires or licensees, the staff physicians.[22] The hospital is not analogous to a landlord or lessor of chattels, who is not ordinarily responsible for the torts of his or her tenant or lessee, because the landlord or lessor is not in the business of treating but only in the business of renting.

Although it thus seems clear as a matter of elementary law that a hospital could be liable for its own negligence in the selection or retention of incompetent physicians on its medical staff, *Darling* was an enormous surprise to the medical and hospital community. It has been characterized as undoubtedly "the most significant medical malpractice case of the 1960's,"[23] and it created a furor with overtones continuing to this day.[24] A current text calls it "a hard case,"[25] an expression lifted from lawyers' old aphorism, "Hard cases make bad law." The rejoinder to this, which is less frequently heard, is "Bad law makes hard cases."[26] But quips aside, *Darling* was a departure, "a revolutionary decree,"[27] if viewed in terms of the tradition of hospital immunity from liability for physicians' conduct. The Yale Law Journal cited, years before *Darling*, "the failure of the courts to require observance by the hospital of what would seem to be an obvious duty—to see that incompetent practitioners are not permitted the use of hospital facilities even under the heading of independent contractors."[28]

The exemption of hospitals from obvious duties began on December 9, 1870, when James McDonald, a construction worker, sustained a fractured femur. He was treated at the Massachusetts General Hospital, a charity, by a student intern supervised by a "visiting surgeon," who would now be called a staff physician. The result was unsatisfactory, and McDonald sued the hospital. He lost because the court, relying on English precedents that had been overruled, announced, for the first time in this country, the doctrine of charitable immunity.[29] Under this doctrine, a charitable hospital would not be liable for the acts of its "inferior agents" if they had been selected with due care. "[T]he funds entrusted to it are not to be diminished by such casualties" as befell the unfortunate McDonald.[30] Charitable immunity became a general rule in this country for many years. Since it applied in most of the cases, it relieved the courts of the burden of considering the relationship between the hospital and its physicians, either staff or employed, its nurses and other professional or lay personnel.

For legal precedent on the relationship between a hospital and its staff physicians, one must review cases in which charitable immunity did not apply. *Glavin v. Rhode Island Hospital*[31] is the archetype. Glavin, a worker in a lumberyard, lost two fingers to a circular saw. He was treated at a charity hospital by an intern, who, in violation of the hospital's rules, neglected to summon a surgeon promptly and applied a tourniquet. The delay and the procedure resulted in the amputation of Glavin's arm, and he sued the hospital. The hospital's defense of charitable immunity was rejected. The argument from English authority contradicted rather than supported the result in *McDonald;*[32] and the argument on policy was "not a question for the court, but for the legislature."[33]

Since it rejected the charitable immunity, the court had to consider whether the intern was a servant for whose violation of the rule the hospital was vicariously liable under *respondeat superior*. As had apparently been argued in *McDonald* but was there not necessary to consider,[34] the Rhode Island Hospital argued that it "undertook merely to provide the plaintiff the shelter, food, warmth and nursing of a hospital," that it "did not undertake the duties of a surgeon in treating the plaintiff's injury, but only to place him in charge of the intern or visiting surgeon," and "not undertaking professional charge of the plaintiff, owed him no professional duty, and would not be responsible for a breach of professional duty on the part of the intern."[35] The court found it easy to conceive a case in which a hospital might agree to do "no more than furnish hospital accommodations, leaving the patient to find his own physician." The hospital would then not be liable because the physician was not its servant. But here the hospital had undertaken to select a physician. Nevertheless, the hospital was not liable because mere selection did not make the physician its servant.[36] The court used what can be called the helpful neighbor analogy:

If A out of charity employs a physician to attend B, his sick neighbor, the physician does not become A's servant, and A, if he has been duly careful in selecting him, will not be answerable to B for his malpractice. The reason is that A does not undertake to treat B through the agency of the physician, but only to procure for B the services of the physician. The relation of master and servant is not established between A and the physician. And so there is no such relation between the corporation and the physicians and surgeons who give their services at the hospital. It is true the corporation has power to dismiss them, but it has this power not because they are its servants, but because of its control of the hospital where their services are rendered. They would not recognize the right of the corporation while retaining them, to direct them in their treatment of patients.[37]

The case of the intern, however, was different. He acted not only as a physician but also, under the hospital's rules, as the person appointed to "send for the surgeon of the day." The court stated, "Here then we have the relation of principal and agent, or master and servant. If the intern neglects to call the surgeon in the class of cases designated, his neglect is the neglect of the corporation."[38] And so the hospital lost and "the case was subsequently settled."[39]

Glavin was remarkably modern in its rejection of charitable immunity and in the concurring opinion that would have held that the hospital treated the patient and furnished a physician to him for whose competence it was responsible.[40] But these ideas were in advance of their times and disapppeared for seven or eight decades. What endured from *Glavin* was the notion that hospitals were liable only for some of the acts of their employees in the course of their employment. They were liable for their "administrative" or "ministerial" acts but not for their "professional" or "medical acts" because they could not control acts of the latter descriptions. If they could not control and hence were not liable for the professional or medical acts of employees, it followed even more certainly that they were not liable for the acts of nonemployees such as private staff physicians. But, although ability to control may be made the basis of liability, absence of the ability to control is not necessarily a basis for nonliability.[41]

At the time of *McDonald* and *Glavin*, hospitals were just emerging from the period when they had been exclusively institutions for sheltering the poor without a connotation of medical care.[42] It is no coincidence that both were cases of humble laborers; they were the sort of people for whom hospitals were intended. The well-to-do were cared for at home. Only a small minority of the doctors practiced in hospitals, and, as the years advanced, those who did not decried the idea that surgery should be done only in hospitals rather than on kitchen tables at home. Those who did practice in hospitals constituted a medical elite who used hospital experience for education and prestige.[43] It was not until the 1890s when the pressure of finances forced hospitals to rely on paying patients and, therefore, on private physicians who could supply such patients that "hospitals became more clearly defined as places for medical treatment rather than shelters for the poor and homeless."[44] Only after substantial numbers of doctors treated paying patients in hospitals did the movement for improving the quality of hospital care begin. Until then "Hospitals (were) in many instances walk-in garbage cans, which people entered reluctantly as a last resort before death."[45]

The impetus for the improvement of the quality of hospital care must be attributed to a desire for medical excellence rather than to any legal compulsion. The impetus of the law was to encourage the private benefactions on which the hospitals were so dependent. Thus, within nine months after *Glavin*, the Rhode Island Legislature exempted charitable hospitals from liability for the negligent and even malicious acts of their officers, agents, or employees, a statute not changed for almost a century.[46] *Glavin's* denial of charitable immunity was derided by courts, which refused to follow it.[47]

Glavin had another effect equally devastating to the concept of hospital liability for the quality of patient care by physicians. The King's Bench in England used it as a precedent for *Hillyer v. Governors of St. Bartholomew's Hospital*.[48] *Hillyer*, in turn, became a precedent for a case of utmost importance in American law, *Schloendorff v. Society of New York Hospital*.[49] *Hillyer* and *Schloendorff* are prime examples of how the courts tinkered with the ordinary rules of responsibility to reach the result of charitable immunity in cases where it did not apply.

Hillyer, a "medical man" at "the end of his resources" and a charity patient, sustained paralyzing injuries to his arms during surgery on his leg, an obvious case of negligent positioning. Present during the surgery were a "consulting surgeon," "house surgeons," "certified nurses," and "box carriers." All except the consulting surgeon seem to have been employees of the hospital. Nevertheless, the hospital was not held liable. The court picked up *Glavin's* helpful neighbor analogy and applied it to the nurses and house surgeons. The only duty the hospital undertook was that the patient should be treated by "experts, whether surgeons, physicians or nurses of whose professional competence the governors have taken reasonable care to assure themselves."[50] There was no evidence of improper selection,[51] and the hospital was not liable "if members of its professional staff, of whose competence there is no question, act negligently towards the patient in some matter of professional care or skill. . . ."[52] The court expanded on the distinction made in *Glavin* between the intern's role as a physician and his role as a messenger. The hospital could not be made liable for matters of "professional skill, in which the governors of the hospital neither can nor could properly interfere either by rule or supervision," although they might be liable for their servants' performance of "purely ministerial or administrative duties," such as attending on the wards, summoning aid (i.e., *Glavin*), or supplying food.[53] The question of the liability for the nonprofessional box carriers was "conveniently forgotten."[54] In short:

> The legal duty which the hospital authority undertakes towards a patient
> . . . *is not the ordinary duty* of a person who deals with another through
> his servants or agents and undertakes responsibility to that other person
> for damage resulting from any injury inflicted upon him by the neg-
> ligence of those servants or agents.[55]

Hillyer did not consider charitable immunity because, despite *McDonald*, it was
not applied in England. But many years later the extraordinary exemption from
ordinary duties was recognized as "a desire to relieve the charitable hospitals
from liabilities which they could not afford."[56]

The fear of prejudicing hospital finances was, however, an express rationale
of *Schloendorff v. Society of New York Hospital:*

> A ruling would, indeed be an unfortunate one that might constrain
> charitable institutions, as a measure of self-protection, to limit their
> activities. A hospital opens its doors without discrimination to all who
> seek its aid. . . . In this beneficent work, it does not subject itself to
> liability for damages, though the ministers of healing whom it has
> selected have proved unfaithful to their trust.[57]

Although New York recognized charitable immunity, the court had to abridge
the ordinary duties to protect the hospital in *Schloendorff* because the immunity
did not apply in that case. Mrs. Schloendorff claimed that she had been operated
on by a "visiting physician" and a "house physician" under circumstances that
should have suggested to the hospital's nurses that she had not consented. Since
the trial court had directed a verdict for the hospital, "her narrative, even if
improbable, must be taken as true."[58] Thus Mrs. Schloendorff was the victim
of a battery, an intentional tort. Charitable immunity did not apply to intentional
torts, and without it the court, as in *Glavin* and *Hillyer,* had to consider the
relationship between the hospital and its staff physicians and employees. Judge
Cardozo, then on the Court of Appeals for but three months, relied on *Glavin*
as extended by *Hillyer* and articulated it further:

> [T]he truc ground for the defendant's exemption from liability is that
> the relation between a hospital and its physician is not that of master
> and servant. The hospital does not undertake to act through them, but
> merely to procure them to act on their own responsibility.[59]
>
> The wrong was not that of the hospital; it was that of physicians,
> who were not the defendant's servants, but were pursuing an inde-
> pendent calling, a profession sanctioned by solemn oath, and safe-
> guarded by stringent penalties. If, in serving their patient, they violated
> her commands, the responsibility is not the defendant's; it is theirs.

> There is no distinction in that respect between the visiting and the resident physicians. Hillyer v. St. Barth. Hosp., supra. Whether the hospital undertakes to procure a physician from afar, or to have on the spot, its liability remains the same.[60]
>
> It is true I think, of nurses, as of physicians, that in treating a patient, they are not acting as servants of the hospital. . . . The hospital undertakes to procure for the patient the services of a nurse. It does not undertake, through the agency of nurses, to render those services itself. The reported cases make no distinction in that respect between the position of a nurse and that of a physician . . . and none is justified in principle.[61]

Judge Cardozo recognized the possible liability for negligent selection of the physician as an independent contractor and for negligence of nurses in relation "to the administrative conduct of the hospital," but he did not develop these because they were not shown by the record.[62]

In *Schloendorff*, the hospital had selected the physician but, nevertheless, escaped liability. Had the patient chosen her own doctor, the case would have been even stronger, for according to *Glavin*:

> It is quite conceivable that a corporation might not agree to do more than furnish hospital accommodations, leaving the patient to find his own physician or surgeon. In such a case the corporation would plainly not be liable for the torts of the physicians or surgeons, for in such a case they would not be its servants and it would not have assumed any responsibility in their selection.[63]

When coupled with cases such as *Hillyer* and *Schloendorff*, what had been only "conceivable" in *Glavin* turned into common understanding among both lawyers and doctors. Lawyers described a hospital as "really not much more than a specialized hotel" or workshop where a doctor chosen by the patient could do as he saw fit without subjecting the hotelier or proprieter of the workshop to any liability for the quality of the physician's care.[64] The attitude of doctors was the same. A surveyor for the American College of Surgeons in 1917 reported the doctors considered a hospital as:

> a more convenient place . . . than the home in which to perform an operation and for the patient to remain during his convalescence. The hospital's sole obligation was to furnish space with proper heat, light and food for the patient. When these services were paid for by the patient and he was discharged, the hospital's interest and obligation to the patient ceased.[65]

This is almost a paraphrase of the hospitals' argument in *Glavin*.[66]

But change was in the wind. Dr. Ernest Amory Codman of Boston, a man of astonishing prescience, had already recognized that "charitable hospitals have become businesses. . . ."[67]—an idea that was not to begin to be generally accepted by the courts for some 35 years.[68]

Codman was to serve as a precursor of legal thinking in another way. He was the "grand-daddy of efforts in evaluation in this country."[69] In 1913 he told the Philadelphia County Medical Society that the main product of a hospital was the patient who had been treated there and that the skill of a hospital's staff could be judged only by the "common sense notion that every hospital should follow every patient it treats, long enough to determine whether or not the treatment has been successful and then to inquire, if not, why not?"[70] What is important to note here is that at the time Judge Cardozo was announcing as a matter of law that hospitals merely procured physicians for the patient to act on their own responsibility,[71] the workshop idea, Codman was recognizing that a hospital treated patients—an idea that was resisted in court as late as 1967.[72]

Codman's efforts were initially unsuccessful. He was branded an eccentric and had to leave the Massachusetts General Hospital and establish his own hospital to develop a systematic means of evaluating what he called "end-results."[73] A survey for the American College of Surgeons in 1918 showed that only 89 of 692 hospitals investigated could meet even the simplest requirements, a statistic so embarrassing that the report was suppressed and the printed copies were destroyed.[74]

Nevertheless, in 1919, the American College of Surgeons, in an effort to create an organization "devoted completely to the evaluation of professional and hospital standards which would benefit the patient," adopted its "minimum standard" that each hospital have an organized staff of competent physicians who would adopt rules governing their professional work and who would "review and analyze at regular intervals their clinical experiences." This was a "goal to seek" so that the public could know to which hospitals they could go with safety.[75] The "minimum standard" evolved eventually into the accreditation standards of the Joint Commission on Accreditation of Hospitals beginning with a statement of the "minimum essential" in 1951 and currently stating the "optimal achievable."[76] The most important standards for present purposes are those requiring hospital medical staffs to ensure that each member is qualified and that staff "strive to maintain the optimal level of professional performance" and "provide mechanisms for the regular monitoring of medical staff practice and functions."[77]

The 40-year gap between the beginnings of Codman's efforts and those of the Joint Commission has been ascribed to attitudinal, sociological, and political factors rather than to technological difficulties.[78] Two facts are clear: (1) between 1910 and 1965 the evaluation of patient care by private staff physicians was not compelled by court opinions; and (2) the eventual infiltration into the courts of the concept that a hospital had some responsibility for a staff physician's conduct resulted from their recognition that a hospital's changed role had made the old precedents obsolete. But abandonment of old learning is hard for lawyers. Holmes stated, "[J]ust as the clavicle in the cat only tells of the existence of some earlier creature to which a collarbone was useful, precedents survive in the law long after the use they once served is at an end and the reason for them has been forgotten."[79]

The English cases are particularly illustrative. After *Hillyer* and *Schloendorff* the English and American cases do not refer to each other,[80] but they reach parallel results for parallel reasons. Thus, comparison of the two groups demonstrates the futility of resisting an idea whose hour has come, and they are cited for their analytical rather than precedential value.

The notion from *Glavin* and *Hillyer*, adverted to in *Schloendorff*, that a hospital was not liable for the professional negligence of its employees such as nurses, interns, or physicians but only for their administrative or ministerial negligence leads to absurd results. A hospital would be liable if a nurse, in her capacity as a waitress, scalded a patient by spilling hot tea on him but would not be liable if, as a nurse, she negligently dosed him with poison.[81] This was a paradox that could not be tolerated forever. Although a standard legal encyclopedia, *Halsbury's Laws of England*, had said, citing *Hillyer*, that a hospital was not liable for the professional negligence of its nurses, the statement was refuted by none other than Arthur Lehman Goodhardt, Professor of Jurisprudence at Oxford and later Master of University College, who suggested "the law is almost exactly the opposite" and a "hospital is liable for the negligence of its trained nurses."[82] Nothing from his pen was to be taken lightly, nor was it. Despite the traditional aversion of English courts to cite the works of living authors, Goodhardt's article, *Hospitals and Trained Nurses* became a basis of *Gold v. Essex C.C.*[83]

In *Gold* a little girl's face was disfigured through the negligence of a competent but careless radiographer, an employee. The court rejected the professional-administrative dichotomy, held the hospital liable, and set the stage for the erosion of the idea that the relationship between a hospital and its professional employees did not impose "the ordinary duty of a person who deals with another through his servants or agents."[84] In *Collins v. Hertfordshire County Council*,[85] a hospital was held liable for the combined negligence of a student nurse and a pharmacist in the injection of a lethal dose of cocaine instead of the procaine that had been ordered. "The case of *Hillyer* . . . is no longer a binding authority."[86] And in *Cassidy v. Ministry of Health*,[87] a hospital was held liable for the negligence of an employed physician who received a patient with two stiff fingers and sent him out with four—a useless hand. *Cassidy* repudiates the idea that a hospital cannot be responsible for the acts of physicians simply because it cannot control them and adopts the principle that hospitals have responsibilities for the treatment of patients:

[A]uthorities who run the hospital . . . are in law under the selfsame duty as the humblest doctor; whenever they accept a patient for treatment they must use reasonable care and skill to cure him of his ailment. The hospital authorities cannot, of course, do it by themselves; they have no ears to listen through the stethoscope, and no hands to hold the surgeon's knife. They must do it by the staff they employ; and if their staff are negligent in giving treatment, they are just as liable for that negligence as is anyone else who employs others to do his duties for him. . . .

It is no answer for them to say that their staff are professional men and women who do not tolerate any interference by their lay masters in the way they do their work. The doctor who treats a patient in the Walton Hospital can say equally with the ship's captain who sails his ship from Liverpool, and with the crane driver who works his crane in the docks, 'I take no orders from anybody.' That 'sturdy answer,' as Lord Simonds described it, only means in each case that he is a skilled man who knows his work and will carry it out in his own way; but it does not mean that the authorities who employ him are not liable for his negligence. . . . The reason why the employers are liable in such cases is not because they can control the way in which the work is done—they often have not sufficient knowledge to do so—but because they employ the staff and have chosen them for the task and have in their hands the ultimate sanction for good conduct, the power of dismissal.

This all seems so clear on principle that one wonders why there should ever have been any doubt about it. Yet for over thirty years— from 1909 to 1942—it was the general opinion of the profession that hospital authorities were not liable for the negligence of their staff in the course of their professional duties.[88]

Some American jurisdictions had ignored the professional-administrative dichotomy,[89] but it survived in New York until *Bing v. Thunig*[90] in 1957, that "brilliant opinion,"[91] "the fall of the citadel" of hospital immunity.[92] In *Bing,* a patient was burned during surgery because nurses had negligently not removed sheets on which an inflammable antiseptic was spilled. The hospital defended on two grounds: (1) that the nurses had acted in a medical or professional capacity; and (2) that it had charitable immunity. The Court of Appeals rejected both defenses. The dichotomy had become so riddled with distinctions from which there could be deduced "neither guiding principle nor clear delineation of policy,"[93] as shown by what has been called a "perhaps colored catalog of (its) anomalous results."[94] This disparagement seems undeserved because some of the examples, such as employers' liability for the conduct of uncontrollable employees (i.e., airplane pilots and locomotive engineers), are no more extreme than those that already occurred to the English judges and are the sort that would occur to any objective inquirer who asked why hospitals were the beneficiaries of special rules. And, as in *Gold v. Essex, C.C.*, the court proceeded, contrary to *Hillyer,* to impose "the ordinary duty of a person who deals with another through his agents."[95] Starting from the proposition that a hospital treats patients and does not merely procure professional employees to act on their own responsibility or provide facilities in which someone else may act,[96] the court reached the conclusions that:

> The doctrine of *respondeat superior* is grounded on firm principles of law and justice. Liability is the rule, immunity the exception. . . .[97]
>
> Hospitals should, in short, shoulder the responsibilities borne by everyone else. There is no reason to continue their exemption from the universal rule of *respondeat superior.*[98]
>
> The rule of nonliability is out of tune with the life about us, at variance with modern-day needs and with concepts of justice and fair dealing. It should be discarded. . . .[99]
>
> In sum, then, the doctrine according the hospital an immunity for the negligence of its employees is such a rule, and we abandon it.[100]

Of course, until hospitals were held liable for the professional negligence of their employees, they would not be liable for the acts of nonemployees such as staff physicians. But liability for the acts of employees does not mean that they are also liable for the acts of nonemployees. *Bing v. Thunig* was thus an indispensable, but not a complete, basis for the decision on the liability for acts of staff physicians retained by the patient.[101] Under *Schloendorff,* a staff physician selected by the patient could, despite *Bing,* still be considered "an independent contractor, following a separate calling . . . involving the hospital in no liability. . . ."[102] Unless it is recognized that the hospital treats patients, i.e., that the doctor is not following a "separate calling" from that of the hospital, this would be a routine invocation of the old idea that the employer of an independent contractor is not liable for the latter's negligence. But this conventional rule is subject to many exceptions "whose very number is sufficient to cast doubt upon the validity of the rule."[103] For example, the employer of an independent contractor may be liable for its own negligence in selecting an incompetent,[104] or for failure to supervise a concessionaire,[105] or for its own breach of a nondelegable duty of care. A hospital has a nondelegable duty to keep its premises safe. Thus, when a patient fell in a bath because she was alarmed by a rat, the hospital did not escape liability simply because it had employed an exterminator as an independent contractor.[106] It would be a strange rule of law that would make a hospital more liable for rats than for accepting or retaining deficient physicians on its medical staff. Delegation to the staff of the duties of selection and retention of its own members is no defense because the medical staff is an agent of the hospital, and the hospital, therefore, remains responsible for the staff's negligence.[107] And the staff itself, as an unincorporated association, may be liable and sued as an entity.[108]

These examples are intended to make obvious the distinction between the vicarious liability of hospitals for the acts of employees and their liability for their own, or corporate, negligence. The hospital is liable for the acts of an employee whether or not it was itself negligent. But it is not liable for the act of a staff physician merely because he commits malpractice within the hospital.[109] It is liable if it knew or should have known that he or she was liable to commit an act of malpractice such as by negligently appointing him or her to the staff or failing to review his or her work.[110] The qualifying phrase "should have known" is necessary because if liability were restricted to cases of actual knowledge, "the less a hospital (knew) about a patient's condition, the safer it (would be) against charges of negligence."[111]

Darling was startling not because it invented any new rules of law; it was startling because it applied the ordinary rules to hospitals and deprived them of the special privileges they once enjoyed, privileges that were designed to ameliorate the financial burdens of charities in cases where charitable immunity did not apply. When the immunity disappeared, the privileges were also destined for oblivion.

Despite the apprehensions it caused, *Darling* has not been the forerunner of a great number of other cases. The relatively few cases up to 1978 have been variously listed and analyzed,[112] and repetition here is unnecessary. However, *Fiorentino v. Wenger*[113] should be noted. It held only that a hospital was not liable for failure to ascertain that a surgeon had obtained the informed consent of a patient to a novel, indeed unique, surgical procedure.[114] Otherwise, there was no claim of negligence on the part of the hospital.[115] The court, however, delivered a dictum described as a "significant stride in developing" the *Darling* theory that a hospital has a "duty to monitor the quality of care rendered within its walls."[116] "[A] hospital will not be held liable for an act of malpractice performed by an independently retained healer, unless it had reason to know that the act of malpractice would take place."[117]

At least two trial courts have acted on this dictum. In *Corleto v. Shore Memorial Hospital*,[118] it became a basis for allowing an action against not only the hospital but also its administrator, board of directors, and medical staff based on allegations that they should have known that the operating physician was incompetent and nevertheless permitted him to remain on a case obviously beyond his control. The author relied on it in *Gonzales v. Nork*, which, although unreported, received much publicity.[119] The *Nork Case*, as it is usually called, was one of allowing a surgeon to perform a laminectomy despite a history of bad results in the hospital. It has been described as the first case in which "a hospital was held liable for failure to adopt procedures to monitor the quality of medical care provided by a physician in the hospital."[120] In retrospect, the author views it as also a case of the hospital's neglect in failing to use even the inadequate review procedures available in the late 1960s[121] or, to paraphrase Southwick, its liability for failure to "stimulate" its medical staff to perform its peer review responsibilities.[122] Whichever characterization is correct, as a result of *Nork,* the Joint Commission on Accreditation of Hospitals is said to have adopted new accreditation standards,[123] now found in its manual under "Quality Assurance."[124]

The hospitals settled in both *Corleto* and *Nork.*[125] If these settlements were efforts to suppress awkward holdings, they have been unsuccessful as shown by the three latest opinions to come to hand: *Johnson v. Misericordia Community Hospital;*[126] *Fridena v. Evans;*[127] and *Bost v. Riley.*[128] *Johnson* held a hospital liable for the malpractice of an incompetent surgeon whom it had appointed to the staff without investigation. *Fridena* held a hospital liable for negligent supervision of a surgeon. *Bost,* in effect, applied the ordinary rules to a hospital to its benefit. The hospital had failed to enforce its rule requiring surgeons to keep progress notes, which would be at least evidence of negligence. But there was no showing that this failure contributed to the patient's death from complications of a splenectomy. Therefore, under the ordinary rules of legal causation, the negligence was not actionable.[129] "Negligence in the air, so to speak, will not do."[130]

In addition to these cases, "the view espoused in *Darling* has been embodied in the statutory law of several states."[131] Elsewhere, as in California, it may be found in administrative regulations having the force of law that make a hospital, through its medical staff, responsible for the quality of care of its patients.[132] It is also reflected in the requirements of the Joint Commission[133] and hospital rules,[134] but these may be only a grudging acceptance of the inevitable. For a while, after *Nork,* the Joint Commission's standard on Quality of Professional Services was imperative,[135] but it has since been qualified by prefatory phrases.[136] Some patients' bills of rights state that hospital patients are entitled to "considerate and respectful care,"[137] but only the pediatric bill of rights states expressly that they are entitled to "competent health care."[138] And although the prefatory statement to the American Hospital Association's version of the bill states, "Legal precedent has established that the institution itself . . . has a responsibility to the patient," at the end of the bill is the added statement, "No catalogue of rights can guarantee for the patient the kind of treatment he has a right to expect."[139] Unless the word "guarantee" is read in a strict technical sense, the last sounds like a disclaimer. Standard consent forms continue to recite that "all physicians furnishing services to the patient . . . are independent contractors and are not employees or agents of the hospital" but are the patient's "agents, servants, or employees."[140] Even if the patient read and understood what such phrases are intended to mean, i.e., that his or her consent was "informed," they would not exculpate the hospital from liability for its own negligence in appointment of incompetents or in failure to monitor the care delivered by its medical staff.[141]

Johnson refers to "the common law duty of care owed to patients by the hospital,"[142] and *Fridena* to its "inherent responsibilities regarding the quality of medical care furnished to patients within its walls."[143] What these mean are that the courts, not the medical profession nor the custom of the community, will ultimately determine the standards of care. Custom may be evidence of due care but it is not conclusive, for "there are precautions so imperative that even their universal disregard will not excuse their omission."[144] The courts will not determine those precautions solely by a logical process; they will determine them by the experience and felt necessities at the time of the decision. They now recognize that:

> the public's perception of the modern day medical scientific research center with its computed axial tomography (CAT-scan), radio nucleide imaging thermography, microsurgery, etc., formerly known as a general hospital, (and that the) public is indeed entitled to expect quality care and treatment while a patient in our highly technical and medically computed hospital complexes.[145]

In short, hospitals having shown what they can do have themselves established a standard of what they should do. And since what they can and should do depends on constantly changing facts, no effort has been made here to give a catalogue of hospitals do's and don'ts. What has been shown is one example of the malleability of the law in response to changes in society and technology. This is not peculiar to the law relevant to medicine. Former Justice Potter Stewart, speaking of United States Supreme Court decisions generally, says, "They reflect nothing more than what was on the mind of contemporary America. Those decisions are a reflection of American morality with a time lag."[146] If this discussion provides a sense that the law is unpredictable, it is no more unpredictable than the society it depicts. "[C]ertainty generally is illusion, and repose is not the destiny of man."[147]

NOTES

1. Bing v. Thunig, 2 N.Y.2d 656, 666, 143 N.E.2d 3, 8, 163 N.Y.S.2d 3, 11 (1957).

2. Cassidy v. Ministry of Health, [1951] 2 K.B. 343, 36 (Denning, L.J.).

3. The first use of "corporate negligence" found in this connection is Note, *Torts—Hospital's Liability—Standard of Care*, 43 N.C.L. Rev. 469, 471 (1965). It may come from the "corporate act" exception to charitable immunity; see Note, *Charitable Hospitals' Liability for Negligence: Abrogation of the Medical-Administrative Distinction*, 7 Duke L.J. 127, 130 n.15 (1958).

4. Darling v. Charleston Community Memorial Hospital, 33 Ill.2d 326, 211 N.E.2d 253 (1965), *aff'g* 50 Ill. App.2d 253, 200 N.E.2d 149 (1964).

5. *Darling,* 50 Ill. App.2d at 268, 284, 200 N.E.2d at 158, 165 (1964). California requires the medical staff to have such a rule. 22 Cal. Admin. Code § 70703, ¶ (g) (1975). See also, JOINT COMMISSION ON ACCREDITATION OF HOSPITALS, ACCREDITATION MANUAL FOR HOSPITALS 24, lines 31–37 (1982) [hereinafter cited as AMH].

6. "An odor of decaying flesh" that one witness had not smelled since World War II. *Darling,* 50 Ill. App.2d at 287, 200 N.E.2d at 167 (1964).

7. *Darling,* 50 Ill. App.2d at 283, 200 N.E.2d at 165 (1964). California requires the medical staff to develop criteria for consultation. 22 Cal. Admin. Code § 70703, ¶ (j) (1975). See also AMH, *supra* note 5, at 104–05 (requirement in medical staff bylaws).

8. *Darling,* 33 Ill.2d at 331, 211 N.E.2d at 257; 50 Ill. App.2d at 309, 200 N.E.2d at 177.

9. *Id.* at 333, 211 N.E.2d at 258; 50 Ill. App.2d at 306, 200 N.E.2d at 166 (the hospital administrator "knew the patient was a problem").

10. *Id.* at 332, 211 N.E.2d at 257.

11. A catalog by jurisdiction of the various modes and qualifications of the abolition of both charitable immunity and governmental immunity appears in 2 D. LOUISELL AND H. WILLIAMS, MEDICAL MALPRACTICE ¶¶ 17.01–17.57 and *id.* 1981 Supp. 3–34.

12. President and Director of Georgetown College v. Hughes, 130 F.2d 810, 814–15, 828 (D.C. Cir. 1942) (special nurse injured by student nurse allowed recovery against hospital). The leading case.

13. Note the two aspects. The "locality rule" could not apply because many communities have but one hospital. Since there is no other to which to compare it, in effect, it would set its own standards. Shilkret v. Annapolis Emergency Hospital Ass'n, 276 Md. 187, 194, 349 A.2d 245, 253 (1975). A hospital may not escape liability merely by doing what all other hospitals are doing. A calling may not set its own tests to the exclusion of the courts, because the whole calling may be negligent. The T.J. Hooper, 60 F.2d 737, 740 (2d Cir. 1932), cited in *Darling,* 33 Ill.2d at 332, 211 N.E.2d at 257, and Gonzales v. Nork in S. LAW AND S. POLAN, PAIN AND PROFIT 244 (1978).

14. Bing v. Thunig, 2 N.Y.2d 656, 143 N.E.2d 3, 163 N.Y.S.2d 3 (1957).

15. RESTATEMENT (SECOND) OF TORTS § 286 and Comment f, § 288B (1965).

16. RESTATEMENT (SECOND) OF TORTS §§ 299A, 323, 324A (1965); W. PROSSER, TORTS § 56 at 344–47, 350 n. 52 (4th ed. 1971). See Glavin v. Rhode Island Hospital, 12 R.I. 411, 430 (1879) (concurring opinion). See generally James v. United States, 483 F. Supp. 581, 584–85 (N.D. Cal. 1980) and Coffee v. McDonnell-Douglas Corp., 8 Cal.3d 551, 557–58, 503 P.2d 1366, 1370, 105 Cal.Rptr. 358, 362 (1972).

17. Glavin v. Rhode Island Hospital, 12 R.I., 411, 422, 425 (1879) (intern's violation of hospital rule that he summon surgeon in difficult cases); Collins v. Hertfordshire County Council, [1947] 1 K.B. 598, 608–09, 614 (nurse's and pharmacist's violation of hospital rule requiring medical officer's signature on order for drugs). See generally Dillenbeck v. City of Los Angeles, 69 Cal.2d 472, 481, 446 P.2d 129, 135, 72 Cal.Rptr. 321, 327 (1968) and W. PROSSER, TORTS § 33 at 168 (4th ed. 1971). *Cf. Darling,* 33 Ill.2d at 332, 211 N.E.2d at 257.

18. *Darling,* 33 Ill.2d at 333, 211 N.E.2d at 258. The evidence supported the verdict on the alternative grounds of negligence of the nurses or violation of the hospital's rule on consultation.

19. *E.g.,* Schloendorff v. Society of New York Hospital, 211 N.Y. 125, 129, 105 N.E. 92, 93 (1914).

20. *Cf.* Volpicelli v. Jared Sydney Torrance Memorial Hospital, 109 Cal. App.3d 242, 167 Cal.Rptr. 610 (1980).

21. AMH, *supra* note 5, at 104, lines 39–41; 22 Cal. Admin. Code § 70703, ¶ (d) (1975).

22. RESTATEMENT (SECOND) OF TORTS §§ 318, 344 Comment c, 415 (1965).

23. W. CURRAN AND E. SHAPIRO, LAW, MEDICINE AND FORENSIC SCIENCE 368 (3d ed. 1982).

24. Copeland, *Hospital Responsibility for Basic Care Provided by Medical Staff Members: "Am I My Brother's Keeper?"*, 5 N. KY. L. REV. 27, 33 n. 30 (1978); Dunn, *Hospital Corporate Liability: The Trend Continues*, 8 MEDICOLOGICAL NEWS, no. 5, October, 1980, at 16. Copeland is both a hospital administrator and a lawyer and wrote from both points of view. His article is particularly comprehensive and interesting.

25. A. SOUTHWICK, THE LAW OF HOSPITAL AND HEALTH CARE ADMINISTRATION 411 (1978) [hereinafter cited as SOUTHWICK].

26. Hayes, *Crogate's Case: A Dialogue in ye Shades on Special Pleading Reform* in 9 W. HOLDS-WORTH, A HISTORY OF ENGLISH LAW at 423 (3d ed. 1944).

27. Note, *Hospital's Liability for Poor Medical Treatment*, 39 HOSPITALS, JAHA, Dec. 1, 1965, at 118. "A major disappointment . . . a potent blow."

28. Note, *Liability of Hospital for Injuries to Patients Using Hospital Facilities*, 48 YALE L.J. 81, 85 (1938).

29. McDonald v. Massachusetts General Hospital, 120 Mass. 432 (1876).

30. *Id.* at 436. The exception to charitable immunity was frequently stated but seldom held. It was denied in Roosen v. Peter Bent Brigham Hospital, 235 Mass. 66, 70, 126 N.E. 392, 396 (1920). Note, *supra*, note 3, 7 DUKE L.J. at 129–30 n. 15. It was applied in Norfolk Protestant Hospital v. Plunkett, 162 Va. 151, 173 S.E. 363 (1934) (bladder injured by vaginal douche administered by incompetent nurse). Like the "captain of the ship" doctrine, *infra* note 88, it served "the obvious practical purpose of cutting down an immunity that promises more harm than good." Comment, 37 HARV. L. REV. 263, 264 (1923).

31. Glavin v. Rhode Island Hospital, 12 R.I. 411 (1879).

32. *Id.* at 422–23, 426–29.

33. *Id.* at 425–26.

34. *McDonald*, 120 Mass. at 434.

35. *Glavin*, 12 R.I. at 417. Glavin was charged only for "board, washing, warmth, and the services of nurses and ward tenders," $21.47, at the rate of $8 per week. *Id.* at 421.

36. *Id.* at 423–24.

37. *Id.* at 424. See also 430–31 (concurring on negligent selection).

38. *Id.* at 425.

39. *Id.* at 435.

40. *Id.* at 433.

41. See the discussion of Cassidy v. Ministry of Health, [1951] 2 K.B. 343, 360, *infra* at note 88.

42. "The legal sense of the word *hospital* is a corporate foundation, endowed for the perpetual distribution of the founder's charity, in the lodging and maintenance of a certain number of poor persons, according to the regulations and statutes of the founder. Such institutions are not necessarily connected with medicine or surgery, and in their original establishment had no necessary reference to sickness or accident." GRANT, CORPORATIONS (ed. 1850) 567, in 9 W. HOLDSWORTH, A HISTORY OF ENGLISH LAW 45 n. 2 (3d. ed. 1944).

43. Vogel, *The Transformation of the American Hospital, 1850–1920* in HEALTH CARE IN AMERICA 109–09 (S. Reverby and D. Rosner eds. 1979). One judge recognized this in *Glavin* as follows, "In the present case the services were gratuitous to the person injured, but the agent [physician] is indirectly compensated by the corporation: *i.e.*, by the opportunities for acquiring skill, experience, reputation, and subsequent practice in the profession." 12 R.I. at 431 (concurring opinion).

44. Rosner, *Business at the Bedside: Health Care in Brooklyn, 1890–1915* in HEALTH CARE IN AMERICA 124 (S. Reverby and D. Rosner eds. 1979).

45. Schlicke, *American Surgery's Noblest Experiment*, 106 ARCHIVES OF SURGERY 379 (1973).

46. 1880 R.I. Pub. Laws c. 802, p. 107; R.I. GEN. LAWS § 7-1-22 (1956); repealed 1968 R.I. Pub. Laws c. 43, § 2, and replaced by R.I. GEN. LAWS § 9-1-26 (Cum. Supp. 1981) (charitable hospitals liable as "at common law"). Hodge v. Osteopathic General Hospital of Rhode Island, 107 R.I. 135, 136, n.2, 145, 265 A.2d 733, 735 n.2, 739 (1970) (repeal not retroactive). Fournier v. Miriam Hospital, 93 R.I. 299, 308, 175 A.2d 298 302, (1961), aff'd on rehearing, 93 R.I. 308, 179 A.2d 578 (1962) (statute of 1880 constitutional because remedy against negligent actors preserved).

47. Flagiello v. Pennsylvania Hospital, 417 Pa. 486, 499, 208 A.2d 193, 199–200 (1965) (rejecting charitable immunity, the rule for 77 years, and holding hospital liable to patient for negligence of employees). Apparently unaware of the 1880 Rhode Island statute, the Pennsylvania court lauded Rhode Island as "a state . . . with wisdom and courage in inverse proportion to its geographical size." 417 Pa. at 499, 208 A.2d at 199.

48. Hillyer v. Governors of St. Bartholomew's Hospital, [1909] 2 K.B. 820.

49. Schloendorff v. Society of New York Hospital, 211 N.Y. 125, 105 N.E. 125 (1914).

50. Hillyer, [1909] 2 K.B. at 829.

51. Id. at 826, 830.

52. Id. at 829.

53. Id. at 829.

54. Goodhardt, Hospitals and Trained Nurses, 54 LAW Q. REV. 553, 556 (1938). But see Hillyer, [1909] 2 K.B. at 828.

55. Hillyer, [1909] 2 K.B. at 828–29 (emphasis added).

56. Cassidy v. Ministry of Health, [1951] 2 K.B. 343, 361. Goodhart, supra note 54, 54 LAW Q. REV. at 561, 574.

57. Schloendorff, 211 N.Y. at 135, 105 N.E. at 95. By relieving a hospital of a "grave responsibility and a budgetary item [it] would have had to assume," Judge Cardozo played a "favourite among competing social forces." B. LEVY, CARDOZO AND FRONTIERS OF LEGAL THINKING 103, 104 (1938). As late as 1939 Schloendorff was listed among the "tort cases which illustrate his permeating influence and his wisdom in decision," particularly as delineating "the extent of immunity of eleemosynary institutions and the reasons for granting it." Seavey, Mr. Justice Cardozo and the Law of Torts, 52 HARV. L. REV. 372, 405, 406, 390 YALE L.J. 390, 423, 424, 39 COLUM. L. REV. 20, 53, 54 (1939). But "In lapidary inscriptions a man is not upon oath." 2 J. BOSWELL, LIFE OF JOHNSON 407 (7 Apr. 1775).

58. Schloendorff, 211 N.Y. at 128, 105 N.E. at 93. Nevertheless, Cardozo seems to have disbelieved the plaintiff. "[I]f we are to credit the plaintiff's narrative." 211 N.Y. at 131, 105 N.E. at 94.

59. Schloendorff, 211 N.Y. at 130, 105 N.E. at 94.

60. Id. at 131–32, 105 N.E. at 94.

61. Id. at 132, 105 N.E. at 94.

62. Id. at 129, 105 N.E. at 93 (care in selection); Id. at 132, 105 N.E. at 94 (administrative conduct "not established by this record").

63. Glavin, 12 R.I. at 423.

64. Smith v. Duke University Hospital, 219 N.C. 628, 634, 14 S.E.2d 643, 647 (1941) (hospital only a provider of room and board); Alden v. Providence Hospital, 382 F.2d 163, 166 (D.C. Cir. 1967) (Berger J., dissenting, "a hotel with special services" but no diagnostic function). The analogy has also been stated only to disagree with it: Fridena v. Evans, 127 Ariz. 516, 518, 622 P.2d 463, 465 (1980) ("a physical structure and furnishings in which physicians practiced their art"); Yepremian v. Scarborough General Hospital, 88 D.L.R.3d 161, 172 (Ont. 1978) (a "specialized kind of hotel" if physician is private but not if employed); S. LAW AND S. POLAN, PAIN AND PROFIT 54 (1978) (hotel for the sick, workshop for physician); SOUTHWICK, supra note 25, at 346 ("a mere facility or hotel. . . . a 'doctor's workshop' "); Koskoff and Nadeau, Hospital Liability: The Emerg-

ing Standard of Care, 48 CONN. B.J. 305, 309 (1974) (more than a hotel or workshop). But see even the defense testimony in *Darling:* "[A] hospital is more than just bricks and mortar. . . . [T]he governing board is responsible for the proper care of the patient . . . it has the power to choose the standard of medicine that will be practiced in its hospital. . . ." 50 Ill. App.2d at 300, 200 N.E.2d at 173.

65. L. DAVIS, FELLOWSHIP OF SURGEONS 205 (1960).

66. *Glavin*, 12 R.I. at 417.

67. Rosner, *supra* note 44, at 124. "[T]oday's hospital . . . operates . . . in a businesslike fashion." Bing v. Thunig, 2 N.Y.2d 656, 664, 143 N.E.2d 3, 7, 163 N.Y.S.2d 3, 9 (1957).

68. 2 D. LOUISELL AND H. WILLIAMS, MEDICAL MALPRACTICE ¶¶ 17.01–17.57 and *Id.* 1981 Supp. 3–34 and President and Directors of Georgetown College v. Hughes, 130 F.2d 810, 814–15, 828 (D.C. Cir. 1942).

69. S. JONAS, MEDICAL MYSTERY 147 (1978). The idea of review did not originate with Codman. It had been suggested as early as 1732. *Id.* at 147. Dr. John Gregory, professor of medicine at Edinburgh and author of a work on medical ethics, suggested independent reviewers in 1770. J. BERLANT, PROFESSION AND MONOPOLY 88, 92 (1975). But Percival's Medical Ethics became dominant in this country, and they called only for moral sanctions and left "accountability for mistakes to individual conscience rather than collective professional action." *Id.* at 78. A variation of this idea of moral rather than coercive enforcement was to reappear. It is said to have been argued in *Darling* that "if licensing and accrediting bodies are satisfied that their regulations are being met," the courts should not interfere. Foster, *Illinois Case Extends Hospital Liability*, 103 MODERN HOSPITAL, Sept. 1964, at 95. In Corleto v. Shore Memorial Hospital, 138 N.J. Super. 302, 309, 350 A.2d 534, 538 (1975), the New Jersey Hospital Association argued that competence should be determined exclusively by the "hospital and its related personnel," not by the courts. And in Johnson v. Misericordia Community Hospital, 99 Wis.2d 708, 733, 301 N.W.2d 156, 169 (1981), the hospital argued unsuccessfully that a statutory declaration of its "moral obligation" negated its common law duty of care. Such faith in conscience and contrition might call for recitation of the General Confession in the Book of Common Prayer, "We have left undone those things we ought to have done; And we have done those things which we ought not to have done; And there is no health in us."

70. L. DAVIS, *supra* note 65, at 116; Goldberg, *The Duty of Hospitals and Hospital Medical Staffs to Regulate The Quality of Patient Care*, 129 W.J. MEDICINE 443, 445–46 (1978).

71. *Schloendorff*, 211 N.Y. at 131–32, 105 N.E. at 94.

72. Alden v. Providence Hospital, 328 F.2d 163, 166 (D.C. Cir. 1967) (hospital liable for negligence of employed physician, chief medical resident; dissent that hospital did not treat patient). Flagiello v. Pennsylvania Hospital, 417 Pa. 486, 519, 521, 208 A.2d 193, 209, 210 (1965) (charitable immunity abolished; dissent, "Hospitals and public charities are, next to the Church, the greatest benefactors known to mankind. . . . [and] are and always have been favorites of the law. . . .").

73. C. JACOBS, T. CHRISTOFFEL, AND N. DIXON, MEASURING THE QUALITY OF PATIENT CARE 24 (1976).

74. L. DAVIS, *supra* note 65, at 221. Goldberg, *supra* note 70, at 445.

75. L. DAVIS, *supra* note 65, at 204; Goldberg, *supra* note 70, at 445–46.

76. AMH, *supra* note 5, at ix–xi. There is no adequate work on the standardization movement which grew out of the scientific orientation that is marketed in the medical and surgical "specialties." M. Vogel, *The Invention of the Modern Hospital 1870–1930*, AMH, note 34, at 148.

77. AMH, *supra* note 5, at 93, 106.

78. C. JACOBS, *supra* note 73, at 24–25.

79. O. HOLMES, THE COMMON LAW 31 (M. Howe ed. 1963).

80. But see Rabon v. Rowan Memorial Hospital, Inc., 269 N.C. 1, 5, 152 S.E.2d 485, 488 (1967) (charitable immunity abolished; hospital liable for medical negligence of nurse), and Comment,

Private Hospital Held Liable for Medical Negligence of Professional Staff, 57 COLUM. L. REV. 1041, 1043 n. 23 (1957). Neither develops the references to English authority.

81. Gold v. Essex C.C. [1942] 2 K.B. 293, 302–03, 312–13.

82. Goodhart, *supra* note 54, at 553. This is said to be the most famous of Goodhardt's articles. Baker, *A.L.G.: An Editor's View,* 91 LAW Q. REV. 463, 464 (1975).

83. *Gold,* [1942] 2 K.B. at 297.

84. Hillyer v. Governors of St. Bartholomew's Hospital, [1909] 2 K.B. 820, 828–29.

85. Collins v. Hertfordshire County Council, [1947] 1 K.B. 598.

86. *Id.* at 616.

87. Cassidy v. Ministry of Health, [1951] 2 K.B. 343.

88. *Id.* at 360 (Denning, L.J.). Denning relates the pathetic circumstances of *Gold* and *Cassidy* in his little memoir, A. DENNING, THE DISCIPLINE OF LAW 237–41 (1979). His reference to a ship's captain is not to the "captain of the ship" doctrine known to American malpractice law. See J. KING, THE LAW OF MEDICAL MALPRACTICE 243 (1977). Denning was referring to the general rule that the employer of a ship's captain is responsible for the negligence of the captain despite the owner's inability to control him. The critical issue is employment, not control. See Hibbs v. Ross, 1 L.R.-Q.B. 529, 542 (1866). Although ability to control may be a basis of liability, inability to control does not inevitably lead to nonliability. *Cf.* River Wear Commissioners v. Adamson, 2 A.C. 743, 751 (1877). The irrelevance of control is very old. *Cf.* Boson v. Sandford, 91 Eng. Rep. 382 (K.B. 1691). See generally, 35 HALSBURY'S LAWS OF ENGLAND, Shipping and Navigation ¶ 1056 at 703 (3d ed. 1961). The American law is the same. See The Steamboat New World v. King, 57 U.S. (16 How.) 469, 475–76 (1853). *Glavin's* dictum that liability depended on control (*supra* see note 37) resulted in the special rule for hospitals. Exemption from liability by "reason of superior knowledge and skill of the servant has never been applied in other situations." Skill is a test "without legal or logical basis." Bobbé, *Tort Liability of Hospitals in New York,* 37 CORNELL L. REV. 419, 421, 428 (1952). See also Cunningham, *infra* note 92, at 534–35. "[T]he modern and proper basis of vicarious liability of the master is not his control or fault but the risks incident to his enterprises." See Hinman v. Westinghouse Electric Company, 2 Cal.3d 956, 960, 471 P.2d 988, 990, 88 Cal.Rptr. 188, 190 (1970). Continental law is said to be similar. See Kahn-Freund, *Servants and Independent Contractors,* 14 MOD. L. REV. 504, 508 (1951).

The "captain of the ship" doctrine is typically a device to impose liability on a surgeon for negligence of operating room personnel. McConnell v. Williams, 361 Pa. 355, 362 n.*, 65 A.2d 243, 246 n.1 (1949). It is a way of obtaining recovery from a physician when a hospital is protected by charitable immunity. Note that the immunity was not abolished in Pennsylvania until 16 years after *McConnell.* Flagiello v. Pennsylvania Hospital, 417 Pa. 486, 208 A.2d 193 (1965).

89. Silva v. Providence Hospital of Oakland, 14 Cal.2d 762, 781, 97 P.2d 978, 808 (1940) (charitable immunity abolished; hospital liable in bed-rail case without regard to whether decision to omit rails was by nurse or doctor; *Schloendorff* cited in dissent); Brown v. La Societe Francaise de Bien Faisance Mutuelle, 138 Cal. 475, 71 P. 516 (1903) (hospital liable for negligence of employed physician); see Rice v. California Lutheran Hospital, 27 Cal.2d 296, 304, 163 P.2d 860, 865 (1945) (hospital liable for professional acts of nurses and physicians despite argument based on *Schloendorff*). Garfield Memorial Hospital v. Marshall, 204 F.2d 721, 725 (D.C. Cir. 1953) (hospital liable for acts of employed physician; California dictum followed).

90. Bing v. Thunig, 2 N.Y.2d 656, 143 N.E.2d 3, 163 N.Y.S.2d 3 (1957).

91. Brown v. Moore, 247 F.2d 711, 717 (3d Cir. 1957) (hospital liable for negligence of employed physician). As a premonition of *Bing* see Moeller v. Hauser, 237 Minn. 368, 376–77, 54 N.W.2d 639, 645–46 (1952).

92. Cunningham, *The Hospital-Physician Relationship: Hospital Responsibility for Malpractice of Physicians* in HOSPITAL LIABILITY 532 (M. Bertolet and L. Goldsmith eds., 4th ed. 1980) (detailed

analysis of Brown v. La Societe Francaise etc., *supra* note 89, at 536–40 and 551–52).

93. *Bing*, 2 N.Y.2d at 661, 143 N.E.2d at 5, 163 N.Y.S.2d at 6.

94. Note, *Hospital Liability in New York Court of Appeals: A Study in Judicial Methodology*, 61 COLUM. L. REV. 871, 881 n. 50 (1961). *Bing* should also dispose of the "antiquated [and] rather meaningless notion that a corporation cannot practice medicine." SOUTHWICK, *supra* note 25, at 197, 412; Cunningham, *supra* note 93, at 530 nn. 31 and 33. Inability to do an act does not preclude liability for another's doing of the act. "Otherwise it is difficult to see how any corporate body could ever be liable for the acts of their servants." Gold v. Essex C.C., [1942] 2 K.B. 293, 312.

"If we were to rule that *respondeat superior* does not apply because the hospital is not licensed as a Nurse, then it would seem to follow that an airline should not be liable for the negligence of its pilot because the airline is not licensed to fly an aircraft." Bernardi v. Community Hospital Association, 166 Colo. 280, 291, 443 P.2d 708, 713 (1968) (applying *Bing*).

95. *Cf. Hillyer*, [1909] 2 K.B. at 828–29.

96. *Schloendorff*, 211 N.Y. at 130–132, 105 N.E. at 105.

97. *Bing*, 2 N.Y.2d at 666, 143 N.E.2d at 8, 163 N.Y.S.2d at 10.

98. *Id*. at 666, 143 N.E.2d at 8, 163 N.Y.S.2d at 11.

99. *Id*. at 667, 143 N.E.2d at 9, 163 N.Y.S.2d at 11.

100. *Id*. at 667, 143 N.E.2d at 9, 163 N.Y.S.2d at 12. But the language in *Schloendorff*, "Every human being of adult years and sound mind has a right to determine what shall be done with his own body, and a surgeon who performs an operation without his patient's consent commits an assault for which he is liable in damages," 211, N.Y. at 129, 105 N.E. at 93, lives on as a basis for the present law of informed consent. J. KATZ AND A. CAPRON, CATASTROPHIC DISEASES: WHO DECIDES WHAT? 80 (1975).

101. No English case on liability of a hospital for negligence of a physician selected by a patient has been found. The dicta say that there is no liability. See Cassidy v. Ministry of Health, [1951] 2 K.B. 343, 362 (liability said to depend on who pays the physician); Gold v. Essex C.C., [1942] 2 K.B. 293, 302 (hospital not liable for negligence of consulting physicians and perhaps not liable for that of house physicians). See also Kahn-Freund, *supra* note 88, at 508; 30 HALSBURY'S LAWS OF ENGLAND, The Medical Profession and Medical Practice ¶ 40, n.7 at 36 (4th ed. 1980). But HALSBURY'S is not infallible. See Goodhart, *supra* note 54, at 553. And the further dictum in *Gold*, that a hospital might not be liable for house physicians, was not followed in Cassidy.

102. *Schloendorff*, 211 N.Y. at 129, 105 N.E. at 93; Johnson v. Misericordia Community Hospital, 99 Wis.2d 708, 722, 301 N.W.2d 156, 163 (1981).

103. W. PROSSER, TORTS § 71 at 468 (4th ed. 1971). RESTATEMENT (SECOND) OF TORTS §§ 409–29 (1965). Section 409 states a general rule of nonliability, and the following 20 sections state exceptions thereto. Indeed, the Restatement says its "general rule" of nonliability of employers of independent contractors "is now primarily important as a preamble to the catalog of its exceptions." *Id*. § 409, Comment b. PROSSER, *supra*, says there are 24 exceptions. Whichever number is correct, the statement in SOUTHWICK, *supra* note 25, at 350, that the courts have "circumvented" the defense of independent contractor, has an unwarranted pejorative quality. What the defense now seems to mean is that a hospital is not liable for a staff physician's "collateral negligence." RESTATEMENT, *supra* § 426 and Illustration 3; Cassidy v. Ministry of Health, [1951] 2 K.B. 343, 364–65. Thus if an employee scalds a patient with hot tea, the hospital is liable. But if a private physician, as a gracious act, serves a patient and scalds him, the hospital is not liable, unless of course, it had reason to know he was often careless. RESTATEMENT, *supra*, § 411.

104. RESTATEMENT (SECOND) OF TORTS § 411 (1965).

105. *Id*. at § 415 (1965).

106. Hill v. James Walker Memorial Hospital, 407 F.2d 1036 (4th Cir. 1969); SOUTHWICK, *supra* note 25, at 404; W. PROSSER, TORTS § 93 at 624 n. 41 (4th ed. 1971).

107. Joiner v. Mitchell County Hospital Authority, 125 Ga. App. 1, 12, 186 S.E.2d 307, 308 (1971), aff'd, 229 Ga. 140, 142, 189 SE.2d 412, 414 (1972). SOUTHWICK, supra note 25, at 196, 349. The administration of the hospital must "stimulate the medical staff" to review "the professional qualifications and performance of each individual staff physician." Id. at 411. Denning rebuked himself for failing as counsel in Gold v. Essex C.C. to make clear the nondelegability of the duty of care. Cassidy v. Ministry of Health, [1951] 2 K.B. 343, 363.

108. Corleto v. Shore Memorial Hospital, 138 N.J. Super. 302, 350 A.2d 534 (1975); St. John's Hospital M.S. v. St. John Reg. M.C., 245 N.W.2d 472, 474 (S.D. 1976) (capacity of medical staff to sue hospital).

109. Fiorentino v. Wenger, 19 N.Y.2d 407, 227 N.E.2d 296, 280 N.Y.S.2d 373 (1967); Mayers v. Litow, 154 Cal.App.2d 413, 316 P.2d 351 (1957). Cf. Pogue v. Hospital Authority of DeKalb County, 120 Ga. App. 230, 170 S.E.2d 53 (1969) as explained by Mitchell County Hospital Authority v. Joiner, 229 Ga. 140, 141, 189 S.E.2d 412, 414 (1972) (hospital not liable for negligence of independent contractor operating emergency service where failure to supervise contractor was not raised as hospital's own negligence).

110. "[A] hospital has a direct and independent responsibility to its patients, over and above that of the physicians and surgeons practicing therein, to take reasonable steps to (1) ensure that its medical staff is qualified for the privileges granted and/or (2) to evaluate the care provided." Johnson v. Misericordia Community Hospital, 99 Wis.2d 708, 725, 301 N.W.2d 156, 165 (1981).

111. Foley v. Bishop Clarkson Memorial Hospital, 185 Neb. 89, 94, 173 N.W.2d 881, 884 (1970); Johnson v. Misericordia Community Hospital, 99 Wis.2d 708, 739–44, 301 N.W.2d 156, 171–73 (1981).

112. E.g.: W. CURRAN, supra note 23, at 364–90, 474–81 (3d ed. 1982) (with copious references to periodicals); HOSPITAL LIABILITY (M. Bertolet and L. Goldsmith eds., 4th ed. 1980), passim; SOUTHWICK, supra note 25, passim; Copeland, supra note 24. The two Wisconsin opinions seem to list all the relevant cases. Johnson v. Misericordia Community Hospital, 99 Wis.2d 708, 301 N.W.2d 156 (1981), aff'g, 97 Wis.2d 521, 294 N.W.2d 501 (1980).

113. Fiorentino v. Wenger, 19 N.Y.2d 407, 227 N.E.2d 296, 280 N.Y.S.2d 373 (1967).

114. For similar holdings see Cox v. Hayworth, 54 N.C. App. 328, 262 S.E.2d 391 (1980), 283 S.E.2d 392, 395 (1981), and Cooper v. Curry, 92 N.M. 417, 589 P.2d 201, 204 (1979).

115. Fiorentino v. Wenger, 26 A.D.2d 693, 694, 279 N.Y.S.2d 557, 559 (1966) (dissent).

116. Dunn, supra note 24, at 16.

117. Fiorentino, 19 N.Y.2d at 415, 227 N.E.2d at 299, 280 N.Y.S.2d at 278. The holding of nonliability for allowing the experimental surgery has been questioned. W. CURRAN, supra note 23, at 480. But Wenger had outstanding qualifications and was a vice president of the Euthanasia Society of America. NEW YORK TIMES, Feb. 11, 1975, p. 42, col. 3.

118. Corleto v. Shore Memorial Hospital, 138 N.J. Super. 302, 311, 350 A.2d 534, 538 (1975).

119. Most of the opinion is reprinted in S. LAW AND S. POLAN, PAIN AND PROFIT 215–45 (1978). The references to Fiorentino are at 241 and 244. Other extracts are in Copeland, supra note 24, 5 N. KY. L. REV. at 74–75. For general references see SOUTHWICK, supra, note 25, and HOSPITAL LIABILITY, supra note 112. Accounts of the case are in 29 Citation 18 (1974) and Goldberg, The Duty of Hospitals and Hospital Medical Staffs to Regulate the Quality of Patient Care, 129 W. J. MEDICINE 443 (1978). The reference to reversal by the intermediate appellate court for holding Nork had waived a jury trial in SOUTHWICK, supra note 25, at 421 n. 188, is wrong. The correct citation is Gonzales v. Nork, 20 Cal.3d 500, 573 P.2d 458, 131 Cal.Rptr. 240 (1978) (affirming waiver of jury). See S. LAW, supra at 215 n.*. For an example of the notoriety of the case see S. BOK, LYING 155 (1978). The first California appellate opinion upholding corporate responsibility of a hospital appeared after this chapter had been prepared for the press. Elam v. College Park Hospital, 132 Cal. App.3d 332, 183 Cal. Rptr. 156 (1982). The author's opinion in Nork is said to "articulate almost precisely the same standard as the Elam opinion." CALIFORNIA MALPRACTICE TOPICS n.3 (D.

Rubsamen ed. June 1982); Loveridge & Kimball, *Hospital Corporate Negligence Comes to California: Questions in the Wake of Elam v. College Park Hospital*, 14 PAC. L.J. 803 (1983).

120. S. LAW, *supra* note 119, at 52.

121. S. LAW, *supra* note 119, at 245.

122. SOUTHWICK, *supra* note 25, at 349 and 411.

123. S. LAW, *supra* note 119, at 65; Copeland, *supra* note 24, at 75.

124. AMH, *supra* note 5, at 151.

125. S. SHARPE, S. FISCINA AND M. HEAD, LAW AND MEDICINE 658 N. 18 (1978) (*Corleto*); 29 Citation 19 (1974) (*Nork*).

126. Johnson v. Misericordia Community Hospital, 99 Wis.2d 708, 301 N.W.2d 156 (1981), *aff'g*, 97 Wis.2d 521, 294 N.W.2d 501 (1980).

127. Fridena v. Evans, 127 Ariz. 516, 622 P.2d 463 (1981).

128. Bost v. Riley, 44 N.C. App. 638, 262 S.E.2d 391 (1980).

129. Thus failure to investigate competence is not a basis of liability where investigation would have disclosed no reason for refusal of staff appointment. *See* Ferguson v. Gonyaw, 64 Mich. App. 685, 698, 236 N.W.2d 543, 550 (1976).

130. Renslow v. Mennonite Hospital, 67 Ill.2d 348, 355, 367 N.E.2d 1250, 1254 (1977) (hospital liable for preconception injury caused by transfusion of Rh positive blood).

131. SOUTHWICK, *supra* note 25, at 413, lists Michigan, Indiana and Arizona. See Beeck v. Tucson General Hospital, 18 Ariz. App. 165, 170, 500 P.2d 1153, 1158 (1972).

132. 22 Cal. Admin. Code §§ 70701, 70703 (1975).

133. AMH, *supra* note 5, at 56.

134 *E.g.*, UNIVERSITY OF CALIFORNIA SAN FRANCISCO HOSPITALS AND CLINICS, BYLAWS, RULES AND REGULATIONS OF THE MEDICAL STAFF 5, 21–22 (1979).

135. "The hospital shall demonstrate that the quality of care provided to all patients is consistently optimal by constantly evaluating it through reliable and valid measures. Where the quality of patient care is shown to be less than optimal, improvement in quality shall be demonstrated." JOINT COMMISSION ON ACCREDITATION OF HOSPITALS, ACCREDITATION MANUAL FOR HOSPITALS 143 (1979).

136. "The hospital shall demonstrate a consistent endeavor to deliver patient care that is optimal within available resources and consistent with achievable goals. A major component in the application of this principle is the operation of a quality assurance program." AMH, *supra* note 5, at 151.

137. W. CURRAN, *supra* note 23, at 750, 753, 762–63, 764.

138. W. CURRAN, *supra* note 23, at 757.

139. W. CURRAN, *supra* note 23, at 750, 751.

140. *E.g.*, CALIFORNIA HOSPITAL ASSOCIATION, CONSENT MANUAL 21 (conditions for admission), 41 (consent to surgery etc.) (10th ed., revised May, 1981).

141. Tunkl v. Regents of University of California, 60 Cal.2d 92, 383 P.2d 441, 32 Cal.Rptr. 33 (1963); but *cf.* SOUTHWICK, *supra* note 25, at 423.

142. *Johnson*, 99 Wis.2d at 733, 301 N.W.2d at 169.

143. *Fridena*, 127 Ariz. at 516, 622 P.2d at 466.

144. *Darling*, 33 Ill.2d at 331, 211 N.E.2d at 257.

145. *Johnson*, 99 Wis.2d at 724, 301 N.W.2d at 164.

146. As quoted in Reeves, *A Reporter at Large (Along Tocqueville's Path—Part I)*, THE NEW YORKER, April 5, 1982, at 77. For quite different examples of this phenomenon see Holman, *The Time Lag Between Medicine and Law*, 9 LEX ET SCIENTIA 102 (1972), reprinted in W. CURRAN, *supra* note 23 at 2.

147. Holmes, *The Path of the Law*, 10 HARV. L. REV. 457, 466 (1897).

Chapter 3

The Role of JCAH in Assuring Quality Care

*John E. Affeldt, M.D., and Regina M. Walczak, M.P.H.**

INTRODUCTION

For over 60 years, the health care industry has participated in a voluntary accreditation process designed to improve the quality of services provided in health and health-related facilities. Voluntary accreditation is founded on the philosophy that health care professionals should assess the quality of patient care they provide. The Joint Commission on Accreditation of Hospitals (JCAH), organized by health care professionals to support and maintain this philosophy, is committed to establishing and improving standards that suggest the optimal structure in which care can be delivered. The introduction of a quality assurance standard in 1979 illustrates the evolution of quality appraisal mechanisms and establishes parameters for evaluation of patient care within the context of other JCAH standards.

This chapter will describe the roots of voluntary accreditation; the evolution of quality assurance activities in the context of JCAH standards; and the research and social, economic, and political forces that shaped quality assurance program evaluation and risk management activities. Finally, it will discuss JCAH's role in quality assurance and in the future directions of quality assurance.

THE ROOTS OF VOLUNTARY ACCREDITATION

The concept of voluntary accreditation grew out of a resolution made at the Third Clinical Congress of Surgeons of North America in 1912 that "some system of standardization of hospital equipment and hospital work should be developed, to the end that those [sic] institutions having the highest ideals may

*The authors wish to thank Maryanne Shanahan, Director, Department of Publications, JCAH, for her assistance in preparing this material.

49

have proper recognition before the profession, and that those of inferior equipment and standards should be stimulated to raise the quality of their work. In this way patients will receive the best type of treatment, and the public will have some means of recognizing those institutions devoted to the highest ideals of medicine."[1]

As a result of this resolution, the American College of Surgeons (ACS) was established in 1913, and it developed a one-page set of minimum essential standards in 1917. The *Minimum Standard* focused on the medical staff and its responsibility for assuring quality care.

In 1918, the ACS inaugurated the Hospital Standardization Program, and the quality of the care provided in hospitals that participated in the program improved noticeably. As the success of the program became known, more and more hospitals voluntarily sought the educational and consultative benefits of the program. The number of approved hospitals increased from 89 during the first year of operation to more than 3,000 in 1951—over one-half of the hospitals in the country.

As the size of the standardization program increased, so did its costs. By 1950, the annual cost of operating the program exceeded two million dollars. Unable to continue sole support of the program, ACS sought the participation of other national professional organizations. In 1951, the ACS, the American College of Physicians, the American Hospital Association, the American Medical Association, and the Canadian Medical Association established the Joint Commission on Accreditation of Hospitals. (The Canadian Medical Association withdrew in 1959 to participate in its own national hospital accreditation program. The American Dental Association became a corporate member in 1979, and in 1981 the JCAH Board of Commissioners appointed a public member.)

In 1953, JCAH published *Standards for Hospital Accreditation*, an updated and expanded edition of the *Minimum Standard* of the Hospital Standardization Program. This edition included standards on a hospital's governing body, bylaws, buildings, food preparation, drug control, and dietary and nursing services. The standards emphasized that

> the medical staff is responsible to the governing body of the hospital for the quality of all medical care rendered. . . . This will depend upon the medical staff's effectiveness in selection of those recommended for staff appointments and hospital privileges, constant check upon the character and quality of medical care rendered, preparation of adequate medical records, and conduct of conferences in clinical pathology. The medical staff organizational duties shall include maintenance of the proper quality of all medical care and treatment in the hospital.[2]

From its inception in 1951, JCAH has maintained the principle promulgated in the *Minimum Standard*—that the medical staff is responsible for analyzing, reviewing, evaluating, and, when necessary, improving the quality of clinical practice. JCAH also responded to the results of research in quality assessment, to changes and advances in technology, and to social, economic, and political forces that affected the health care industry by refining and expanding quality protective mechanisms of the medical staff as the state of the art of medical care and medical care evaluation evolved. From the late 1950s through the mid-1970s, considerable research in quality assessment, as well as social, economic, and political forces, stimulated the evolution of JCAH quality assurance requirements. During that time, JCAH also expanded its accreditation activities and programs. Today, JCAH has four accreditation programs: (1) the Hospital Accreditation Program (HAP); (2) Accreditation Program/Psychiatric Facilities (AP/PF); (3) Accreditation Program/Long-Term Care (AP/LTC); and (4) Accreditation Program/Ambulatory Health Care (AP/AHC).

EVOLUTION OF QUALITY ASSURANCE REQUIREMENTS

Research

Although research in the quality of medical care can be traced to the Flexner report, which condemned standards of medical education in 1910,[3] such research did not become rigorous until the 1950s and 1960s. In 1956, Lembke received national recognition as a pioneer in the development of scientific methods of medical audit. He attempted to make judgments on the quality of care objective by establishing criteria for physician performance.[4] A number of other studies were conducted in the mid-1960s. Payne and Lyons proposed a similar system that advocated self-assessment by providers of care.[5] Williamson, Alexander, and Miller explored the relationship of process and outcome measures of quality.[6] Sanazaro and Williamson classified elements of physician performance and its effects on patients.[7] Brown and Fleisher introduced the bi-cycle concept, which proposed linking quality assurance efforts to continuing education.[8]

Social, Economic, and Political Forces

The socioeconomic and political climate of the 1960s triggered major alterations in American thinking, and the nation's traditional value systems came under considerable scrutiny. Public consensus supported the concept that every American was entitled to a reasonable degree of health care services. Consumer activists demanded that health care professionals be held accountable for their activities and services.

In 1965, Public Law 89-97 (Medicare)[8a] was enacted. Written into the Medicare Act was the provision that the hospitals participating in that program were to maintain the level of patient care that had come to be recognized as the norm.

The standards of JCAH are specifically referred to in the law, and the *Conditions of Participation for Hospitals,* subsequently promulgated and published by the Social Security Administration,[8b] reflected the 1965 standards of JCAH.

Public financing of health care stimulated an unprecedented inflation in the cost of care and use of services. Business, industry, government agencies, and third party payers became increasingly concerned about the use and quality of health care services and sought a more active role in determining the appropriateness of these services. In 1972, Congress directed the then Department of Health, Education, and Welfare to develop its own program to ensure the necessity, quality, and cost-effectiveness of care financed under federal health programs. Through the legislation, professional standards review organizations (PSROs) were established.

Case Law

Before the mid-1960s, case law recognized that hospitals had only limited responsibilities to patients. In 1965, however, the *Darling v. Charleston Community Memorial Hospital* decision (211 N.E. 2d 253) clarified the roles of hospital trustees, hospital administration, and medical staffs by ruling that "the hospital was liable for direct duties owed to the patient."[9a] The *Darling* decision made the hospital the focal point for the provision and coordination of medical care and for controlling and improving standards of care. The decision affected statutory law in several states.

In 1972, in *Purcell and Tucson General Hospital v. Zimbelman* (500 P. 22 335), the court found the hospital negligent because it failed to ensure that only competent professionals were on its staff. The hospital was held responsible for controlling medical staff privileges.[9b]

In 1974, in *Gonzales v. Nork and Mercy Hospital* (Cal. Super Ct, Sacramento Cal, Docket No. 228566), the court found that the hospital "was liable for the breach of its duty to the patient to protect him from acts of malpractice by an independent or privately retained physician. The duty was breached if the hospital knew, had reason to know, or should have known of the surgeon's incompetence." Although the hospital argued that it had a medical staff peer review system in place, the court found the system "casual, random, and uncritical."[9c]

The trend in these cases is clear. The organized medical staff and its committees act on behalf of the hospital, which is accountable for the medical staff's negligent omissions.

JCAH Response

During these years, JCAH revised its standards several times to reflect the rapid advancements in the health care industry that were the result of the research and social, economic, political, and legislative changes just described. A major revision of the standards was initiated in 1965, partly as a response to the Medicare legislation. The revised standards were introduced in 1970 in the *Accreditation Manual for Hospitals*. A landmark achievement, these standards elaborated on medical staff responsibilities for the "analysis, review, and evaluation of clinical practice that exists within the hospital."[10] For the first time, medical care evaluation was described as a fact-finding and educational function—an analysis of medical practice based on criteria established by the medical staff. This evaluation included periodic review of the use of a facility's beds and a review of medical, surgical, and obstetrical functions (including tissue review and analysis of necropsy reports).

Further revisions in 1972 related the quality of care to use of services and required a more prescriptive approach to medical care evaluation. Although JCAH standards had specifically required clinical privileging and patient care evaluation since 1951, utilization review since 1965, and continuing medical education since 1970, the methods by which these functions could be accomplished were not explicitly stated. Because of increased concern that the assessment and improvement of care be demonstrated, medical care evaluation became a critical element of JCAH's accreditation decision process. JCAH maintained that:

> one of the most important obligations of an organized medical staff of a hospital is to provide a continuing, objective, critical, and corrective analysis of the clinical work performed by its members. The steps involved are several. . . . Develop and refine the most useful possible patient data bank. . . . Develop working norms . . . to permit the careful analysis of variations from usual practice, and [to] facilitate the rational assessment of justification for them. . . . Establish an efficient method of reviewing all or an equitable and representative sample of all clinical work. . . . Provide for systematic utilization of the findings from medical care evaluation activities to identify areas of need for medical staff education, [to] counsel with practitioners displaying frequent variation from the norms, [to] make recommendations to medical staff authority concerning suspensions, curtailment or removal of clinical privileges, or separation from staff of those members who display an inability to benefit from educational efforts.[11]
> (p. 186)

By 1975, these principles had been refined, and the performance evaluation procedure for auditing and improving patient care (PEP) had been developed. The procedure provided a method for an objective, systematic approach to patient care evaluation and focused primarily on measuring the outcome of care rather than the process of care. JCAH became known as the proponent of "outcome audit."

During the same time, other standards of the Hospital Accreditation Program were refined and expanded. In 1976, JCAH introduced standards for antibiotic review, utilization review, and infection control. JCAH also developed standards for the Accreditation Program for Psychiatric Facilities that addressed clinical privileging, utilization review, professional growth and development, individual case review, audit, and program evaluation. The accreditation programs for ambulatory health care and long-term care facilities adopted the principles of patient care audit, as well as other quality related mechanisms.

By 1978, emphasis on audit activities had caused other essential quality related activities to be overshadowed. All too frequently, efforts to meet audit requirements were a matter of paper compliance. Data collection was heavily emphasized, and few results could be used for follow-up activities. Although the objectives of audit were desirable and many hospital staffs had conducted successful audits that were useful in analyzing patterns of care, the activity was often regarded as tedious, costly, and unproductive. Facilities frequently lost sight of the purpose of evaluation and paid little heed to whether improvement occurred as a result. It also had become apparent that review and evaluation activities in hospital departments and services had proliferated to the extent that they required purposeful integration if patient care and clinical performance were to improve.

Responding to survey information and research data that demonstrated lack of improvement in patient care and clinical performance to the extent anticipated, the Board of Commissions directed staff to examine alternate methods for assessing the quality of care. After an extensive review of the literature and discussion with researchers and health care professionals involved in quality assessment, a broadened approach to quality assurance was proposed.

The New Quality Assurance Standard

In 1979, the Board of Commissioners approved a new quality assurance standard for hospitals. At the same time, the board eliminated the numerical requirements for patient care audit. This action emphasized JCAH's broader, more flexible approach to quality assurance. In this approach, audit becomes just one of many useful methods for assessing and monitoring quality of care.

The intent of the standard is to allow greater flexibility in quality assurance activities; to encourage innovation and creativity in the evaluation process; to encourage elimination of duplicate committees, activities, and functions; to encourage coordination of fragmented activities throughout the facility; to promote systematic and effective evaluation of overall patient care; and to encourage communication of the results of evaluation so that improvement in patient care and clinical performance can be assured.

Recognizing that the principles of quality assurance apply to all areas of health care delivery, the Board of Commissioners directed all accreditation programs to develop similar standards for quality assurance. Between 1979 and 1981 all four accreditation programs had adopted similar quality assurance standards. Although the functional, or quality related, components may differ, the fundamental principles are the same: (1) an effective problem-solving process that identifies and resolves important problems in patient care; and (2) integration and/or coordination of all quality related activities in an organized, comprehensive program.

Problem Identification and Resolution

Improvement in patient care through the identification and resolution of problems is the heart of quality assurance. To be effective, the problem-solving process should be an integral part of the management of the facility or department and the medical staff organization. Response to problems frequently requires the involvement and support of administration, departmental managers, or medical staff leaders. Through management channels, problems often can be addressed by modifying policies or changing staffing patterns or equipment. Performance-related problems can be addressed through staff performance appraisals or medical staff reappraisal and reappointment.

Once corrective actions have been taken, monitoring the status of the problem should verify its resolution or reduction to an acceptable level.

Organized, Comprehensive Programs

An organized quality assurance effort or program is necessary to ensure appropriate communication of findings and appropriate action to correct identified problems. Organizing the quality assurance program also should ensure that all relevant data are being used in individual quality assessment functions. For example, data gathering or monitoring functions such as infection control, surgical case review, incident reporting, drug utilization review, preventive maintenance programs, medical staff department review, support service review, utilization review, and audit have existed in most facilities for many years. Under the auspices of a quality assurance program, these activities can be designed to identify or assess patient care problems.

In organizing a quality assurance program, facilities should define the responsibilities and relationships of committees, functions, and departments and refine sources of information on patient care problems. Once this is accomplished, problem identification and assessment become the focus of various quality assurance activities, and findings can be channeled to the appropriate authority in the department or facility for response.

Risk Management and Program Evaluation

Risk Management

Risk management refers to those activities designed to reduce or eliminate the potential of financial loss due to damage, theft, misplacement of property, or patient injury. The concept of risk management developed as a result of the malpractice crisis in the mid-1970s, which demonstrated the need to respond to or prevent patient injuries that might result in hospital liability. In 1976, the California Medical Feasibility Study examined the types and severity of adverse events that occurred in 23 hospitals. Results indicated that nearly five percent of patients hospitalized in 1974 had experienced a potentially compensable event (i.e., an occurrence that could have resulted in litigation against the facility and/or medical staff).[12] As part of the study, generic screening criteria were developed to detect serious adverse effects.

The process of general screening for, evaluating, and responding to adverse events is known by a variety of terms, including risk management, loss control, risk control, and risk monitoring. By whatever name it is called, the main focus of the process is to identify, respond to, or prevent potentially compensable events. The conduct of risk management activities varies dramatically from facility to facility. Many facilities maintain a traditional safety program that focuses on environmental hazards and merely screens incident reports. Others have established formal programs that anticipate risk by using screening criteria and claims analysis to detect and analyze adverse events. Findings are used to plan corrective measures and prevent further occurrences.

Although there is no standard that requires establishment of a risk management program, JCAH recognizes the importance of identifying and responding to untoward events or incidents. Whether the activity is part of the safety program or a separate department in the facility, risk prevention and response can be considered a component of the overall quality assurance program. Just as infection control is a facility-wide function aimed at minimizing nosocomial infection, risk management can be considered a facility-wide function aimed at minimizing risk to patients and to the facility. Operationally, both may be discrete programs, although each has a specific, narrow focus. Data from each function can be assimilated with data from other quality related functions as part of the overall quality assurance program.

Program Evaluation

Program evaluation was introduced in 1975 in the standards for alcoholism facilities to provide management a tool for examining the degree to which program goals and objectives are achieved. As described in the *Consolidated Standards Manual,* facility and program evaluation is a systematic process for analyzing progress in attaining the goals and objectives of a facility's programs or their components.[13] In psychiatric and substance abuse facilities, quality related activities, such as patient care monitoring and infection control, focus on clinical aspects of care. Program evaluation is similar to management by objectives. Just as quality assurance does not require an elaborate design methodology, a separate committee, or an individual with specific academic requirements, neither does program evaluation. It can be accomplished within the organizational structure of a facility. Like quality assurance, the mission of program evaluation should be described in writing, and its effectiveness should be appraised.

Problems identified through program evaluation may have an impact on patient care and may be addressed through mechanisms established by the facility's quality assurance program. From this perspective, program evaluation can be considered a component or function of the facility-wide quality assurance program. At the same time, because its scope includes operational or administrative functions and because it focuses on achieving defined objectives, program evaluation can provide management and department heads with a system of management accountability. As a management tool, program evaluation can be used to evaluate functioning programs, including the quality assurance program.

The Relationship between Risk Management, Program Evaluation, and Quality Assurance

Because their scope is facility-wide and their approaches to problem solving are similar, risk management and program evaluation have been linked with quality assurance in some facilities. The key distinction among these three functions lies in the nature and impact of the problems they address.

Quality assurance encompasses the detection, evaluation, and resolution of problems directly related to patient care. That is, quality assurance deals with the identification of and response to problems that affect the care and treatment of patients. Only some problems identified through risk management or program evaluation have a direct impact on the care provided to patients. When risk management or program evaluation activities detect such problems, they are a source of data for the quality assurance program. Because risk management and program evaluation have other objectives, they operate outside the scope of quality assurance, with only limited interaction. For example, program evaluation may address budget, community goals, or management deficiencies in implementing a program. Similarly, some activities of a risk management program may focus on detection of problems, such as loss of property or the safety of employees. Because these areas do not have a direct impact on patient care, they can be addressed without involving the quality assurance program. (For an illustration of interaction with and action without the quality assurance program, see Figure 3-1.)

Figure 3-1 Illustration of the Relationship between Risk Management, Program Evaluation, and Quality Assurance

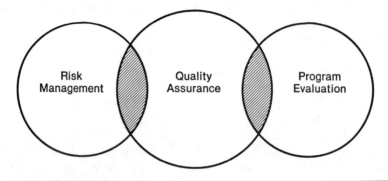

ROLE OF JCAH IN QUALITY ASSURANCE

Throughout its history, JCAH has represented the health care professions and served as their voice for quality. JCAH responded to technological, scientific, political, legal, social, and economic forces by revising and improving its standards. JCAH also has been a leader in improving health care by developing new standards that assist health care facilities to improve their operations. By working with experts in specialty areas and keeping pace with research activities, JCAH has strengthened the quality of health care services in this country. In 1976, for example, the JCAH Board of Commissioners approved an infection control standard that outlined an organized approach to infection surveillance. Today, infection control programs are essential functions in health care facilities. Moreover, as prophylactic use and overutilization of antibiotics grew to untoward proportions, JCAH established specific standards for medical staff antibiotic review.

The quality assurance standards are yet another example of JCAH's leadership in the health care field. The standards shifted emphasis from broad-based review of diagnoses to focused assessment of known or suspected problems in patient care. In defining the problem-solving goal of quality assurance, JCAH has established the direction of quality assurance for the 1980s.

Progress in Implementing the Standards

Implementing change can be a difficult process fraught with resistance. Response to the new latitude and flexibility of the quality assurance standards has thus been relatively slow and uneasy. Because many staffs had become adept at conducting audits and felt secure in meeting previous JCAH requirements, the opportunity to implement alternate approaches and become creative in problem-solving efforts left many without direction and support from facility administration and the medical staff hierarchy. Consequently, many facilities deferred implementation of the problem-focused approach and began organizing a quality assurance program, examining the roles and functions of various committees, defining levels of authority and responsibility, and developing an implementation plan. Obtaining approval for a quality assurance plan and allocating personnel to manage the program typically took between six months to one year. For most facilities that began implementing quality assurance activities shortly after the standards were announced, results are only now becoming apparent.

Although implementation has progressed slowly, the principles of the new approach to quality assurance have been applauded. However, it is premature to expect empirical data to substantiate the impact of quality assurance in facilities. To date, this impact can be ascertained only through observations during on-site surveys and anecdotal descriptions of problems that individual facilities have solved.

Since JCAH began surveying quality assurance programs in late 1980, accreditation data have been evaluated to determine facilities' progress in implementing the standards. As benchmarks of initial progress, JCAH looked at three basic aspects of quality assurance programs:

1. assignment of authority and responsibility for quality assurance;
2. progress toward integration or coordination of quality related activities; and
3. a written quality assurance plan describing the program's operation.

Survey data[14] indicate that in mid-1981, two years after the standards were first introduced, only 20 percent of facilities surveyed by the hospital and psychiatric accreditation programs had not met these basic requirements. By mid-1982, only 10 percent of the hospitals surveyed did not meet the basic requirements, although noncompliance among psychiatric, substance abuse, long-term care, and ambulatory care facilities remained at 20 percent.

Because a basic tenet of the quality assurance standards is flexibility, many different organizational approaches to quality assurance have emerged. For example, most facilities established quality assurance committees. In many of those facilities, utilization review or audit committees simply changed their names and adopted a broader scope. In others, new committees were formed.

Quality assurance appears to work best when senior management and senior medical staff members assume responsibility for oversight. Placing authority for quality assurance with those empowered to bring about change facilitates the problem-solving process. Frequently, the quality assurance committee reports to the medical staff executive committee. In some facilities, members of the governing body sit on quality assurance committees that report directly to the governing body.

In many facilities, a quality assurance director or coordinator has been appointed to perform day-to-day functions in conjunction with the committee. In others—although the percentage is small—a quality assurance coordinator or director may be the primary authority for quality assurance, working with the facility's management and existing committee structure.

Though organizational issues have, for the most part, been addressed, facilities still face several challenges in developing effective quality assurance programs. Perhaps the greatest of these challenges is obtaining and maintaining physician involvement in and support of the quality assurance program. Although quality assurance programs frequently will be found operating with the support and involvement of administration and nursing and support services, the organized medical staff often will provide only perfunctory support. Physicians may be hesitant to accept the ramifications of a hospital-wide quality assurance effort; they may be skeptical of such a program's success because of previous experience with audit; and/or they may not wish to address problems openly. In general, however, physicians have been reluctant to embrace the concept of an integrated, facility-wide quality assurance function. But, because of the nature of physicians' responsibilities for patient care, their involvement in quality assurance is essential if it is to succeed.

Another challenge that facilities face is the shift from general evaluation of care to a specific, objective mechanism for problem identification and assessment. Although many facilities continue to use the audit method, existing data sources must be refined and used, and broader data collection instruments must be developed. Moreover, data from these sources must be used more effectively in privilege delineation, in reappraisal and reappointment, and in continuing education activities and management systems revisions. In addition, greater emphasis should be placed on "closing the loop" by taking action and monitoring problem status, major functions of an effective quality assurance program.

Finally, facilities must develop a strong commitment to defining and addressing real problems in patient care. Health care professionals frequently confuse patient care problems with management problems and often use the quality assurance program to confront management issues, such as interpersonal or interdepartmental conflicts or system deficiencies, that do not have direct impact on patient care. For example, a nursing unit in one facility focused on ensuring that charge slips for services and supplies were accurate, rather than on ensuring that nursing care assessments were performed appropriately.

Resolution of systems problems such as the timely communication of diagnostic reports or patient waiting time can be addressed, but on balance the detection and resolution of problems in the actual provision of care should be the major goal of the quality assurance program. The intent of quality assurance activity is to ensure that competent health care professionals provide quality care to all patients.

FUTURE GOALS

For more than 30 years, JCAH has been the recognized leader in quality health care, establishing and revising progressive standards as the state of the art of medical care and evaluation evolved. The quality assurance standards are the culmination of an evolutionary process that links all other quality related standards. From a minimum standard in 1918 that required medical staffs to "review and analyze their clinical experience at regular intervals,"[15] standards for infection control, surgical case and antibiotic usage review, and evaluation of nursing and support services have evolved. The quality assurance standards complete the circle by linking these quality related standards in a manner that allows information to be communicated and accountability for problem resolution to be established.

The quality assurance standards mark a turning point in the purpose and focus of quality review. Rather than focusing strictly on broad diagnostic categories, quality assurance goals are now aimed at identifying and resolving patient care problems by strengthening all appraisal and response mechanisms. However, although the quality assurance standards have helped health care professionals coordinate efforts to identify and assess facility-wide problems, objective and thorough scrutiny of discrete areas of care has not improved. In fact, 33 percent of hospitals surveyed in 1981 received recommendations in medical staff monitoring activities (e.g., antibiotic usage and surgical case review) and clinical privileging; 39 percent of psychiatric and substance abuse facilities surveyed in 1981 received recommendations in clinical privileging, patient care management, and program evaluation.[14] One of JCAH's essential goals for the future, therefore, is to help facilities achieve a balance between problem-focused review of facility-wide concerns and in-depth review of critical indicators or single parameters of care.

JCAH will guide facilities in these efforts and will also monitor their progress. Now that the structure for quality assurance in the 1980s has been defined, JCAH, working with health care professionals, will refine and strengthen the process for conducting all quality appraisal activities. Because the outcome— improved patient care and clinical performance—remains to be achieved, JCAH will seek to strengthen objective, valid measurements of care by encouraging more definitive application of clinical criteria. It will strive to keep pace with and lead change in the field of quality assessment and assurance.

NOTES

1. L. Davis. *Fellowship of Surgeons: A History of the American College of Surgeons* (Chicago: Charles C Thomas, Pub., 1960), p. 476.

2. Joint Commission on Accreditation of Hospitals (JCAH), *Standards for Hospital Accreditation*, 1953 ed. (Chicago: JCAH, 1953), p. 22.

3. A. Flexner, *Medical Education in the United States and Canada*, Bulletin no. 4. (Boston: Merrymount, 1910).

4. P.A. Lembke, "Medical Auditing by Scientific Methods," *Journal of the American Medical Association* 162 (1956):646–655.

5. B. Payne and T.F. Lyons, *Method for Evaluating and Improving Personal Medical Care Quality: Episode of Illness Study* (Ann Arbor, Mich.: University of Michigan School of Medicine, 1972).

6. J.W. Williamson, M. Alexander, and C.E. Miller, "Priorities in Patient-Care Research and Continuing Medical Education," *Journal of the American Medical Association* 204 (1968):303–308.

7. P.J. Sanazaro and J.W. Williamson, "Physician Performance and Its Effects on Patients: A Classification Based on Report by Internists, Surgeons, Pediatricians and Obstetricians," *Medical Care* 8 (1970):299–308.

8. C.R. Brown and D.S. Fleisher, "The Bi-cycle Concept—Relating Continuing Education Directly to Patient Care," in *Continuing Medical Education in Community Hospitals: A Manual for Program Development*, N.S. Stearns, M.E. Getchell, and R.A. Gold, eds. Massachusetts Medical Society (published as a supplement to *New England Journal of Medicine* 284, May 20, 1971), 1971, pp. 88–97.

8a. Public Law 89-97, 1965.

8b. Conditions for participation—original published.
      31 CFR 134.24 Oct. 18, 1966
      32 CFR 136, Jan. 7, 1967
    Republished as:
      42 CFR 405.1011 through 405.1041.

9a. A.F. Southwick, *The Law of Hospital and Health Care Administration* (Ann Arbor, Mich.: University of Michigan Press, 1976), p. 413.

9b. Ibid., p. 419.

9c. Ibid., p. 422.

10. Joint Commission on Accreditation of Hospitals (JCAH): *Accreditation Manual for Hospitals*, 1970 ed. (Chicago: JCAH, 1970), p. 43.

11. Joint Commission on Accreditation of Hospitals (JCAH): *Accreditation Manual for Hospitals*, 1973 ed. (Chicago: JCAH, 1973), p. 186.

12. J.W. Craddick, "The Medical Management Analysis System: A Professional Liability Warning Mechanism," *Quality Review Bulletin* 5 (April 1979):2–8.

13. Joint Commission on Accreditation of Hospitals (JCAH): *Consolidated Standards Manual of Child, Adolescent, and Adult Psychiatric, Alcoholism, and Drug Abuse Facilities*. 1981 ed. (Chicago, JCAH, 1981), p. 39.

14. Joint Commission on Accreditation of Hospitals (JCAH), "Tabulated Results of JCAH 1981 Surveys," Unpublished data, JCAH, 1982.

15. Minimum Standards for 1918, *American College of Surgeons Bulletin*, 4, no. 1 (1920):4.

Part II

Quality Assurance and Cost Containment

Chapter 4

An Integrative Model of Quality, Cost, and Health*

Avedis Donabedian, M.D., M.P.H., John R.C. Wheeler, Ph.D., and Leon Wyszewianski, Ph.D.†

INTRODUCTION

Much of the current concern about the health care field has come to center on the rapid rise in health expenditures that has taken place over the last 20 years. Another area that has attracted increasing attention in the past 10 years has been the quality of health care services. The two sets of concerns—health expenditures and quality of care—are not, of course, independent of one another. As expenditures have grown, so has the interest in the quality of the services being purchased, not only because of the increasing pressure to ascertain that those services are, in fact, of satisfactory quality, but also because of growing unease with the size of some expenditures relative to the corresponding increments in quality.

The passage, in 1972, of the Social Security Amendments mandating the establishment of Professional Standards Review Organizations (PSROs)[1] was a visible manifestation of the concern with quality of care in the face of rapidly escalating health care expenditures. Through this legislation, the federal government, which by 1972 had become a major third party payer, was to establish a mechanism for ensuring that payments would be made only for care that was

*This article is reprinted with permission from *Medical Care*, October 1982, vol. 20, no. 10. © J.B. Lippincott Co.

†The authors' choice of the particular graphic representation of the effect of health care on health status was reinforced by the collaboration of Professor Donabedian and T.M. Kashner, one of his doctoral students, in developing a model of health services utilization that employed an index of health based most directly on the work of Rosser and Watts.[29] Donabedian's more recent work on quality assessment and monitoring has been supported by the National Center for Health Services Research (Grant 1-R01-HS-0281) and by the Commonwealth Fund. The authors gratefully acknowledge their indebtedness to these organizations. In this paper, however, the authors speak only for themselves and must, therefore, absolve everyone else of any complicity in the errors they may have made.

necessary, provided at the least costly site, and of satisfactory quality. As is well known, the PSRO legislation did not challenge basic prevailing notions or forms of practice. The methods of the PSROs were based on traditional peer review mechanisms and well-established procedures, such as utilization review, statistical "profiles," and medical audits. The implementation of these methods remained where it had always been, in the hands of local physicians and hospitals. But, most fundamentally, the PSRO legislation did not (indeed could not) define what was necessary care of good quality, beyond stipulating that it comply with practices and standards that were acceptable to the profession itself.

However, at the time the PSRO legislation was passed, more fundamental questions about the value of much of medical practice were being raised from other quarters. Cochrane pointed to the many practices in medicine that are widely accepted even though their effectiveness has never been definitively established.[1a] Later, Illich went even further, arguing that, on balance, medical care is more harmful than beneficial,[2] and thus advocating what Starr, in a cogent critique, refers to as a new kind of "therapeutic nihilism."[3] Similar doubts about the efficacy of medical care appear in the work of Fuchs, although he placed his primary emphasis on questions of allocative efficiency and equity.[4,5]

Drawing on the work of Fuchs and Cochrane, as well as that of others, Havighurst and Blumstein examined in some detail the broad area of "quality/ cost trade-offs in medical care."[6] The relation between costs and quality has also been examined, from a perspective more closely rooted in quality of care considerations, by Donabedian[7,8,9] and Vuori[10] and from yet another perspective by Phelps, who proposed a method for benefit/cost evaluations of quality assurance programs.[11] Focusing more specifically on ambulatory care, Brook and Davies-Avery have also discussed the tradeoff between cost and quality.[12,13]

The following discussion presents a framework within which the relation between resource expenditures and quality of care is systematically examined. The proposed framework integrates salient concepts from the works just cited, as well as other relevant concepts, such as those related to health status measurement.

THE SPECIFICATION AND MEASUREMENT OF HEALTH STATUS

Following Donabedian, the discussion will begin with a working definition of medical care quality in terms of outcomes associated with care received.[8] Specifically, the highest quality of care is defined as that which yields the greatest expected improvement in health status, health being defined very broadly to include physical, physiological, and psychological dimensions. While this definition seems simple enough, and perhaps even obvious, its explication requires consideration of some complex interrelationships and subtle distinctions. The notion of quality has two basic components: (1) a definition and measurement of health status and of changes or differences in health status; and (2) a specification of the medical care associated with any given health status outcome. This section and the next deal with these relationships.

A reasonably complete characterization of health status recognizes both the multidimensional nature of health and the relationship between current health and the probabilistic level of future health. Following Fanshel and Bush,[14] if health is measured in terms of mutually exclusive levels of function or performance in various functional areas, a person's multidimensional health status can perhaps best be represented by a matrix, such as shown in Figure 4-1.

For present purposes, the precise functional areas or the levels of functioning or performance need not be specified. As an illustration, according to Breslow and his associates, health has "three axes: the physical, the mental and the social well-being of the WHO definition."[15] The scales of functional performance that Breslow and his associates constructed for each of these functional areas might then be adopted.[16,17] A more complex formulation is illustrated by the "sickness impact profile" that recognizes 14 areas of behavior, each of which is described by a multiposition scale of performance or function.[18-21] Brook and his associates developed four sets of measures corresponding to the four dimensions of health status they identified: physical, mental, and social health, and "general health perceptions."[22] This same group of investigators has more recently dealt with the issues of aggregating the several scales that represent physical health, while at the same time advocating a more parsimonious model that only includes two major components of health status: the physical and the mental.[23,24]

Given a matrix of functional areas, on the one hand, and of levels of functioning or performance, on the other, two courses are open. One of these is to attach numerical values to each of the possible health states that make up the matrix,

---

Figure 4-1 Health Status Matrix

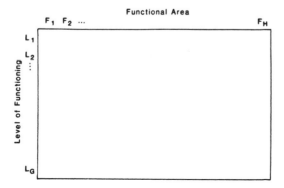

based on the preferences of individuals or groups for: (1) the functional areas relative to each other; and (2) the levels of functioning within each area relative to other levels in that same area. In this way, a single numerical value can be derived for the entire matrix. This value has built into it the utility of each health state to an individual or group.[25]

The alternative procedure is to first reduce the multidimensional matrix into a unidimensional representation of it, as advocated by Bush and his coworkers,[14] as well as others. Once this is done, it is possible to use a variety of methods to assign a numerical value to each state in a manner that represents the preferences (and, therefore, utilities) of a person or a group.[14,25-30] In this way, the original matrix of health states can be summarized by a vector S_t, whose elements indicate measures of possible health status levels for a person at time t:

$$\begin{bmatrix} S_{1t} \\ S_{2t} \\ \vdots \\ S_{jt} \end{bmatrix}$$

In either of the two procedures described, death, which is the absence of all function, is quite reasonably assigned a value of zero. The highest definable level of performance is assigned a more arbitrary value, such as 1 or 100. It is assumed that health status is measurable on a ratio scale, that is, a scale characterized by equal intervals and an absolute zero point.[31] This means that an $S_{jt} = 20$ represents twice the health status of an $S_{jt} = 10$. This is not an unreasonable assumption since it seems that death represents an acceptable zero point for the ratio scale. If there are health states less desirable than death these would be assigned a negative value.

There is evidence that groups of professionals and "consumers" are able to indicate, rather reliably, the relative values of the several levels of the vector of health states on a scale of equal-seeming intervals, although the levels themselves are not necessarily at equal "distances" from each other.[25,28] The ratio properties of this measure of health status, of course, simplify the task of arriving at mathematically manipulable numerical values of the outcomes of health care. It is also important to recognize that measurement of health status on a ratio scale derived from people's preferences for levels of functioning implies that the total utility of health will increase by a constant amount for each increment in the measure of health status. That is, the marginal utility of health is constant if health is measured in terms of preferences.

Future expected health can be included in the assessment of a person's health status by taking the sum over time of expected health states in the future, where expected health in a future year is the probability weighted sum of possible health states in that year. Let S = current plus future expected health; then

$$S = \sum_t \sum_j p_{jt} S_{jt},$$

where p_{jt} = the probability that the person will have health state j in period t. To simplify the notation and exposition ignore, for now, the time preference for health and assume that current health states have the same values as similar health states in the more distant future. The period of time over which expected health status is evaluated could be either a normatively defined life span, as proposed by Fanshel and Bush,[14] or the average expectation of life, as proposed by Sullivan.[32]

Many difficulties, both conceptual and operational, might be encountered in the implementation of either of the procedures described above. Others have argued in favor of using a profile of functional states or of one or more measures that directly or indirectly represent health status in specific, often clinically defined, situations.[22,23,33] The authors have, nevertheless, chosen to envisage a more comprehensive, integrative measure of health status because it is a necessary ingredient in a correspondingly comprehensive definition of quality, which, in particular, includes the technical and interpersonal aspects of the quality of care discussed by Donabedian.[9] Less inclusive measures of health status can be used. To do so would imply a less than comprehensive definition of quality but would not alter in other ways the properties of the model that will be presented. In any event, the model will demonstrate the intimate relationship between the definition and measurement of health, on the one hand, and the definition and measurement of quality, on the other.

THE RELATIONSHIP BETWEEN MEDICAL CARE AND HEALTH

The definition and measurement of health status developed above can be employed to examine the relationship between medical care received and health status. Consider a person who has become ill. In the event that he or she receives no medical care, the illness will follow its "natural" course, which is probabilistic in its progression and which produces an expected health status over time. Let S_o represent expected health over time without medical intervention; then:

$$S_o = \sum_t \sum_j p_{jto} S_{jt}$$

where p_{jto} is the probability that the person will have health state j in period t if strategy o, no medical care, is adopted. Note that the probability of being in any health state in the future depends upon the medical strategy adopted.

There are many types of disease courses that can be identified.[34] In one case, the disease is self-limiting in the sense that as time passes the person's health

Figure 4-2 Possible Course of a Self-Limiting Disease in the Absence of Medical Intervention

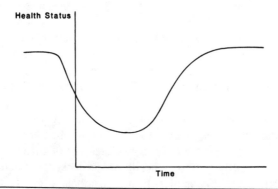

status can be expected to return to a level close to the person's level of health before the onset of the disease even though no treatment has been received. The expected course of this type of disease, and hence the person's expected level of health over time, might appear as in Figure 4-2, where time = 0 corresponds to the period of time immediately after the appearance of overt symptoms of the disease and where health status = 0 indicates death. Note that the points on the vertical axis correspond to the elements in the S_t vector discussed earlier. Note also that S_o, the expected value of health in the absence of medical care, is described by the disease course in the diagram in the sense that S_o is the summation over time of the expected health levels at each point in time.

In other cases, the disease may persist and become chronic, or it may ultimately result in death. The passage of time does not, in the absence of medical treatment, return the person to the predisease state. These cases might take the general forms indicated in Figure 4-3. For purposes of the exposition to follow, only

Figure 4-3 Possible Courses of Non-Self-Limiting Diseases in the Absence of Medical Intervention

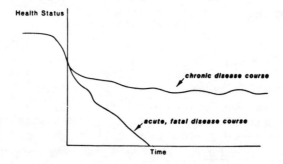

the case of the self-limiting disease will be considered. The relationships developed can be extended to other cases without difficulty.

In most instances, receipt of medical care can be counted upon to alter the course of expected health states following the onset of a disease. The magnitude of the alteration and whether it is for better or worse depends on the expertise of the health care providers, the availability of resources, the state of the science and technology of medicine, and a number of factors that influence the severity of the disease and the recuperative powers of the patient. Under the best circumstances, the case will be managed by an expert or "ideal" physician operating in a setting where resources are not constrained.* The authors conceive of management as a "strategy" of care and assume that a "strategy" can be specified in terms of the kinds and amounts of services rendered, the succession and timing of these services, and the decision rules that eventuate in particular choices being made, out of the much larger set of possible courses of action. The authors define the ideal physician as one who selects and implements that strategy of care that maximizes health status improvement without wasting resources. The authors also make the simplifying assumption that the strategies of care selected by the ideal physician—as well as those selected by "non-ideal" physicians—are *executed* with optimal efficiency. That is, no resources are wasted due to underutilization of facilities, improper performance of tasks, inadequate coordination, or any other such factors. A subsequent section will consider the implications of this assumption.

The expected, time-summated health status associated with case management by the ideal (I) and unconstrained (U) physician, S_{IU}, is given by:

$$S_{IU} = \sum_t \sum_j p_{jt|IU} S_{jt}$$

where $p_{jt|IU}$ is the probability that the person will have health state j at time t if the case is managed by the ideal physician whose treatment decisions are unconstrained. Graphically, the progression of health states in a self-limiting disease subjected to this ideal, unconstrained treatment might appear as the top curve in Figure 4-4. The area between the two progressions of health states shown in Figure 4-4, which may be found by integrating the expressions for S_{IU} and S_o over t and taking the difference, represents the expected improvement in health status resulting from care provided by the ideal, unconstrained physician. Let ϕ_{IU} represent this expected improvement, where:

---

*For clarity of exposition, the authors use the physician as the prototype of the independent practitioner who decides on the course of treatment for the patient. This analysis is meant to apply equally well to any other practitioner who makes analogous determinations about the overall course of treatment.

Figure 4-4 Possible Progressions for a Self-Limiting Disease When Untreated and When Treated by the Ideal, Unconstrained Physician

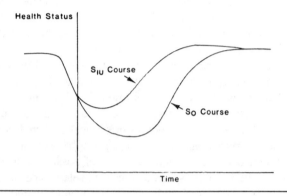

$$\Phi_{IU} = S_{IU} - S_o$$

Using the more traditional terminology of quality assessment, this is the health "outcome" of the care provided by the ideal, unconstrained physician.

Now, if the dollar value of the resources available to the ideal physician is constrained to R_{IC}, without constraining the *types* of resources that may be used and the physician is asked to manage the care of the same patient, the expected time-summated health state, given by:

$$S_{IC_1} = \sum_t \sum_j p_{jt|C_1} \, S_{jt}$$

will be somewhat lower. In the case of a self-limiting disease, recovery may be slower, as indicated by the middle curve in Figure 4-5.

The area between the disease course leading to S_{IC_1} and the course leading to S_o represents the expected health improvement, Φ_{IC_1}, in this first resource-constrained case; while the area between the course of illness leading to S_{IC_1}, and that leading to S_{IU} represents the total decrement attributable to this level of resource constraint.

By successively constraining the resources available to the ideal physician more and more, a series of points relating expected health outcome (Φ) to resource expenditure is generated. Although the actual curve described by these points is unknown, it may have the general parabolic shape of OI in Figure 4-6. Other shapes, such as a classical S-shape or an exponential shape, are of course possible. In fact, due to the indivisible nature of medical care services, the relationship may appear as a step function over some range of resource expenditures. For convenience of exposition, the authors make the assumption

Figure 4-5 Possible Progressions for a Self-Limiting Disease When Untreated and When Treated by the Ideal Physician with and without Resource Constraints

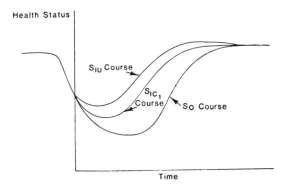

that the relationship between resource expenditure and expected health improvement can be approximated by a continuous parabolic curve indicating that marginal improvements in health diminish at a constant rate as resource expenditure rises. The following exposition does not depend on this simplifying assumption. The presentation can be readily extended to curves with shapes different from OI in Figure 4-6.

Curve OI in Figure 4-6 shows the relationship between medical care and health outcome when treatment is managed by the ideal physician. The ideal physician is, of course, a myth created in order to define the upper bond of possible outcomes under specified resource inputs. In everyday circumstances, the large majority of points corresponding to the "observed" relationship between ex-

Figure 4-6 Hypothetical Relationship between Resource Expenditure and Expected Health Improvement for Strategies of Care Selected by the Ideal Physician

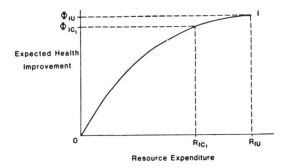

pected health status and resource expenditure lie below and to the right of OI, because most episodes of illness are not managed by the ideal physician.

To see how deviations from OI occur, consider what might happen if a typical or nonideal physician were asked to care for a hypothetical patient. First assume that the nonideal (N) physician has unlimited (U) resources. The expected health outcome of the patient in this situation is given by:

$$S_{NU} = \sum_t \sum_j p_{jtNU} \, S_{jt}$$

where p_{jtNU} is the probability that the person will have health state j at time t if the person's care is managed by a nonideal physician whose decisions are unconstrained. In the case of a self-limiting disease, the progression of health states might have the shape given in Figure 4-7.

Obviously, the nonideal physician has achieved a smaller increment of time-summated health, as compared to the ideal physician, when no limits are placed on the resources used by either. Furthermore, it can be postulated that, when resources *are* constrained, the nonideal physician will achieve smaller health outcomes than the ideal physician for each specified dollar value of resource inputs. Alternatively, the nonideal physician will use more resources than would the ideal physician in order to achieve any specified health outcome. These relationships between resource inputs and health outcomes are shown in Figure 4-8.

In Figure 4-8, the curve OI shows the performance of the ideal physician. Curve ON shows the performance of the typical or average nonideal physician in a given community. In addition to portraying the relationships already described, a comparison of the two curves shows another major distinction. The

Figure 4-7 Possible Progression for a Self-Limiting Disease When Untreated and When Treated by the Ideal and Nonideal Unconstrained Physician

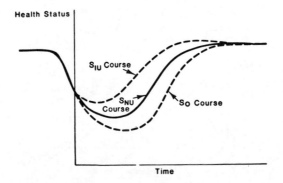

Figure 4-8 Hypothetical Relationships between Resource Expenditure and Expected Health Improvement for Strategies of Care Selected by the Ideal Physician and by Nonideal Physicians

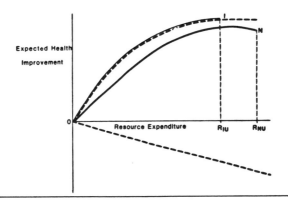

ideal physician will use no resources in excess of those that are required to bring about the largest attainable benefit to health. By contrast, the average, nonideal physician is shown to have been induced by the excessive availability of resources to apply strategies of care that have larger elements of risk to the patient's health. For that reason, curve ON actually takes a downward turn beyond a certain level of resource inputs.

Needless to say, any large community is served by a relatively large number of less-than-ideal physicians who vary widely in knowledge, judgment, and skill. The health outcomes achieved by this population of physicians in the treatment of any specified condition in a community of patients can be shown by a large set of points that are postulated to fall, in varying degrees of density, within the space bounded by the dotted lines in Figure 4-8. As already described, all these points fall below and to the right of OI. Furthermore, Figure 4-8 provides for the occurrence of actually harmful care at all levels of resource input, though it is postulated that both the magnitude and the probability of harm are larger when resource inputs are excessive. Although the occurrence is probably rare, a physician can exist who usually does his or her patients more harm than good at any level of resource input. The performance of this physician would be approximated by the lower of the two dotted lines in Figure 4-8. By contrast, the performance of the best physician in the community might approximate that of the hypothetical ideal. Strictly speaking, however, the two dotted lines in Figure 4-8 do not represent the performance, respectively, of the best and worst physicians in a community. Rather, they are the upper and lower bounds of the therapeutic outcomes achieved by all the physicians in the community as they care for all patients with any given illness. The performance of the "average" physician, as shown by curve ON in Figure 4-8, is also a statistical construct that represents the mean, median, or modal performance of all the physicians in the community as they care for all patients of a particular kind. The performance of any individual physician, especially when observed for a relatively short time, is likely to be much more erratic, and the curve of average performance generated by that physician would be very difficult to specify in advance.

This distinction between the care provided by the ideal physician and that provided by the nonideal physician has some similarities to the distinction between "efficacious" care and "effective" care. As defined by Williamson, *efficacy* refers to "the extent to which a health care intervention can be shown to be beneficial under optimal conditions of clinical care," while *effectiveness* refers to "the extent to which benefits achievable under optimal conditions of clinical care are actually achieved in practice."[35]

COST AND THE DEFINITION OF QUALITY

Point I on curve OI in Figures 4-6 and 4-8 indicates the greatest possible improvement in health status achievable through medical intervention, given existing medical knowledge and technology. Earlier, the highest quality of care was defined as that which yields the greatest improvement in health status. Therefore, in terms of that definition, the strategy of care employed to produce Φ_{IU} at a resource cost of R_{IU} represents the maximal quality of medical care. This concept of quality is a purely medical one in the sense that it reflects what is maximally feasible to do for the patient given current medical knowledge. A more comprehensive conceptualization of quality requires some consideration of the relationship between the value of health status improvements and the resource expenditure necessary to produce such improvements.

This definition of health status reflects a set of preferences for one level of functioning over another, but it does not reflect preferences for health relative to preferences for other valued commodities and activities. Curve OI in Figure 4-8 can be considered a total product curve for medical resources expended to improve health. Figure 4-9 shows the marginal product analog to the total product relationship, where marginal product is defined as the *change* in expected health improvement associated with the additional dollar of resource expenditure. Mathematically, marginal expected health improvement, or Marginal Φ, is the slope of the total expected health improvement curve. Therefore, at the peak of curve OI in Figure 4-8, where resource expenditure is R_{IU}, the marginal expected health improvement associated with employing additional resources is zero in Figure 4-9.

The value to a sick person of a marginal improvement in the person's expected health status, as indicated by the price the person is willing to pay for that improvement, depends upon the relationship between the utility of health and the utility of other commodities and activities to the person. Specifically, the

Figure 4-9 Relationship between Resource Expenditure and Marginal Expected Health Improvement

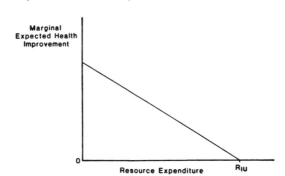

price a person is willing to pay for a marginal improvement in expected health status, that is, its value in dollars, is given by the relationship:

$$\text{Value} = \frac{\text{marginal utility of expected health improvement}}{\text{marginal utility of money}}$$

The marginal utility of money represents the utility of other commodities and activities that money can purchase; it is assumed to be a decreasing function of the individual's wealth. The marginal utility of expected health improvement is assumed to be constant, given the definition and measurement of health status presented earlier in the paper. Specifically, by defining health in terms of people's preferences for levels of functioning, a linear utility function for health can be specified, providing a constant marginal utility of health.* Hence, the value a person places on a marginal improvement in expected health depends upon the person's: (1) wealth; and (2) preference for health relative to other commodities and activities.† Therefore, the relationship between the value of a marginal improvement in expected health status and resources expended has the general shape depicted in Figure 4-10. The slope of the curve is steeper for wealthier persons and for persons who assign a high relative value to health and more gradual for those with lower incomes and for those who assign a lower relative value to health. The y-axis of Figure 4-10 is most precisely defined as the dollar value of the additional increase in expected health status resulting from a $1

---

*If health is measured in some other way, independent of peoples' preferences, the utility function for health would in general be nonlinear. In this case, the more common assumption of diminishing marginal utility of health would be invoked. The subsequent analysis presented would show the same results, although the graphical representations would be more complex.

†For simplicity, risk aversion is ignored here. Its inclusion would have no effect on the relationships developed in this section.

Figure 4-10 Resource Expenditure, Value of Marginal Expected Health Improvement, and Optimal Strategy

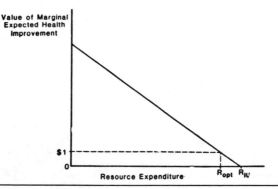

increase in resource expenditure. The cost of a $1 increase in resource expenditure is of course $1. Therefore, the marginal costs and benefits of medical treatment are balanced at a resource expenditure of R_{opt}, so that the employment of additional resources in treatment will benefit the individual less than would the spending of those additional resources on some other commodity or activity. From the perspective of individual welfare, as opposed to individual health status, the optimal strategy of care results in an expenditure of R_{opt}, a lower level of resource expenditure than R_{IU}. The highest quality medical care, in terms of its effect on individual welfare, is therefore that strategy of care associated with a resource expenditure of R_{opt}.

It should be noted that this specification of optimality depends on the relationship between resource employment and health outcome when treatment is managed by the ideal physician. Since this relationship differs from physician to physician, the optimal strategy of care will also vary, but the optimum for the ideal physician remains the standard of comparison.

Figure 4-11 combines the previous figure with two other figures to show the effect of employing the level of resources that corresponds to R_{opt} on both expected health improvement and the net value of total expected health improvement. This latter is determined by multiplying expected health improvement (Φ) by the value per unit of improvement, given by the expression above, and subtracting from this product the resource expenditure. Notice that while at a resource expenditure of R_{opt} expected health improvement can be increased somewhat by the expenditure of additional resources, the value of that increase is quite small. In fact, the value of the expected health improvement is less than the value of the resources that would be employed to produce the improvement, so that the net value of total expected health improvement declines. Therefore, it is not worthwhile to undertake the additional expenditure. From this more comprehensive perspective, a strategy of care that produces an expected health

Figure 4-11 Effect of Employing Optimal Strategy on Expected Health
Improvement and on Net Value of Total Expected Health
Improvement

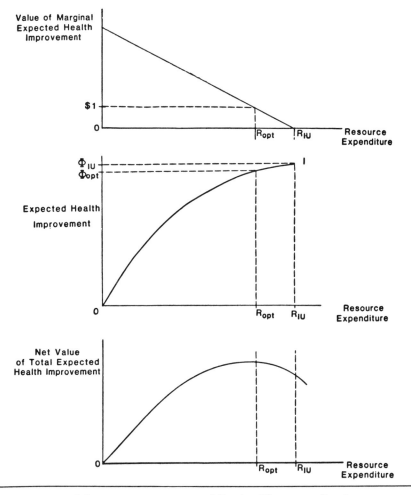

improvement of Φ_{IU} at a resource cost of R_{IU} is of lower quality than a strategy that produces an expected health improvement of Φ_{opt} at a cost of R_{opt}.

QUALITY, COST, AND THE EFFICIENCY OF PRODUCTION

In developing the model of the relationship between quality and cost the authors have assumed, so far, that cost varies according to the strategy of care used by the physician. The ideal physician always combines, times, and sequences services in the most efficient manner possible so as to produce the greatest increment of health, given a specified available or permissible expenditure. Other physicians use less efficient strategies, so that they produce less health per dollar spent on care.

The efficiency of the strategies of care may be called *clinical efficiency.* Another kind of efficiency, termed *production efficiency,* pertains to the manner in which the services are produced. For example, care is inefficiently produced if the hospital is half empty, if the laboratory does not report a finding promptly, or if highly trained personnel are used to do work that can be done just as well at lower cost by less trained personnel. It follows that it is possible to obtain larger increments of health (or more quality) per dollar of expenditure by: (1) combining, timing, and sequencing services into more efficient strategies, that is, by increasing clinical efficiency; and (2) producing services more efficiently, in other words, increasing production efficiency.

While clinical efficiency is a fundamental component of the definition of quality, the authors prefer to exclude production efficiency from the definition of quality because it does not involve the use of clinical judgment. The authors do, however, recognize the central importance of production efficiency to the organization and delivery of health care services. Improvements in production efficiency will allow the achievement of current levels of quality at lower cost. Alternatively, larger quantities of care could be produced in which the mix of quality remains as it is now. To improve quality beyond that would require a change in the strategies of care. Therefore, while production efficiency is a component of the quality of the system that produces care, it is not a component of the quality of care itself.

QUALITY, INCOME, AND PREFERENCES FOR HEALTH

The implications of defining quality in terms of the patient's ability and willingness to incur expenditures to improve expected health outcome have been discussed above. The patient's income and preferences for health influence the specification of the optimal strategy of care. Given stable preferences, lower income implies a reduced willingness to pay for improvements in expected health status. Therefore, the curve indicating the value of marginal improvement in expected health status for a low-income person is below the same curve for a high-income person, and it has a flatter slope, as shown in Figure 4-12. Hence, when consideration is given only to maximizing the person's utility, the optimal strategy of care for a low-income person suggests a lower level of resource expenditure (R_{opt}) and a smaller expected health status improvement (Φ_{opt}) than does optimality for a high-income person. In other words, this analysis leads to the disquieting, even unacceptable conclusion that the specification of optimal quality depends upon a person's ability to purchase services.

Figure 4-12 Effect of Income on Optimal Strategy of Care

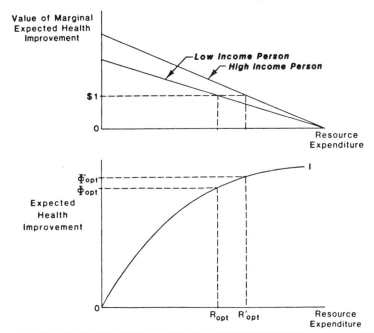

The same sort of reasoning applies when relative preferences for health are allowed to vary and income is held constant. If person A prefers material possessions to health relatively more than person B, optimality requires that A have fewer resources devoted to the improvement of health than B. Again, the definition of quality is rooted in the person's valuation of health. Of course, in actuality, both the valuation of money and the valuation of health vary simultaneously, and they depend on many factors, such as income, education, and occupation. As a result, if this perspective is adopted, the optimal strategy of care, and hence the definition of quality, will vary from one person to another, depending on the preferences of the individual.

In addition to the relative preferences for health and money at any given time, variability in individual preferences for these over time also enters into the specification of optimality. Specifically, the discounting of future health benefits at a high rate, to reflect a significant preference for current well-being over future well-being, has the effect of lowering the value of the marginal expected health improvement and hence of reducing R_{opt} and Φ_{opt}. Perhaps even more important is the influence of time preferences on the choice among strategies that differ in the timing of their risks and expected benefits. McNeil and his associates have reported an instructive example of the effect of such preferences on the choice between medical and surgical treatment for lung cancer.[36]

It is apparent from the above that there are two kinds of definitions of quality. The first kind, just discussed, corresponds to what Donabedian has called the "individualized" definition.[9] It assumes that all costs are borne and all benefits are enjoyed by the individual, and it reflects each individual's valuations of health and other goods and each individual's time preferences. This approach to defining quality implies that there is no single best strategy, but that there is a best strategy for each person in each situation. It may be contrasted with the approach to defining quality that ignores cost, as described earlier in this paper. Vuori has referred to this as "absolute" quality,[10] and Donabedian has called it the *absolutist* definition.[9] These descriptors are particularly apt if the physician makes an independent valuation of the desirability of alternative health outcomes, without consultation with the patient. Under these circumstances, it may be possible, at least theoretically, to specify the one best strategy, as the criteria and standards of quality assessment sometimes seem to do.

INDIVIDUAL OPTIMUM AND SOCIAL OPTIMUM IN THE DEFINITION OF QUALITY

The interest of persons other than the patient, including the physician, the patient's family and friends, and society in general, may appropriately enter into the consideration of what is the best strategy of care. The inclusion of the interests of these others in the health of the individual person leads to yet another possible definition of quality, what Donabedian terms the "social definition."[9] The social definition of quality differs from the individualized definition in including a number of considerations. Each of these, in its turn, alters the optimum outcome, and the level of corresponding resource inputs.

In the discussion of the individualized definition of quality, it is assumed that each person bears all the costs and enjoys all the benefits of decisions regarding strategies of care. As one consequence of this definition, the specification of optimal quality varies according to the individual's ability to pay for health services. But in many cases neither all the costs nor all the benefits accrue entirely to the individual person.

The cost of care is shared partly because of the existence of insurance programs to spread risk and of public assistance programs to address social inequities. The presence of these mechanisms creates a divergence between individual costs and social costs and consequently a disparity between social and individual optimums. The disparity arises because, as many investigators have pointed out, the sick person considers only individual costs in the decision about which strategy to adopt, whereas society must be concerned with total social costs.[37,38,39] Therefore, if some or all of the person's care is financed through insurance or social assistance, the person may prefer a strategy of care that is both more costly and more beneficial than society would. As a result, there is a conflict of interests, at least in the short run, that places the physician in the difficult position of reconciling the individual's immediate preferences with the long-range interests of society.[9]

The presence of shared or external benefits is a second factor that produces a difference between individual and social optimums. When an individual receives care, there is often a benefit to society over and above that which accrues to the individual. Therefore, the social valuation of care becomes the sum of individual valuation and external valuation. The result is that society is willing to spend more for care than is the individual, and the magnitude of the disparity depends on the magnitude of external valuation as compared to individual valation.

Figure 4-13 shows how these two factors can influence resource expenditure and expected health outcome. In the absence of external benefits and insurance, both individual and social optimums occur at R_{opt}. Now, if because of insurance the individual pays less than the full cost of the resources employed in treatment, so that individual cost is less than social cost, resource expenditure will exceed R_{opt}, the socially optimal amount. In the limiting case of free care to the patient, expenditure will approach R_{IU}. In this situation, social costs exceed social benefits on the margin. Hence, from a social perspective, too many resources are

Figure 4-13 Effect of Considering Social Valuation in Specifying Optimal Strategies of Care

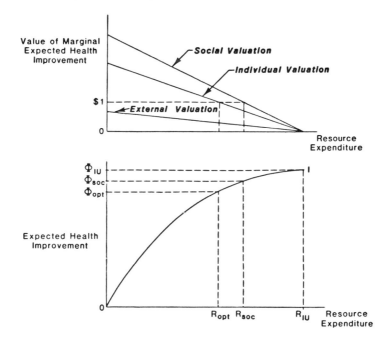

devoted to treatment, and the additional health improvement cannot justify the additional expenditure.

Consideration of external benefits, on the other hand, alters the specification of social optimality from R_{opt} to R_{soc}. The problem here is that the patient, in the absence of insurance or assistance, will prefer to spend R_{opt}. Therefore, from a social perspective, too few resources are devoted to treating the patient. The expenditure of additional resources would be justified by the resultant additional expected health improvement.

A third factor that brings about a difference between the individualized and social specifications of quality is a social preference for a particular distribution of quality or of increments of health status among subgroups in the population distinguished by one or more of a set of factors, including age, sex, ethnic origin, geographic location, income, and the like. Some of the pertinent considerations are illustrated in Figure 4-14, using as an example the distribution of health among four income groups.

Figure 14-4 incorporates a number of reasonable postulates. The first is that the present level of health is lower than it could be and that it is inversely related to income. The second postulate is that unlimited personal health care would improve the general level of health but would not bring it up to the ideal. It

Figure 4-14 Hypothetical Distribution of Health Status by Income Group

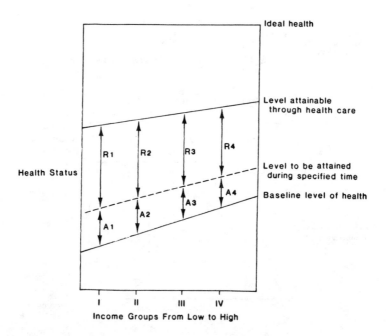

would reduce, but not eliminate, income-related disparities in health. The inability of personal health services either to achieve "ideal" health or to totally eliminate the differences among income groups at less than an ideal level of health, flows from a third postulate. This recognizes the influence of many other factors on health and posits that these factors are systematically more adverse in lower income groups. The authors do not know the relative importance of personal health services as compared to those other influences on health and do not intend Figure 4-14 to make a statement on that point. The authors also do not presume to define what "ideal" health might be.

The authors do postulate, however, that in some way society assesses the current level and distribution of health relative to a set of social values and preferences. It then allocates resources so as to make progress in a manner congruent with socially defined objectives. For example, the objective could be to achieve, within ten years, an equal increment of health of specified magnitude in each income class. Alternatively, under the influence of a perverse egalitarianism, society could aim to actually lower the level of health in the higher income groups until all groups are equally burdened with ill health. The authors assume that our own society would choose to make progress in all income groups, while it moves more rapidly in the lower income groups, so as to make the distribution of health status less unequal.

What implications this social decision will have on resource allocation will depend on the magnitude of change in the level and distribution of health that an individual wishes to achieve and on the amenability of health status to improvement through personal health care. It is quite likely that this amenability is also not equal across income groups, though it is not easy to say how the income groups differ in this respect. In some ways, the illnesses in the lower income groups may be easier to prevent and treat. In other ways, they may be more recalcitrant, partly because of their nature and partly because the social situation of the poor makes the effective delivery of care more difficult and costly. Whatever the net consequence of these factors might be, the object is to provide the mix and distribution of resources that most efficiently achieves the socially desired change in the current level and distribution of health. In a sense, this is a social strategy of care that takes account of and includes the strategies of clinical management that were used earlier in the formulation of the model.

It is assumed that the cost of whatever social strategy of care is chosen and applied can be determined. For each income group, the outcome of the strategy is the sum of all the changes in health that are attributable to personal health care in all members of that group. Obviously, costs include all social costs, and health benefits take account of individual as well as external valuation. What remains to be specified is a method for expressing the value of health gains across income groups.

If society were neutral with regard to the income-related distribution of health, the gains in each income group would simply be weighted by the number of persons in each group. But if, as postulated, there is a preference for a specific degree of redistribution among income groups, that preference must be introduced as weights that attach to the health product in each income group.

Donabedian has offered a simple, hypothetical example of how a system of weights might be derived.[40] Using the notation in Figure 4-14, the sum of the health products for all income groups would be:

$$A_1 P_1 (A_1 + R_1)^n + A_2 P_2 (A_2 + R_2)^n + A_3 P_3 (A_3 + R_3)^n + A_4 P_4 (A_4 + P_4)^n$$

where P is the number of persons in each group, and the exponent n is the social preference function. By setting $n = 0$, society expresses neutrality with regard to the distribution of increments of health by income group. When $n = 1$, there is a preference that is inversely related to income, assuming the current distribution of health status to be as shown. By increasing the value of n, the slope of the preference is rapidly increased in favor of the rectification of the current inequality in the distribution of health. Of course n could also be a negative number, but most people would not want to live in a society that has a negative n on its banner, despite seeming endorsement of this principle in Holy Writ.[41]

CONCLUSION

By means of an admitted hypothetical construct, a specification of quality has been developed that relates increments of total inputs into personal health care to increments in a measure of health status that includes personal valuation and external valuation and is further weighted according to preferences for a specified social distribution of health. The optimum point on the curve that describes this relationship corresponds to the optimum social strategy of care.

By taking into account social costs as well as individual costs, society will tend to settle for a smaller net gain in health than individuals might want. By taking into account external as well as individual valuations, society will tend to devote more resources to care than individuals would want to do. By aiming to redistribute health among population subgroups, society would take away from some in order to give to others. In all these ways, we are reminded, yet another time, of the contingent nature of the specification of quality. But, while the precise specification of quality is variable, the authors regard the underlying conceptual and analytic framework to be firm, consistent, and valid.

NOTES

1. Public Law 92603 Amendments to the Social Security Act, Section 2491, October 30, 1972.

1a. A.L. Cochrane, *Effectiveness and Efficiency: Random Reflections on Health Services* (London: The Nuffield Provincial Hospitals Trust, 1972).

2. I. Illich, *Medical Nemesis: The Expropriation of Health* (New York: Pantheon Books, 1976), pp. 24–30.

3. P. Starr, "The Politics of Therapeutic Nihilism," *Working Papers for a New Society* 4 (1976):48–52.

4. V.R. Fuchs, "Health Care and the United States Economic System—An Essay in Abnormal Physiology," *Milbank Memorial Fund Quarterly* 50 (1972):211–244.

5. V.R. Fuchs, *Who Shall Live? Health, Economics and Social Choice* (New York: Basic Books, 1974).

6. C.C. Havighurst and J.F. Blumstein, "Coping with Quality/Cost Trade-offs in Medical Care: The Role of PSROs," *Northwestern University Law Review* 70 (1975):6–68.

7. A. Donabedian, *Needed Research in the Assessment and Monitoring of the Quality of Medical Care*, DHEW Publication No. (PHS) 78-3219 (Hyattsville, Md., 1978).

8. A. Donabedian, "The Quality of Medical Care: A Concept in Search of a Definition," *Journal of Family Practice* 9 (1979):277–284.

9. A. Donabedian, *The Definition of Quality and Approaches to its Assessment* (Ann Arbor, Mich.: Health Administration Press, 1980).

10. H. Vuori, "Optimal and Logical Quality: Two Neglected Aspects of the Quality of Health Services," *Medical Care* 18 (1980):975–985.

11. C.E. Phelps, "Benefit/Cost Analysis of Quality Assurance Programs," in *Quality Assurance in Health Care*, R.H. Egdahl and P.M. Gertman, eds. (Rockville, Md.: Aspen Systems Corporation, 1976), pp. 289–329.

12. R.H. Brook and A. Davies-Avery, "Quality Assurance and Cost Control in Ambulatory Care," in *Ambulatory Medical Care Quality Assurance 1977: Issues, Directions and Applications*, G.A. Giebink and N.H. White, eds. (La Jolla, Calif.: La Jolla Health Science Publications, 1977), pp. 46–69.

13. R.H. Brook and A. Davies-Avery, "Trade-off between Cost and Quality in Ambulatory Care," *Quarterly Review Bulletin* 3, no. 11 (1977):4–7.

14. S. Fanshel and J.W. Bush, "A Health-Status Index and Its Application to Health Services Outcomes," *Operations Research* 18 (1970):1021–1066.

15. L. Breslow, "A Quantitative Approach to the World Health Organization Definition of Health: Physical, Mental and Social Well-Being," *International Journal of Epidemiology* 1 (1972):347–355.

16. N.B. Belloe, L. Breslow, and J.R. Hochstim, "Measurement of Physical Health in a General Population Survey," *American Journal of Epidemiology* 93 (1971):328–336.

17. P. Berkman, "Measurement of Mental Health in a General Population Survey," *American Journal of Epidemiology* 94 (1971):105–111.

18. B.S. Gilson et al., "The Sickness Impact Profile: Development of an Outcome Measure of Health Care," *American Journal of Public Health* 65 (1975):1304–1310.

19. M. Bergner et al., "The Sickness Impact Profile: Validation of a Health Status Measure," *Medical Care* 14 (1976):57–67.

20. W.E. Pollard et al., "The Sickness Impact Profile: Reliability of a Health Status Measure," *Medical Care* 14 (1976):146–156.

21. M. Bergner et al., "The Sickness Impact Profile: Development and Final Revision of a Health Status Measure," *Medical Care* 19 (1981):787–805.

22. R.H. Brook et al., "Overview of Adult Health Status Measures Fielded in Rand's Health Insurance Study," *Medical Care,* 17 (July Suppl. 1979).

23. J.F. Ware et al., "Choosing Measures of Health Status for Individuals in General Populations," *American Journal of Public Health* 71 (1981):620–625.

24. A.L. Stewart et al., "Advances in the Measurement of Functional Status: Construction of Aggregate Indexes," *Medical Care* 19 (1981):473–488.

25. W.B. Carter et al., "Validation of an Interval Scaling: The Sickness Impact Profile," *Health Services Research* 11 (1976):516–528.

26. D.L. Patrick et al., "Methods for Measuring Levels of Well-being for a Health Status Index," *Health Services Research* 8 (1973):228–245.

27. W.R. Blischke et al., "Successive Intervals Analysis of Preference Measures in a Health Status Index," *Health Services Research* 10 (1975):181–198.

28. R.M. Kaplan et al., "Health Status Index: Category Rating Versus Magnitude Estimation for Measuring Levels of Well-being," *Medical Care* 17 (1979):501–525.

29. R.M. Rosser'and V.C. Watts, "The Measurement of Hospital Output," *International Journal of Epidemiology* 1 (1972):361–368.

30. G.W. Torrance, "Toward a Utility Theory Foundation for Health Status Index Models," *Health Services Research* 11 (1976):349–369.

31. H.M. Blalock, *Social Statistics* (New York: McGraw-Hill Book Co., 1972).

32. D.E. Sullivan, "A Single Index of Mortality and Morbidity," *HSMHA Health Reports* 86 (1971):347–354.

33. R.H. Brook et al., "Assessing the Quality of Medical Care Using Outcome Measures: An Overview of the Method," *Medical Care* 15 (Sept. Suppl. 1977).

34. A. Donabedian, *Aspects of Medical Care Administration: Specifying Requirements for Health Care* (Cambridge, Mass.: Harvard University Press, 1973).

35. J.W. Williamson, *Improving Medical Practice and Health Care: A Bibliographic Guide to Information Management in Quality Assurance and Continuing Education* (Cambridge, Mass.: Ballinger, 1977).

36. B.J. McNeil et al., "Fallacy of the Five-Year Survival in Lung Cancer," *New England Journal of Medicine* 290 (1978):1397–1401.

37. K. Arrow, "Uncertainty and the Welfare Economics of Medical Care," *American Economic Review* 53 (1963):941–973.

38. D.S. Lees and R.G. Rice, "Uncertainty and the Welfare Economics of Medical Care: Comment," *American Economic Review* 55 (1965):140–153.

39. M.V. Pauly, "The Economics of Moral Hazard: Comment," *American Economic Review* 58 (1968):531–537.

40. A. Donabedian, "Models for Organizing the Delivery of Personal Health Services and Criteria for Evaluating Them," *Milbank Memorial Fund Quarterly* 50 (1972):103–154.

41. Matt. 25:29.

Chapter 5

Cost versus Quality

James W. Holsinger, Jr., M.D., Ph.D.

Underlying the concepts of the cost and the quality of health care lies the problem of defining health and health care. To define health requires a systematic effort to reach a reasonable definition. In 1946, the World Health Organization (WHO) defined health as "... a state of complete physical, mental, and social well-being and not merely the absence of disease or infirmity."[1] It is no wonder that "our society is unsure of what it expects from its health care system, since such a far reaching definition places all of society under the aegis of health care."[2] When looking at this definition, it is difficult to expect that any health care system could provide the care required to reach the goals implicit in the WHO statement. Even if a society could or would strive to reach the essence of this definition, it is doubtful that it could afford the cost. Therefore in order to rationally consider the concepts of the cost and quality of health care, an attainable definition of health must be devised.

Various authors have defined and developed the concept of health in a variety of ways. For example, Twaddle states that health first must be understood as a biophysical status.[1] He finds that illness is any such state that has been so defined by a competent physician. He also notes that some authors suggest that anyone who feels ill should be considered sick; i.e., not in a state of health. Haggerty seems to agree with this latter concept in that while stating that health is difficult to define, he notes it is somehow the reciprocal or absence of mortality, morbidity, disability, and distress.[3] Schlenger notes that "the word 'health' is thought to be of Anglo-Saxon derivation and originally denoted 'wholeness' or functional harmony."[4] Mechanic indicates that in the medical view health has usually been seen in the framework of equilibrium and balance.[5] In this discussion, Kass's definition of health will be used, in which "health is a natural standard or norm— not a 'value' as opposed to an obligation—but a state of being that reveals itself in activity as a standard of bodily excellence or fitness, relative to each species and, to some extent, attainable."[6] Thus, "health is the well-working of the organism as a whole, referring to individuals, not the society in which they live."[2]

89

THE COST OF HEALTH CARE

From 1950, when health care costs were $12.7 billion, until 1980, when they reached $247 billion (an amount equal to 9.4 percent of the Gross National Product (GNP)),[7] the cost of health care in the United States has risen at a logarithmic rate.[8] This rate is expected to continue into the 1990s unabated. This 9.4 percent share of GNP in 1980 represents a dramatic increase over the 8.9 percent rate of 1979. These health care expenditures represent an average of $1,067 per person and of this amount 42.2 percent, or $450, came from public funds. Private health insurance premiums provided $64.9 billion while federal payments represented $70.9 billion, with $33.3 billion provided by state and local government funds. In 1980, direct payment by consumers reached $70.6 billion, accounting for 32.4 percent of all personal health care expenditures. When compared to 1979, 1980 hospital care spending represented 40.3 percent of the total, an increase of 16.2 percent above the previous year. Physician services increased 14.5 percent above 1979 reaching a level of $46.6 billion or 18.9 percent of the health care dollar. It is of interest that Medicare and Medicaid outlays totaled $60.6 billion amounting to 27.8 percent of all personal health care expenses. All third parties combined financed 67.6 percent of the total of $217.9 billion spent for personal health care in 1980.[7] No matter how these statistics are viewed, personal health care in the United States is expensive in both dollars spent and time expended. In addition, the costs of health care continue to rise in the number of dollars spent as well as a percentage of GNP.

There are a variety of causes for the observed increase in the expense of the personal health care system in the United States. Not only are these causes numerous but they are also interrelated. Freeland and Schendler state that two factors are of particular note: "(1) a demand-side factor, the role of third-party payments in increasing consumer demand for services; and (2) a supply-side factor, the fee-for-service and cost-based reimbursement systems which lack incentives to provide medical care in the least expensive manner."[8a] Gibson and Waldo suggest that the rate of growth in personal health care expenditures is greater than can be explained by a combination of population growth as well as price growth.[7] They observe that there has been an increase in the intensity of services consumed as well as an increase in the growth of use of services *per capita*. It is of interest that the proportion of expenditures paid out of pocket by consumers for hospital care has remained at 9.0 percent during the period from 1968 to 1980, during a period in which hospital expenditures have increased at an annual average rate approaching 14.0 percent.[8] However, personal health care expenditures have consumed an increasing part of personal income over the past 15 years when viewed in current dollars, but when inflation is considered this apparent share of personal income has not risen by nearly the same magnitude as the dollar figures would indicate.[7]

The increases noted in personal health care expenditures can be determined. For example, in the case of hospital expenditures, which in 1979 accounted for 40.0 percent of national health expenditures, increases in hospital input prices in excess of the GNP deflator were 10.2 percent of the growth, nearly equal to the 12.3 percent growth in admissions *per capita*. Growth in population resulted in 6.4 percent of the increase, with growth in real expenses per admission accounting for 21.9 percent. Three factors specific to the health care industry— admissions *per capita,* intensity per admission, and hospital input prices in excess of the GNP deflator—account for 44 percent of the growth. Of these factors, growth in intensity per admission accounted for half. The major driving force behind the increase in intensity of services per admission is the demand for higher and higher quality of care, which in turn is fueled by a high level of insurance coverage. The latter combined with the retrospective cost-based reimbursement system provides perverse incentives to provide the least expensive care.[8]

The third party reimbursement system used in the United States has resulted in coverage of all but about six million Americans.[9] This system has developed in order to financially protect the individual consumer of personal health services. In addition, health insurance was developed in order to provide a mechanism for individuals to gain access to the system such that the availability of funds would not serve as a bar. The result of the development of the health insurance system has been to place demands on the system that cannot be met within the apparent resources that can be committed to health care.[2] With a reduction in the out-of-pocket expense to the individual as determined by the combination of health care insurance and other medical benefit plans, financial barriers to health care for most individuals in our society have decreased, resulting in a vastly increased demand. Since it is dominated by third party payers, the health care market is atypical of the perfect market for goods and services as envisioned in standard economic theory. As Gibson and Waldo have stated ''consumers of health care tend to be isolated from the true price of health care and tend to consume more care than they would were they to pay directly the full price of the goods and services they receive.''[7a]

Interim results from a controlled trial of cost sharing in health insurance have shown that individuals fully covered for medical services spend about 50 percent more than do similar individuals covered by income-related catastrophic insurance.[10] Newhouse and co-workers have shown that more services per user and more people using services occur with full coverage. They found increases in both ambulatory care and in-hospital services. Interestingly, there were no differences noted for expenditures per admission once the individuals were admitted to the hospital. Three generalizations of their results were developed. First, they determined that if insurance for ambulatory care services were to be immediately extended, a marked increase in demand would occur that could not be handled within current capacity of the personal health care system. Second, they noted that it might be deemed impossible to allow the system to expand to meet any new demand made of it due to constraints enforced by budget limits or rate and fee controls. Third, they deduced that physicians might create additional demand to offset any decline that might be produced by an increase in cost-sharing levels resulting in a fall in demand. These authors contend that "unless budget limits or other regulations constrain the response, a reduction in cost sharing will expand the total volume of resources in medical care and *vice versa*."[10a]

Overall a variety of factors have produced the problem related to the cost of the personal health care system. Several of these include the cost of new technologies as well as the costs associated with the increased number of and types of health care providers. McNerney has pointed out that the principal factors producing increased demand are: (1) increasing insurance coverage; (2) rising personal income; and (3) greater faith in the curative powers of medicine. He also points out that certain factors have affected the supply of health care including: (1) increasing numbers of doctors and hospital beds; (2) advances in science and technology that require increased amounts of equipment and skilled labor; and (3) the inability of a labor-intensive, personal-service industry to achieve increased gains in productivity.[11] He finds, as a part of the underlying problem, that unqualified cost reimbursement stimulates increasing costs and that there is a linear relationship between bed use and bed supply. There has also been noted a relationship between the degree of technological development and its accompanying cost and the supply and utilization of physicians. No one involved in the health care equation is able to weigh the cost of a procedure against its perceived benefit. McNerney summarizes by stating that there is a cost problem that is related to heavy demand as a function of insurance, income, and expectation and that in turn presses on a relatively unproductive supply response that is excited by new technology. It is interesting that the third party reimbursement system discussed above incorporates incentives to increase costs. This system rewards providers who supply larger quantities and more costly services with an increased level of revenue. Therefore, there is an incentive to adopt new diagnostic and therapeutic techniques and technologies rather than to adopt new processes that more efficiently use existing procedures and techniques.

There is little question that new technologies are expensive. The effect of the costs of new technology has been at least arithmetically, if not geometrically, additive.[2] Thomas discusses three quite different levels of technology—nontechnology, halfway technology, and decisive technology.[12] These three types of technology must be kept separate when looking at their costs. Nontechnology is impossible to measure in terms of its capacity to alter the outcome or natural course of a disease. A great deal of the cost of the personal health care system is involved in this level of technology, and it is highly valued by both patients and practitioners. This level of technology is the supportive therapy provided by practitioners, and it is indispensable to the care of sick patients. It is not a real technology but is extremely expensive due to the time involved in its production.

The level of halfway technology represents all those things that must be carried out after the fact in order to compensate for the incapacitating effects of certain diseases. This is technology that is designed to make up for disease or to postpone death. This technology is well represented by the transplantation of organs or the development of artificial organs. It is the lay public's equivalent to the high technology of the physical sciences. Each new advance is seen as a breakthrough and not as the makeshift that it is. It is what must be done until genuine understanding of the nature and mechanisms of disease are understood. It is a characteristic of this kind of technology that it costs an enormous amount of money and requires a continuing expansion of hospital facilities. To move away from this level of technology will require the development of new information that can only be generated by research. The third type of technology is the high technology of medicine and represents the modern methods of immunization and the contemporary use of antibiotics and chemotherapy. It is the technology that is generated by the genuine understanding of disease mechanisms. When it becomes available, it is relatively inexpensive and easy to deliver.

Technology can also be looked at as requiring the biomedical research that has developed the new expensive technology but has contributed to the modern decline of mortality. The problem of the rising costs of health care often blur the distinction between the costs of research, the costs of care, and the costs of disease. A major part of this problem is the absence of a market test for innovations. This line of reasoning does not mean that the new technologies are ineffective since many of those recently developed are of unquestioned value. The problem lies in the newer technologies being too widely diffused within the system. These costly procedures are found in all facilities, not just in regional or specialized facilities. In addition these new innovations are not tested for effectiveness before they are so widely diffused. The cost-based reimbursement mechanisms are partly at fault in that there are no incentives for such testing. Clinical trials of new technologies before their widespread dissemination have been rare. Thus, another way of looking at technology is that it is easier to focus on it than to look at the hard questions that continue to drive the costs of the personal health care system ever higher. [13]

A major impact on the cost of the personal health care system has been the marked increase in the number of individuals employed in the health care industry. During the decade of the 1970s, 2.4 million people were added to the health care work force, representing an increase of 55 percent when compared to the beginning of the decade. During this same period, the total work force of the nation grew by only 23 percent. [14] In addition to the increase in the number of individuals employed, there has been an increase in the median weekly earnings in the industry during the same period of time. In 1970, these earnings represented 82 percent of the national average and rose to 86 percent in 1978.

It is of interest that work weeks are usually slightly shorter for the health care industry. There has also been a trend toward rising skill levels as evidenced by the growth in the proportion of registered nurses and the relative decline in importance of licensed practical nurses and nurses' aides. During the 1970s, the registered nurse group rose by 60 percent, but the LPN and nurses aides group rose by only 20 percent.

Increases in the number of physicians were also seen during the 1970s. As a result of this growth, the number of physicians in the United States reached 424,000 in 1978, a 51 percent increase over 1970. Approximately 380,000 of these physicians were professionally active (91 percent). Since the number of physicians increased faster than the population at large, the ratio of physicians to population increased from 14.2 per 10,000 in 1950 to 17.9 in 1977, with all the increase occurring after 1960. This increase occurred as a direct result of an increase in the number of professional schools that followed a series of federal acts and programs in the 1960s and 1970s.[15] However even this increase in physicians and other health care professionals has not been able to keep up the increase in demand generated by American society. As the cost of health care as a percentage of the GNP has increased, it is estimated that each physician who goes into practice creates an increase of $300,000 per year in additional health care costs.[16] It has recently been estimated that there will be an oversupply of physicians by the year 1990. It is clear why the federal government has determined that capitation grants and other health profession subsidies are no longer warranted.[17]

As an example of the concept that the physician to some extent is responsible for creating demand, Kopstein[18] has provided data indicating that, for a variety of surgical and invasive procedures, there has been a significant increase between 1966–67 and 1976–77, the period of marked increase in the supply of physicians. Cardiac catheterization increased by more than tenfold among men 45 to 64 years of age. Cesarean section doubled in women aged 15 to 44, and dilation and curettage of the uterus increased by 17 to 23 percent depending upon age group. Likewise, hysterectomy increased by 20 to 22 percent depending on age. Prostatectomy increased by 41 percent for men 45 to 64 years old and by 17 percent in those over age 65. "There is a growing concern that surgery is being used excessively in this country. This overutilization may in part be the result of an oversupply of surgeons and the availability of third-party payment for operative services."[18a]

Field has found that, as the medical system becomes more technologically advanced and as more equipment and personnel become involved in the output of the system, the more fragmented and depersonalized the product becomes to the recipient.[19] The patient's understanding of and control over the process decreases, and there is an increase in the alienation of the ill person. He or she finds that this fragmentation not only acts as a deterrent to continuity of care but also detracts from the quality of the care rendered. There is also a substantially increased cost associated with the fragmentation. Field states that there is no substitute for the general practitioner as a method by which some continuity of care can be restored to the system. Potentially therefore, an increase in the number of general practitioners could represent a way in which the costs of the personal health care system could be reduced.

The social costs of the personal health care system in the United States are often overlooked. Malenbaum studied the effects of changes in health status in poor nations where labor is a dominant factor of production.[20] He found that his preliminary statistical analysis suggested that there is a positive effect of health inputs on subsequent outputs. He determined that health improvement means greater vigor and increased energy for the worker. There are fewer days of illness and therefore fewer days away from work. Consequently there is an increase in both the number of hours worked as well as greater product per hour worked. Thus an unhealthy society has a reduction in production and productivity with its resultant social cost. It is interesting, though, that a variety of environmental factors contribute to the health status of the society. Among these are income, diet, recreation, housing, education, urbanization, drinking, and the use of the automobile. The prevailing assumption is that the rise in real income seems to have the most favorable impact on health, quite apart from the fact that it permits the individual to purchase an increased amount of health care services. However, it may be that the benefits of increased per capita income have been overestimated even though a very high correlation between income and the individual's health status has been found.[21]

Historically, the prevention of disease and injury to others has been the most important rationale for coercive public health measures. However, in the developed countries, communicable diseases, the best rationale for public health activities, have been widely replaced by heart disease, cancer, stroke, and accidents as the leading causes of death. Knowles states:

> Prevention of disease means forsaking the bad habits which many people enjoy—overeating, too much drinking, taking pills, staying up at night, engaging in promiscuous sex, driving too fast, and smoking cigarettes—or, put another way, it means doing things which require special effort—exercising regularly, going to the dentist, practicing contraception, ensuring harmonious family life, submitting to screening examinations.[22] (p. 59)

As Courtwright states: "The traditional harm-to-others doctrine, as it is generally applied, is inadequate to justify proscription of personal bad habits. This doctrine has become increasingly outmoded, particularly as the pattern of disease has changed in the developed countries. Grounds for action appear remote since in most cases only the individual's immediate health and well-being are affected."[23]

As twentieth century medicine has evolved in the United States, a certain false expectation has been created that the physician can cure not only physiological impairments but that he or she can and should be able to cope with all kinds of problems. Ivan Illich, in *Medical Nemesis,*[24] indicates that modern medical technology has gained enormous prestige and influence in American society. This has led to a feeling in the population at large that there is no longer a responsibility for the individual's own health and welfare, but that this burden has been passed on to the health care professional. Thus, the professionals originally charged with the prevention and control of disease become increasingly responsible for new types of illness and disorders. Of the three classes of iatrogenic sickness Illich describes, the social illness, according to Morison, is perhaps the most interesting.[25] Thus there is an obvious need to define the limits of the personal health care system in order to establish that health is, in different ways, everyone's business. Each individual must be responsible for his or her own health. The social cost of health may be markedly reduced if each person would follow Breslow's seven rules: (1) don't smoke cigarettes; (2) get seven hours of sleep; (3) eat breakfast; (4) keep your weight down; (5) drink moderately; (6) exercise daily; and (7) don't eat between meals.[26]

THE QUALITY OF HEALTH CARE

The quality of health is usually determined by using various statistical measures of health. Traditionally, the health of a community is measured by using population statistics regarding death or disease. Population statistics are easier to collect than individual measures and are already collected as part of medical care record keeping. Hennes has found that "population measures have the disadvantage of losing information on variation and of making it difficult to study program-consumer interaction."[27] In addition to the normal measures of health there are a variety of areas or functions that are considered basic to healthy humans. Physiological functions include: (1) seeing; (2) hearing; (3) speaking; (4) sleeping; (5) eating; (6) eliminating; (7) moving; and (8) reproducing. Psychosocial functions include: (1) working; (2) playing; (3) thinking; (4) relating to others; (5) relating to self; and (6) being active. Since our personal health care system deals with individuals, a strong case can be made for developing measures of health that deal with individuals and that has the above listed functions as its basis for development.

Fingerhut provides statistics concerning the determinants of health status.[28] She reports that life expectancy at birth reached a record 73.2 years in 1977 in the United States. From 1900 to 1950, the gains in life expectancy were dramatic and have been attributed to decreases in infectious and parasitic diseases. During the next 20 years, 2.7 years were added to life expectancy, while the pace of improvement has accelerated during the past decade with 2.3 years being added since 1970. On the average, individuals reaching age 65 in 1977 would expect to live an additional 16.3 years, 1.1 years more than those individuals reaching this age in 1970. However, a certain controversy surrounds these raw statistics dealing with mortality rates. McKinlay and McKinlay believe that mortality statistics are inadequate and are misleading as indicators of national health status.[29]

A review of McKinlay and McKinlay's paper is revealing. They cite McKeown, who concludes that the decline in mortality in England and Wales during the eighteenth century was largely due to environmental improvements.[30] In the nineteenth century, he found that the decline in mortality was due to reduction in deaths due to infectious diseases, particularly in the second half of the century. He states that "the main influences were: (a) rising standards of living, of which the most significant feature was a better diet; (b) improvements in hygiene; and (c) a favorable trend in the relationship between some micro-organisms and the human hosts."[30a] Interestingly he found that therapy did not contribute to the decline in death rate, and only in the case of smallpox did immunization have an effect. This accounted for about five percent of the reduction in deaths. McKeown, for the twentieth century, argues that "the main influences on the decline in mortality were improved nutrition on airborne infections, reduced exposure (from better hygiene) on water- and food-borne diseases and, less certainly, immunization and therapy on the large number of conditions included in the miscellaneous group" (non-infectious diseases).[30b] He states that the improvement in nutrition was the major influence on the reduction of death rates in the twentieth century.

A significant decrease in overall mortality in the United States has occurred in the period subsequent to 1900. The steady decline in mortality for women began to level off about 1950, whereas for men the beginning of a slight increase in mortality was noticed in 1960. McKinlay and McKinlay state "it is evident that the beginning of the precipitate and still unrestrained rise in medical care expenditures began when nearly all (92 percent) of the modern decline in mortality in this country had already occurred."[29a] They looked at ten common infectious diseases and compared the fall in death rate for each with the use of chemotherapeutic and prophylactic medical measures. They found that reductions in mortality from tuberculosis and pneumonia substantially contributed to the decrease in total mortality during the period from 1900 to 1973. The other eight conditions contributed only 12 percent of the total decrease in mortality during this period. Smallpox was disregarded since its only effective measure was introduced about 1800. Only influenza, whooping cough, and poliomyelitis demonstrated significant decreases in mortality following the introduction of medical measures. Tuberculosis, scarlet fever, pneumonia, diphtheria, measles, and typhoid demonstrated negligible decreases in mortality subsequent to medical intervention. For tuberculosis, typhoid, measles, and scarlet fever, medical measures were introduced at the point when the death rate from these illnesses was already negligible. Only for poliomyelitis did medical measures have any marked impact.

Pneumonia, influenza, whooping cough, and diphtheria have relatively smooth mortality curves that appear to be unaffected by medical measures even though these were introduced rather early while death rates were still high.

> In general, medical measures (both chemotherapeutic and prophy-lactic) appear to have contributed little to the overall decline in mortality in the United States since about 1900—having in many instances been introduced several decades after a marked decline had already set in and having no detectable influence in most instances. More specifi-cally, with reference to those five conditions (influenza, pneumonia, diphtheria, whooping cough, and poliomyelitis) for which the decline in mortality appears substantial after the point of intervention—and on the unlikely assumption that all of this decline is attributable to the intervention—it is estimated that at most 3.5 percent of the total decline in mortality since 1900 could be ascribed to medical measures intro-duced for the diseases considered. . . .[29b] (p. 425)

Since the quality of health care is extremely difficult to measure, particularly since mortality figures are the only data currently available for this purpose on a nationwide basis, the question raised by Auster et al. is a very real one, i.e., "What is the contribution of medical services as opposed to environmental factors and to changes in the health of the population?"[31] It may well be that environ-mental factors are more important than medical care as far as the health status of society is concerned. These investigators have developed several models to study the relationship of medical care to environmental factors. These models indicate that a 1.0 percent increase in the quantity of medical care is associated with a reduction in mortality of about 0.1 percent. Their models indicate that environmental factors are a more important determinant of interstate variation in death rates, with income and education playing the most important role. The impact of income on mortality is positive while that of education is negative. They found that urbanization is not important but that certain labor force variables are. They also found some indication of harmful effects from cigarette smoking. The implications of these studies indicate that there would be a variety of impacts on mortality rates. The real increase in medical care expenditures of 35 percent between 1955 and 1965 should have produced a decline in mortality of about 4 percent. However, this was affected by a variety of environmental factors. The growth in education should have produced another decline of about 3 percent, while increases in per capita income should have produced an increase in mor-tality (6 percent). Increases in cigarette consumption per capita should have led to a 2 percent increase. Their results imply that adverse environmental factors have been offsetting the advantages of increases in the quantity and quality of medical care.[31] Thus, there is a real question whether additional expenditures should be applied to health care or to the various environmental factors that either enhance health status or that, if reduced, would also reduce the mortality rates in our society.

By and large, the major improvements in health have resulted from changes in personal behavior (hygiene and reproductive practices) and in environmental conditions (food supplies, provision of safe milk and water, and sewage disposal). Knowles states that "over 99 percent of us are born healthy and made sick as a result of personal misbehavior and environmental conditions."[22a] It is difficult to hold the health care system responsible for the effects of our way of life upon our health. It has been estimated that well over half of the visits to American physicians are due to deviations from health for which the patient, or his or her way of life, is in some important way responsible. Knowles has stated that "the greatest portion of our national expenditure (for health care) goes for caring of the major causes of premature, and therefore preventable death and/or disability."[22b] As he states, we cannot hope to develop a rational health care system if the parts of the whole that bear on health are moving in irrational ways. It is interesting that treatment of conditions associated with alcohol abuse accounted for 20 percent of all hospitals care costs for adults in 1975, with the bill estimated at $8.4 billion. Other expenditures associated with this problem are estimated at $4.3 billion. Cigarette smoking has long been described as the chief preventable cause of death in the United States. In 1976, it is estimated that cigarette smoking produced direct health care costs of $8.2 billion with indirect costs of $19.1 billion.[32]

Health care can be divided into two types: (1) personal health care; and (2) nonpersonal health care. The latter is perceived to be what is commonly known as public health. In association with personal health care, Clogg[33] finds that endogenous causes of death account for about 80 percent of mortality in Sweden, the United States, England, and Wales.[33] Endogenous causes of death include: (1) malignant and benign neoplasms; (2) cardiovascular diseases; (3) certain degenerative diseases (nephritis, cirrhosis of the liver, ulcers of stomach and duodenum, and diabetes); (4) influenza, pneumonia, and bronchitis; and (5) certain diseases of infancy. Exogenous causes of death include: (1) respiratory tuberculosis; (2) other infections and parasitic diseases; (3) influenza, pneumonia, and bronchitis; (4) diarrhea, gastritis, and enteritis; (5) complications of pregnancy; (6) motor vehicle accidents; and (7) other accidents and violence. Clogg finds:

> withdrawal of personal health services would result in a 57.1 percent increase in cardiovascular mortality, an increase in certain degenerative mortality of 37.5 percent, an increase of 38.3 percent in neoplasm mortality, and an increase of 57.1 percent in influenza-bronchitis mortality . . . the effect of personal health care has been found to be

substantial since 6.4 years loss in life expectation is considerable . . .
the gain in life expectation in the U.S. in the twentieth century has,
by our calculation, been only moderately responsible to the massive
personal health care defense which have been developed. In 1900 life
expectation for males was 45.6; in 1964 it was 66.9, representing a
gain of 21.3 years; 6.4 years, or 30 percent of that gain, is the most
that can be attributed to personal health care.[33a] (p. 22)

The Interaction of the Cost and Quality of Health Care

From the above discussion it is obvious that there is little agreement on the
issues of cost and quality of American health care. There is little doubt that
health care in the United States is expensive. Whether or not this large expenditure
buys high quality health care is another issue. The problem of the high cost of
health care leads almost directly to the question of quality—are we helped or
hurt by what we are paying so much for as a society? What can we expect from
our health care system? As twentieth-century medicine has evolved in the United
States, a certain false expectation has been created that the physician can cure
not only physiological impairments but that he or she can and should be able to
cope with all kinds of problems, "including the prevention of crime, the taming
of juvenile delinquents, the relief of poverty and racial discrimination, the reduction of laziness and philandering, and the rearing of decent and moral men
and women."[6a] It would appear that this expansion of the health "needs" of
our society in conjunction with the development of the concept of the "right to
health care" has produced the marked rise in the cost of delivering health care
over the past 25 years.

However, the two issues of the cost and quality of health care are not unrelated
as the discussion above attests. The question appears to be whether or not these
two issues interact in competition with each other or whether the cost of health
care can be controlled with a concomitant maintenance of the quality of the
health care purchased for fewer dollars. Should the latter hold true, then indeed
the two interact but with a potential synergistic effect, not an antagonistic one.
McClure defines the problem as overelaborate medical care.[34] He states that
over a very wide range of utilization rates, high quality medical care can be
provided to identical populations from the standpoint of health outcomes. McClure[34]
points out that "[f]or example, hospital use rates across excellent medical care
settings have been found to vary from less than 700 hospital days per 1000
population to more than 1400 hospital days per 1000 population for comparable
populations." The average for the United States is 1200 hospital days per 1000
population. These rates are adjusted for sex, age, and risk to assure comparability.
These differences seem to represent legitimate differences in clinical opinion
and style of practice. Practitioners who practice quality medical care can be
found throughout this style spectrum. Some individuals practice a conservative

style while others provide a more elaborate style of care requiring more complex services per capita. For example, the Mayo Clinic practices a conservative style that requires only 800 days of hospital care per 1000 people, 30 percent below the national average.[35] In the city of Boston, where equally high quality medical practice occurs, a more elaborate style of practice is provided with hospital use rates higher than the national average. McClure notes that if the practitioners in the United States were to shift to a more conservative style of practice, approximately 20 percent of the health care expenditures could be saved on a national basis. A shift to a more conservative style would not represent a denial or rationing of services nor would it represent a move from high technology to low. From the standpoint of accepted clinical practice both styles appear equally good. "The key to restraining medical care expenditures without restricting the quality or availability of medical care is to encourage more conservative practice styles and to discourage elaborate styles."[7b] On this basis, it would appear that there is some rationale for the belief that the problems of cost and quality in the health care system can be approached from a synergistic direction and that these problems do not have to be treated in a competitive mode.

NOTES

1. A.C. Twaddle, "The Concept of Health Status," *Society, Science and Medicine* 8 (1974):29–38.

2. J.W. Holsinger Jr., "The Effects of the Evolution of the Health Care System on the Problems of Health Systems Access, Cost and Quality," *Journal of the Medical Association of Georgia* 68 (1979):987–989.

3. R.J. Haggerty, "The Boundaries of Health Care," *The Pharos* 35 (1972):106–111.

4. W.E. Schlenger, "A New Framework for Health," *Inquiry* 13 (1976):207–214.

5. D. Mechanic, *Medical Sociology*. (New York: The Free Press, 1968), p. 2.

6. L.R. Kass, "Regarding the End of Medicine and the Pursuit of Health," *Public Interest* 40 (1975):11–42.

6a. Ibid., p. 20.

7. R.M. Gibson and D.R. Waldo, "National Health Expenditures, 1980," *Health Care Financing Review* 3, no. 1 (1981):1–54.

7a. Ibid., p. 20.

7b. Ibid., p. 16.

8. M.S. Freeland and C.E. Schendler, "National Health Expenditures: Short-term Outlook and Long-term Projections," *Health Care Financing Review* 2, no. 3 (1981):97–138.

8a. Ibid., p. 115.

9. A.D. Bauerschmidt, 1981 personal communication, College of Business Administration, University of South Carolina, Columbia, SC.

10. J.P. Newhouse et al., "Some Interim Results from a Controlled Trial of Cost Sharing in Health Insurance," *New England Journal of Medicine* 305 (1981):1501–1507.

10a. Ibid., p. 1507.

11. W.J. McNerney, "Control of Health-Care Costs in the 1980's," *New England Journal of Medicine* 303 (1980):1088–1095.

12. L. Thomas, "The Technology of Medicine," *New England Journal of Medicine* 285 (1971):1366–1368.

13. S. Schneyer et al., "Biomedical Research and Illness: 1900–1979," *Milbank Memorial Fund Quarterly* 59 (1981):44–58.

14. E.S. Sekscenski, "The Health Services Industry: A Decade of Expansion," *Monthly Labor Review* 104, no. 5 (1981):9–16.

15. S.R. Machlin, "Health Care Resources," in *Health United States 1979* (Washington, D.C.: National Center for Health Statistics, Office of Health Research, Statistics and Technology, DHEW, 1980), pp. 205–210.

16. J.A. Califano Jr., Address to the Association of American Medical Colleges Annual Meeting in New Orleans, La., October 24, 1978 (AAMC Memo 1978; #78-56).

17. A.R. Tarlov and R. Graham, *Interim Report of the Graduate Medical Education National Advisory Committee to the Secretary, DHEW*. DHEW Pub. No. (HRA) 79-633 (Washington, D.C., 1979).

18. A. Kopstein, "Utilization of Health Resources" in *Health United States 1979* (Washington, D.C.: National Center for Health Statistics, Office of Health Research, Statistics and Technology, DHEW 1980), pp. 177–185.

18a. Ibid., p. 183.

19. M.G. Field, "The Medical System and Industrial Society," in *Systems and Medical Care*, A. Sheldon, ed. (Cambridge, Mass.: The MIT Press, 1970), pp. 143–181.

20. W. Malenbaum, "Progress in Health: What Index of What Progress?" *Annals of the American Academy of Political and Social Science* 393 (1971):109–121.

21. V.R. Fuchs, "The Contribution of Health Services to the American Economy," *Milbank Memorial Fund Quarterly* 44, no. 4, part 2 (1966):65–100.

22. J.H. Knowles, "The Responsibility of the Individual," in *Doing Better and Feeling Worse*, J.H. Knowles, ed. (New York: W.W. Norton & Co., Inc., 1977), pp. 57–80.

22a. Ibid., p. 58.

22b. Ibid., p. 95.

23. D.T. Courtwright, "Public Health and Public Wealth: Social Costs as a Basis for Restrictive Policies," *Milbank Memorial Fund Quarterly* 58, no. 2 (1980):270.

24. I. Illich, *Medical Nemesis* (New York: Pantheon, 1976).

25. R.S. Morison, "A Further Note on Visions," *Daedalus* 109, no. 1 (1980):55–64.

26. N.B. Brelloc and L. Breslow, "Relationship of Physical Health Status and Health Practices," *Preventive Medicine* 1 (1972):409–421.

27. V.P. Hennes, "The Measurement of Health," *Medical Care Review* 29 (1972):1271.

28. L.A. Fingerhut, "Health Status and Determinants," in *Health United States 1979* (Washington, D.C.: National Center for Health Statistics, Office of Health Research, Statistics, and Technology, DHEW, 1980), pp. 111–126.

29. J.D. McKinlay and S.M. McKinlay, "The Questionable Contribution of Medical Measures to the Decline of Mortality in the United States in the Twentieth Century," *Milbank Memorial Fund Quarterly* 55 (1977):405–428.

29a. Ibid., p. 414.

29b. Ibid., p. 414.

30. T. McKeown et al., "An Interpretation of the Decline of Mortality in England and Wales during the Twentieth Century," *Population Studies* 29 (1975):391–422.

30a. Ibid., p. 391.

30b. Ibid., p. 422.

31. R. Auster et al., "The Production of Health: An Exploratory Study," *The Journal of Human Resources* 4 (1969):411–436.

32. K.G. Bauer, "The Economic Burden That Prevention Could Reduce," in *Health United States 1980* (Washington, D.C.: National Center for Health Statistics, Public Health Service, DHHS, 1980), pp. 285–290.

33. C.C. Clogg, "The Effect of Personal Health Care Services on Longevity in an Economically Advanced Population," *Health Services Research* 17 (1979):5–32.

34. W. McClure, "The Competition Strategy for Medical Care," Unpublished paper, Center for Policy Studies, Minneapolis, 1982.

35. F.T. Nobrega et al., "Hospital Use in a Fee-for-Service System," *Journal of the American Medical Association* 247 (1982):806–810.

Chapter 6

Cost Containment, Quality Assurance, and Manpower Utilization

Alan M. Leiken, Ph.D. and Edmund J. McTernan, M.P.H., Ed.D.

PUBLIC CONCERN REGARDING HEALTH CARE QUALITY AND COSTS

The increase in the nation's expenditures for health care has increased the public's concern regarding health care quality and costs. In response to these concerns, Congress enacted the Medicare Law, Title XVIII, Social Security Act in 1965. This program's main thrust was cost containment, requiring hospital-based utilization review committees for participation in Medicare reimbursement. The Social Security Amendments of 1967 (PL 90-248) required Medicaid agencies to establish utilization review procedures similar to those required for participants in Medicare reimbursement. The authority to establish utilization procedures was given to the fiscal intermediaries, usually Blue Cross. The United States Department of Health, Education, and Welfare authorized Blue Cross to determine the medical necessity of care provided in select cases and to deny payment when it was determined care was not medically necessary. Significant expansion of review programs occurred with the passage of the 1972 Social Security Amendments (PL 92-603). This established the Professional Standards Review Organization (PSRO) with its stated purpose as follows:

> In order to promote the effective, efficient and economical delivery of health care services of proper quality for which payment may be made (by Medicare or Medicaid) . . . and in recognition of the interests of patients, the public practitioners and providers in improved health care services, it is the purpose of this part to assure . . . that the services for which payment be made . . . will conform to appropriate professional standards for the provision of health care and that payment for such services will be made—
> (1) only when, and to the extent, medically necessary . . .; and
> (2) in the case of services provided by a hospital or other health care facility . . . only when . . . such services cannot, consistent

with professionally recognized health care standards, effectively be provided on an outpatient basis or more economically in an inpatient health care facility of a different type, as determined in the exercise of reasonable limits of professional discretion.[1] (p. 42, Section 11-55)

The primary purpose of this program is somewhat unclear. Optimally, it should be a cost containment and quality assurance program. The AMA maintains that the program is a quality assurance program and that the review process should be used to eliminate poor medical practices rather than to reduce admissions or length of stay.[2] On the other hand, the literature associated with the history of the legislation in Congress notes that legislatures perceived a cost-containment orientation.[3] Others believe that the statute was primarily written "to permit the government to cut, or at least limit the growth of Medicare, and Medicaid costs without forcing medical standards below an acceptable level."[4]

RESEARCH STUDIES

Studies regarding the cost effectiveness of PSROs are inconclusive. The study of the then U.S. Department of Health, Education, and Welfare's Office of Planning, Evaluation, and Legislation found no reduction in utilization variables studied as a result of PSROs.[2] They further report that in order to pay for itself the program would have to reduce utilization of covered groups by 1.6 to 2.05 percent. To date, it has not accomplished this. Researchers studying the effect of PSRO programs upon utilization in Utah and New Mexico found no significant reduction.[5,6] Others, however, have found that PSROs have reduced utilization. Westphal et al. conducted a five-year review at a university hospital. Immediately after the institution of PSRO admission and length of stay review of Medicare-Medicaid patients, a significant decrease in length of stay and average charges generated per patient occurred.[7] Fulchiero et al. found the PSRO to be cost effective, when they studied the effect on utilization of Medicaid patients in Massachusetts hospitals of the Commonwealth Health Agencies Monitoring Program. Over a four-year period they estimated that the program saved $22,128,828. Conversely, the four-year cost of operating the program was only $5,570,852.[8]

Questions regarding the effectiveness of the PSROs as a cost-controlling program also apply to the methods and effectiveness of the program with regard to quality assurance. Programs have been designed and instituted to increase the quality of medical care services through the establishment of ongoing quality assessment programs.[9] All the PSRO programs rely on information regarding the structure, process, or outcome of medical care to assess quality of care.[10] Structural measures are concerned with the characteristics of facilities and status of providers. Process measures evaluate the appropriateness and quality of procedures performed by the provider for a patient. Outcome measures focus on what happened to the patient with regard to treatment, cure, rehabilitation, or death.[11]

Although the ultimate goal of medical care is to favorably affect the outcome of an illness episode, most quality assessment programs have focused upon structure or process. A review of programs that have used these methods to assess quality reveals that the methodology has been employed in a variety of circumstances.

For example, researchers have been interested in studying variations in quality between hospitals. The Stanford Center for Health Care Research has studied variations in quality across 17 short-term care hospitals.[12] Lee et al. and Lipworth compared quality at teaching and nonteaching hospitals.[13,14] Graham and Palovick examined the impact of frequency of cases and how hospitals that treat a given case infrequently compare with those who treat the same cases on a more regular basis.[15]

Lembcke examined hospital medical records at 23 hospital service areas in Rochester, New York to determine the appropriateness of appendectomies.[16] Evaluations have also been conducted to assess the appropriateness of hospital utilization and the necessity of performing ovariectomies in private hospitals in Los Angeles.[17] Similar work has been done with regard to hysterectomies. Trussel et al. evaluated the quality of care rendered to Teamster Union members and their families and concluded that 12.5 percent of all hospital admissions were unnecessarry.[18]

Comparisons of quality in different types of medical care systems have also been made. Much of this work has focused on quality comparisons of group practices versus private fee-for-service practices;[19,20] and group practice versus community practice settings.[21] Some work has focused on attempts to improve quality by intervening to correct identified deficiencies.[22,23]

While it can be argued that the presence of such studies in themselves can be responsible for improving quality, questions regarding the impact of quality assessment programs on costs and quality still remain. Arguments have been made that monitoring quality by examining the process of care will increase the number of procedures and, hence, costs.[24] Others have expressed fears that process standards would lead to "cookbook medicine." This refers to physicians conforming to a set of norms for each diagnosis. This would lead to more expensive care and a reduction in the physician's ability to tailor treatment to fit the special needs of each patient.[25] Bloom et al. raise concerns that PSROs adversely affect quality. They feel that "in a PSRO program where resources are limited, the government's desire to control medicare and medicaid costs will lead it to underfund quality review, leading to an actual reduction in quality, because higher cost services cannot be justified."[26] A Health Care Financing Administration Research Report contradicts these studies. By using the variation rate, defined as "the proportion of patient records audited to a particular criterion of care which do not meet the standard set for the criterion," as a measure of quality they note that variation rates at re-audit are significantly lower than those at audit, indicating improvements in quality of care. Additional work indicates that even small improvements in variation rates have major implications for patient health status.[27]

It is evident from the research performed and concerns expressed about quality assurance programs to date that the cost reduction and quality enhancement effects are at best marginal. Recent studies have also shown that almost 60 percent of hospital costs are consumed by personal expenses.[28] Because there is demonstrably a significant variation in the salaries and wages paid to different categories of health care providers, it is curious that there is little in the literature that compares the cost of performance of different types of service as performed by one category of health care worker in comparison to the performance of that same task by another.

ASSUMPTIONS ABOUT QUALITY OF PROFESSIONAL PERFORMANCE

It is self-evident that many assumptions are made by both providers and consumers concerning the issue of quality when any given task in health care is performed by two or more different categories of worker. In general, the assumption is that the most highly trained individual (who is usually the most highly paid) performs *all* tasks at the highest comparable level of proficiency. For example, most people would assume that the neurosurgeon performs every task in patient care more competently than a licensed practical nurse would perform those same tasks.

In 1980, the average income of all physicians in the U.S. was reported to be $80,900 per year.[29] An estimate of entry salaries of 22 different allied health professions was $14,572.[30] By simple arithmetic, this suggests a per-hour cost for a physician's services that is about five times as expensive as the average cost of services by an allied health professional. To equalize the cost variations of physician-provided services and those same services performed by an allied health professional, the physician would have to be about five times as productive as the nonphysician. While no one would suggest the one-for-one substitution of nonphysician health workers for physicians, only limited interest has been shown in comparing the cost and quality implications of physician and nonphysician health care providers.[31] Given the delivery of comparable quality of services (within reasonable limits), the benefits of substituting the less expensive nonphysician worker whenever safe and efficient, seem obvious.

The minimal impact of the quality assurance program upon cost containment efforts suggests the need for additional and more innovative, perhaps more courageous, approaches to this dilemma. One such potential may rest in testing the folklore that the best care is always available from the providers with the most extensive training. One hypothesis that is in need of scholarly inquiry is the "task-scale phenomenon." The argument for this hypothesis assumes that, considered analytically, patient care (or any other human activity) may be thought of as a series of individual simple steps or tasks to be performed. These tasks may range along a continuum from activities that are entirely intellectual in nature to those that are primarily physical.

As soon as any two or more human beings begin to function cooperatively, a division of labor (a parceling out of the tasks that make up a job to be done) takes place. This process has been carried out with increasing formality, complexity, and institutionalization in the field of patient care over a period of many years.

ROLES AND LEVELS OF TASK PERFORMANCE

With this complex division of labor, formalized roles have been developed. The total job has been divided into areas or disciplines such as nursing, pharmacy, housekeeping, etc. These may be thought of as vertical divisions of labor with responsibility for a total job within the limits of the discipline. Each of these then becomes divided horizontally into levels of responsibility. The top layers have been identified as those with professional responsibility; the next group are at the technological level; the next level is technical; then the vocational; and finally down to the unskilled in one or more additional steps. At each successive ascending step, greater preparation in terms of education and experience is usually required for entrance. Hence, a hierarchy evolved. In our society the layers of hierarchy are usually differentiated primarily in terms of years of education. Level of responsibility usually (but not always) increases in direct proportion to the length of educational preparation required.

In health care, the M.D.s and Ph.D.s are at the highest levels, followed by those with master's degrees, then bachelor's, associates, and so forth down to the unskilled category. For economic reasons, tasks are theoretically reserved to each level commensurate with the appropriate degree of skill and knowledge. Society cannot (yet) afford to pay $20,000 a year to a dishwasher—a minimum skill-level job—nor should a complex procedure in radiotherapy be placed in the hands of a fourth-grade dropout. In life, however, all tasks do not fall neatly into the center of each hierarchy layer, but range through a constant scale. The division between two successive levels is not a neat, thin, sharp line but a gray and irregular area of division. Thus, each person at each level of the pyramid is assigned a range of tasks, some of which fall near the center of his or her responsibility range, some near the top, and some nearer the bottom. Where the division is established between two successive skill levels (for instance, the practical nurse and the aide), there are many tasks that fall into the gray area— tasks that do not clearly belong to either the upper or the lower of the two jobs. Typically, these tasks are assigned rather arbitrarily, depending upon the nature of the manpower available in the given institution. They may also appear in the job descriptions for both levels.

Even when tasks are clearly the responsibility of one or another level, a good deal of "line crossing" occurs in even the most formal institution. This is more likely to be a crossing downward occurrence than a crossing upward. In one hospital, the nursing supervisor with a master's degree may push a patient in a wheelchair to X-ray (an orderly's job) in a rushed situation. In a busy patient care institution, these kinds of occurrences happen every day, everywhere, and involve almost everyone.

Theoretically, the highest level of performance in any given task should be delivered by the individual with the highest level of preparation. In point of fact, this is often not the case. In fact, the authors' hypothesis suggests that, in general, any given task is likely to be performed most competently by that person for whom the task is at or near the top of his or her skill spectrum. This is assuming, of course, that the individual is adequately trained, practiced, and intellectually and physically capable of performing the assigned duties.

AN HYPOTHESIS CONCERNING QUALITY OF PERFORMANCE

The task-scale phenomenon can be demonstrated by numerous examples, such as the surgical technician in the armed services who does a far better job of skin suturing than the surgeon. To that technician, skin suturing is interesting and challenging, while the surgeon is apt to see it as dull, uninteresting "scut work," and may fail to apply his or her full knowledge and training to that particular task. The implications of this phenomenon are obvious. When a task falls in the gray area between two skill levels, it should be assigned to the lower skill level, rather than the higher if at all possible. This rule is expected to yield dividends in terms of higher quality performance as well as in terms of economic advantages. This theory is, as has been noted, a reversal of the popular conception, which holds that better performance is synonymous with a higher level functionary.

"Man doth not live by bread alone" is a cliché, but it is a valid one. Effective performance of any given task depends not only on ability, but on motivation and ego-satisfaction factors. These, in turn, derive not only from tangible rewards (salary), but from social and emotional rewards as well (interest, challenge, sense of achievement, etc.). The worker who is performing a task that challenges him or her because it is near the top of the list of things he or she is permitted to do is very likely to do that task better than if that same task were performed by a higher level person who sees it as dull, routine, and insignificant. The reasons for this are the intangible reward factors that motivate all human activity.

An approach to testing the validity of the task-scale hypothesis in health care might be through the identification of selected specific tasks performed by two or more health workers at different levels of education and qualification, and the evaluation of both cost and quality implications of substituting different workers for the performance of these tasks in the clinical setting. For example, in the clinical laboratory, the isolation and identification of common pathogenic organisms might be performed by a pathologist (M.D.), by a medical technologist (M.T.) or by a medical laboratory technician (M.L.T.). Many other laboratory tasks are commonly performed by two or more of these categories, some of which are presented in Table 6-1.

The pathologist, usually with at least 11 years of postsecondary education and with an average annual income of $114,000, is the most expensive agent for the performance of the tests.[32] The medical technologist, usually with only four years of postsecondary education and a median annual salary of $14,640 requires less than half of this social investment, even with an added factor for necessary supervision by the pathologist. The medical laboratory technician usually enters the work force with just two years of postsecondary preparation. Clearly, this worker requires more supervision by higher level personnel, but with a median salary level in 1979 of only $12,000, the technician represents a far lower cost per test performed than either of the two higher categories.[33] Parts B and C of Table 6-1 present similar situations for two other health professions, physical therapy and respiratory therapy. Situations such as these exist for other health professions and offer ample opportunity to test the task-scale hypothesis.

NEED FOR FURTHER RESEARCH

Legislative activity, such as that which led to the establishment of the PSRO legislation, gives clear evidence of public concern about cost control, quality assessment, and the relationship of the two in contemporary health care. Although there is some difference among the conclusions reached to date by researchers who have studied the effects of PSRO and similar cost/quality control efforts, the bulk of the evidence seems to demonstrate that additional, more imaginative, and (in some cases) perhaps unpopular actions are needed to control the increase in the costs of health care. Clearly, there is a need to carry out such draconian measures only with concomitant efforts to assure that the quality and accessibility of care will not fall below a reasonable standard. One question that has not been studied adequately is which health worker can perform each task needed in patient care at an optimal balance of cost and quality. It has been suggested in this chapter that a need exists for research designed to explore the popular concept that the provider with the most extensive preparation can deliver all services in his or her area of practice best. Preliminary examination of this issue seems to suggest that, in many cases, those with less but adequate preparation may not only perform specific tasks most economically but also with greater care and efficiency. Examples have been cited of specific functions that would lend them-

Table 6-1 Selected Examples of Perceived Professional Tasks

A. Medical Technology

Performed by

Pathologist	Medical Technologist	Medical Technician	Tasks
Yes	Yes	Yes	Isolate and identify routine pathogenic micro-organisms
Yes	Yes	Sometimes	Determine patient and donor blood types and subgroupings
Yes	Yes	Sometimes	Establish compatibility of a donor's blood to a recipient's
Yes	Yes	No	Adapt and establish a new test or instrument for the laboratory
Yes	Yes	Yes	Histologic preparation of tissue for microscopic examination

B. Physical Therapy

Performed by

Physician	Physical Therapist	Physical Therapy Assistant	
Yes	Yes	No	Perform evaluations of pain
Yes	Yes	No	Prescribe treatment regime (i.e., exercise, heat, cold, ultrasound, massage)
No	Yes	No	Teach use of crutches and equipment
No	Yes	No	Evaluate results
No	No	Yes	Observe patients during treatment to gather information and report findings to physical therapist

C. Respiratory Therapy

Performed by

Physician	Respiratory Therapist	Respiratory Therapy Technician	
No	Yes	Yes	Administration of aerosolized drugs
No	Yes	Yes	Incentive spirometry
Yes	Yes	Yes	Drawing arterial blood
Yes	Yes	No	Patient transport with life support
Yes	Yes	No	Cardiopulmonary resuscitation

selves to this kind of investigation. Since personnel costs are the major factor in health care cost escalation, this theory, if valid, might in turn suggest many ways in which costs could be controlled or even reduced without diminishing quality.

SUMMARY

Cost escalation and the maintenance of quality in health care do not necessarily move in conjunction with each other. The issue facing contemporary society is the need to find answers to controlling the first, without deleterious effects upon the other. The answer to this dilemma has not yet been clearly identified. There seems to be a propensity for society to seek sweeping, global solutions in this area of concern; solutions that may very well never be identified. Research designed to identify parts of the problem and potential solutions is urgently needed. Although it is very likely that sweeping legislative programs directed at cost control will continue to be adopted by legislators, history may prove that no action of this type will produce the qualitative and quantitative results that the proponents of such action promise.

NOTES

1. U.S. Congress, House of Representatives, *Social Security Amendments of 1972*, Public Laws 92-603, 92nd Congress, 2nd session, Section 1151, 1972.

2. U.S. Department of Health, Education, and Welfare, Public Health Service, *PSRO: An Evaluation of Professional Standards Review Organizations*, Vol. 1 (Washington, D.C.: Health Services Administration, Office of Planning, Evaluation and Legislation, 1977).

3. D.S. Abernathy and D.A. Pearson, *Regulating Hospital Costs: The Development of Public Policy* (Washington, D.C.: Aupha Press, 1979).

4. J.D. Blum et al., *PSRO's and The Law* (Rockville, Md.: Aspen Systems Corporation, 1977).

5. P. Bonner, "On-Site Utilization Review: An Evaluation of the Impact on Utilization Patterns and Expenditures" (Sc.D. diss., Harvard School of Public Health, 1976).

6. R. Brook and K. Williams, *An Evaluation of New Mexico Peer Review* (Santa Monica, Calif.: The Rand Corporation, 1976).

7. M. Westphal et al., "Changes in Average Length of Stay and Average Changes Generated Following Institution of PSRO Reviews," *Health Services Research* 14 (1979):253–255.

8. A. Fulchiero et al., "Can the PSRO's be Cost Effective?" *New England Journal of Medicine* 299 (1978):574–580.

9. R.H. Brook and A. Davies-Avery, *A Mechanism for Assuring Quality of U.S. Medical Care Services: Past, Present and Future*, R-1939-HEW (Santa Monica, Calif.: The Rand Corporation, 1977).

10. A. Donabedian, "Evaluating the Quality of Medical Care," *Milbank Memorial Fund Quarterly* 44, part 2 (1966):166.

11. R.H. Brook et al., "Assessing the Quality of Medical Care Using Outcome Measures: An Overview of the Method," *Medical Care* 15, no. 9, suppl. (1977):1–165.

12. The Stanford Center for Health Care Research, "Comparison of Hospitals with Regard to Outcome of Surgery," *Health Services Research* 11 (1976):113–127.

13. J.A.H. Lee et al., "Fatality from Three Common Surgical Conditions in Teaching and Non-teaching Hospitals," *Lancet* 2 (1957):785–793.

14. L. Lipworth et al., "Case-Fatality in Teaching and Non-teaching Hospitals. 1956–1959," *Medical Care* 1 (1963):71–76.

15. J.B. Graham and F.P. Palovick, "Where Should Cancer of the Cervix Be Treated?" *American Journal of Obstetrics and Gynecology* 87 (1963):405–408.

16. P.A. Lembcke, "Measuring the Quality of Medical Care through Vital Statistics Based on Hospital Service Areas," *American Journal of Public Health* 42 (1952):276–286.

17. J.C. Doyle, "Unnecessary Hysterectomies: Study of 6,248 Operations in Thirty-five Hospitals during 1948," *Journal of the American Medical Association* 151 (1953):360–368.

18. R.E. Trussell et al., *The Quantity, Quality, and Cost of Medical and Hospital Care Secured by a Sample of Teamster Families in the New York Area* (New York: Columbia University School of Public Health and Administrative Medicine, 1962).

19. J.P. Logerfo et al., "The Seattle Prepaid Health Care Project," in *Quality of Care* (Seattle, Wash.: University of Washington, 1976).

20. S. Shapiro et al., "Patterns of Medical Use by the Indigent Aged under Two Systems of Medical Care," *American Journal of Public Health* 57 (1967):784–790.

21. D.M. Kessner and C.E. Kolk, *Contrasts on Health Status, A Strategy for Evaluating Health Services.* Vol. 2 (Washington, D.C.: Institute of Medicine, National Academy of Sciences, 1973).

22. T.S. Inui et al., "Improved Outcomes in Hypertension after Physician Tutorials: A Controlled Trial," *Annals of Internal Medicine* 84 (1976):646–651.

23. G.H. Escovitz, "The Continuing Education of Physicians: Its Relationship to Quality of Care Evaluation," *Medical Clinics of North America* 57 (1973):1135–1147.

24. F.A. Appel and R.H. Brook, "Quality Assessment: Choosing a Method for Peer Review," *New England Journal of Medicine* 288 (1973):1323–1329.

25. T. Roth and R.B. Russell, Senate Subcommittee on Health, Hearings on Implementation of PSRO Legislation, 1974 (P.L. 92-603) 92nd Congress.

26. J.D. Blum et al., *PSRO s and the Law* (Rockville, Md.: Aspen Systems Corporation, 1977), p. 73.

27. Health Care Financing Administration, Office of Research Demonstration and Statistics, *Professional Standards Review Organization 1979 Program Evaluation* (Baltimore, Md., 1980), p. 73.

28. Health Care Financing Administration, Bureau of Data Management and Strategy, *Health Care Financing Trends*, vol. 2, no. 5, Baltimore, Md., 1982.

29. American Medical Association, Center for Health Services Research and Development, *Profile for Medical Practice* (Monroe, Wisc., 1981), p. 12.

30. American Medical Association, Department of Allied Health and Accreditation, "Program Director's Estimates of Entry Salaries of Graduates," *Allied Health Education Newsletter* 13, no. 41 (1982):8.

31. U.S. Department of Health, Education and Welfare, Public Health Service, Health Resources Administration, *Report of the Physician Extended Workgroup* (Washington, D.C., 1977).

32. Health Care Financing Administration, *Federal Register* (Baltimore, Md., 1982), p. 43586.

33. The American Society for Medical Technology Education and Research Division, "The American Society for Medical Technology 1979 National Compensation Survey," *American Journal of Medical Technology* 46, no. 3 (1980):191–199.

Chapter 7

Insurance and Health Care Cost Containment

James R. Posner, Ph.D.

This chapter discusses how the insurance program of a health care institution can be a significant target for cost-containment efforts. More generally, it examines how insurance expenditures fit in with risk management and quality assurance.

GENERAL DISCUSSION

As a starting point, it is convenient to define cost containment, risk management, and quality assurance as they relate to insurance programs.

Cost containment goes beyond cost minimization, i.e., choosing the least costly alternative for the current year. Effective cost containment involves optimization of costs over the long run. This optimization requires minimizing the direct outlay of cash; reducing jeopardy to the institution's assets and goals; and reducing disruption of management, administrative, and trustee time. Different institutions will select different optimum points on these criteria. For example, "risk-averse" institutions may be willing to pay more money in the short term in order to reduce exposure on the other two criteria, whereas "risk-taking" institutions will accept a certain level of jeopardy to their assets in order to save money in the near term.

There is a further distinction between cost containment in the insurance program and in other areas. The long-run costs and the long-run impact on assets and management time cannot be estimated accurately at the moment when insurance decisions are made. Elsewhere in the institution, the maximum likely expense is known or can be estimated more accurately. For example, differences can be evaluated between the longer useful life or the decreased operating expenses when choosing between pieces of equipment or in the design of new construction. The cost of supplies is known at the time of purchase. By contrast, insurance programs frequently build in the possibility of further expenses or savings in subsequent years, when certain "loss-sensitive" programs are selected. In other words, the analysis of insurance programs differs from other expenditures with regard to cost containment because insurance includes future uncertainty as well as current variations in expenditure. This contrast will emerge throughout the chapter.

A second starting point for the discussion concerns how insurance fits in with the general goals and mission of the health care system. Many health care professionals would state their mission to be: ''Do not harm the patient.'' Based on this injunction, health care providers focus their attention in two directions: (1) to foster the superior care of patients; and (2) to avoid substandard care. This dual focus encompasses many of the key concerns of quality assurance. Another mission of health care organizations is to preserve their own viability— to protect against events that jeopardize their physical, economic, and human assets and to maintain goodwill and the continuity of operations. In other words, effective managers must recognize uncertainties that could have a significant adverse impact on their operations and act so as to minimize their probable effects. This is the essence of risk management.

Both quality assurance and risk management activities typically span a wide range of clinical, organizational, and administrative aspects of patient care services. As a generalization, the focus of quality assurance is to increase the probability of desired outcomes in patient care services. By contrast, risk management activities shift the emphasis more toward the financial and administrative aspects of health care. The focus of risk management is to decrease the probability of adverse outcomes. As illustrated in Figure 7-1, these contrasting statements are not intended to draw a sharp distinction between risk management and quality assurance, nor to make an invidious comparison that one is of broader scope or more central to the health care organization than the other.

Figure 7-1

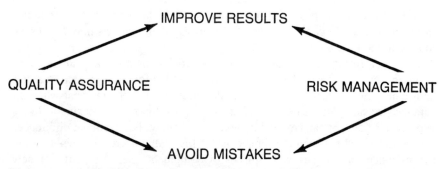

Risk management and quality assurance are both concerned with minimizing adverse outcomes and maximizing desired outcomes.

A third fundamental to this discussion of insurance and cost containment is the concept of risk. Many sources of uncertainty affect the health care organization, ranging from clinical uncertainties in diagnosis and treatment to other organizational concerns, such as finance, labor relations, regulation, and virtually all aspects of operations. This chapter focuses on "pure" risk, namely those uncertainties relating to fortuitous events that can have adverse impact on the organization.

Without giving a lengthy discussion of pure risk, a few points are in order. In contrast to gambling uncertainty, which also includes the probability of favorable outcomes, pure risk typically concerns only the probability of adverse events. Risk concerns fortuitous events, such as "sudden and accidental" occurrences that are "neither intended nor expected" but that result in bodily injury or property damage. Insurance may broaden this concept to include gradual effects, or events that result in "loss of use" or other kinds of harm, such as personal injury and "mental anguish" that extend the traditional definitions of bodily injury. Insurable risks also typically exclude intentional acts by the insured that result in adversity (e.g., arson, assault, fraud, felonies). Another limitation on the definition of risk from the insurance viewpoint is when the adverse events may be of such magnitude as to be uninsurable or are insurable only through special policies (e.g., nuclear accident, earthquake, war).

Key concepts in understanding the insurance mechanism for handling uncertainty are frequency and severity of risk, i.e., the distinction between how often an adverse event occurs, such as a patient falling from bed, and how severe it is, e.g., brain damage resulting from an anesthesia or respiratory problem. Not surprisingly, the health care manager gives less attention to the consequences of high-frequency/low-severity events such as a patient fall, than to the low-frequency/high-severity situation of a brain-damaged patient.

Textbooks identify four general strategies to deal with risk. The first is to avoid the risk altogether. (For example, many institutions do not perform cardiac surgery or transplant.) The second is to reduce the risk. (Plastic surgeons may require counseling and other precautions prior to surgery to reduce the risk of lawsuits. Proper hiring and training of new employees can reduce losses from back injuries.) The third is to retain the risk. (Take a $100 to $250 deductible on automobile physical damage or $25,000 deductible on malpractice.) The fourth is to transfer the risk. (Buy insurance or obtain a hold-harmless agreement from another party.) These strategies are presented in Exhibit 7-1. In general, strategies to avoid or reduce risks concern high-frequency events. Retaining or transferring risks is more appropriate for low-frequency events. The financial implication is straightforward. It makes economic sense to pay an insurance company to take risks where a loss might have a serious effect (high severity).

A last comment in this general discussion concerns the importance of management commitment. The risk management function competes with other pro

Exhibit 7-1 Methods To Treat Risks Are Related to Expected
Frequency and Severity

| | | Severity | |
		Low	High
Frequency	High	Risk reduction	Risk avoidance
	Low	Risk retention	Risk transfer

grams for management attention and a place on the priority list. An example is the widely recognized effectiveness of workplace safety programs in the DuPont Corporation. DuPont's success in this area is not a casual result. It reflects the historical origins of DuPont, a company heavily involved in the manufacture of gun powder and explosives. Any lapse in workplace safety would have had immediate and catastrophic consequences.

By contrast, in many health care institutions, the physicians, other staff, management, and even the trustees have not yet been persuaded that a similar degree of cause and effect exists between the risk management program and the chances of a malpractice disaster or other catastrophe loss.

In summary, it is clear that cost containment must recognize the nature of risk and uncertainty as well as the direct outlay of cash for insurance premiums.

METHODS OF FINANCING

Cost-containment efforts usually begin with an examination of how and when funds are expended. Following this approach, this section covers a number of general methods of financing an insurance program applicable to most health care institutions.

Assumption of Risk

The most direct savings in an insurance program are through assumption of risk: deductibles, self-insurance, and the decision not to insure. These strategies reduce the immediate cash outlay for insurance. They also introduce a whole set of long-run "what-if" questions. Assumption of risk must be analyzed for both short-term cost savings and long-term uncertainty in order to be an appropriate method of cost containment.

Deductibles

Most institutions are familiar with deductibles, whether in their coverage for automobile physical damage, for small property losses, for part of the defense costs in a directors' and officers' liability policy, or perhaps a sizable deductible for malpractice liability. Where an institution accepts a deductible, there is a reduction in premium, but a corresponding need to estimate how many losses are likely to occur within the deductible. The attraction of further savings for high deductibles must be weighed against a monetary estimate of additional losses that will occur and that will be the responsibility of the institution. The general rule is to assume affordable risks (i.e., low severity). A large loss should not be risked for a small saving in premiums.

Quota Share/Coinsurance

Another form of assumption of risk is cost sharing through quota share/ coinsurance arrangements. As in the example of major medical plans, there can be a proportional payment for losses by both the insured institution and the insurance company. There are examples in property insurance and liability insurance where an institution might pay 5 percent, 25 percent, or 50 percent of the loss in order to receive a reduction in premium. With quota share coinsurance, the insured reduces the premium nearly in proportion to the percentage of risks assumed.

With the use of deductibles and coinsurance, the health care institution must take into account the total value of losses expected in the deductible region. One method to make the use of deductibles more attractive is to negotiate a "stop-loss" on the aggregate of all losses in the deductible area. This annual aggregate deductible then permits a financial manager to compute the maximum possible loss, which can be budgeted.

A further refinement is the possibility of aggregate deductibles that extend across different perils or lines of insurance. Where a single carrier writes multiple coverages, this approach can offer further limitation on the exposure to loss within the deductible while still achieving premium credits.

Self-insurance

Self-insurance differs from no insurance because the institution establishes a formal program of services and a financing method for the risks it assumes. The two most frequent examples are hospital malpractice and Workers' Compensation. The hospital ordinarily sets aside funds with an independent fiduciary institution and establishes an explicit program of loss control, claims management, etc. Hospital self-insurance has gained enormous popularity since 1977 when Medicare altered its reimbursement regulations to facilitate this option.

Undoubtedly, most institutions will benefit from their decision to self-insure, some through skillful risk management and others by random good luck. As of the early 1980s, however, the success of self-insurance is still largely unproven because claims experience has not yet matured, especially in the area of malpractice. The real tests will be in the areas of underfunding, catastrophe losses, and litigation. For a small fraction of hospitals, there will be catastrophe losses that will strain their self-insurance programs. If funds are inadequate, then the response of excess insurers, third party payers, and the adequacy of other hospital assets will be critical. At least a few distress situations can be expected over the coming years, even as the picture remains bright for most other institutions.

Another problem area will arise from disputes over the scope of the self-insurance program in terms of questionable claims. Compared with a formal insurance policy, many self-insurance programs are less precise on the exact coverages afforded by their program. A difficult situation could arise, involving both an individual and the institution, when a physician or other individual (or his or her insurer) asserts that coverage was the responsibility of the institution rather than the individual. Some hospitals will find themselves absorbing vicarious liability they did not anticipate.

Like many other programs, self-insurance can create enormous problems for the unwary, the unlucky, or the overly optimistic institution. When the program is carefully defined and monitored, however, self-insurance can be a source of effective long-run savings and cost containment.

Cash-Flow Considerations

In the late 1970s and early 1980s, attention focused on cash-flow savings because of the high prevailing interest rates. There can be significant differences in total long-run cost depending upon the cash flow of a specific program. Premiums may be paid in a single payment up front, spread out during the policy period, or sometimes even deferred until after the policy period has ended. Initial deposit premiums may be raised or lowered, and many forms of security may be used (e.g., letter of credit, promissory note, and so on) as part of the total stream of payments.

The attractiveness of any cash-flow plan will depend upon the alternative uses made of the cash by the institution or by its insurance company. As discussed below, it is also important to keep the reimbursement implications in mind before choosing one or another cash-flow design.

Retrospective Designs

Retrospective designs are most commonly used in Workers' Compensation insurance. Most hospitals above 200 to 300 beds have the number of employees and size of payroll to consider this form of cash-flow program. Retrospective plans offer a wide variety of features, such as the size of initial payment, the time periods when payments are made, the manner of adjustments for credits/debits, and the maximum/minimum payments. Typically, an institution choosing a "retro" assumes that its experience will be better than the underwriting averages and thus will result in lower costs.

Although tax considerations may not be an important consideration for most voluntary or governmental hospitals, reimbursement is usually a critical factor. Retrospective designs may permit a hospital to report a wide range of expenses for reimbursement purposes. In most retrospective plans, there is some security requirement to guarantee the maximum payment under the plan. Even where the cash deposit is depressed, there will be a sizable liability from an accounting viewpoint, which can affect reimbursement.

On the negative side, retrospective plans require more complex recordkeeping over a relatively long time. While the length of time gives flexibility and advantages in the use of funds, it also creates more uncertainty over the total expenditure. Subsequent adjustments, dividends, and return premiums can reduce reimbursable expenses in future years. There is the possibility of additional payments required for prior events occurring three to four years earlier. Thus, some financial managers may resist the use of retros. Nevertheless, with careful analysis, there can be significant savings.

Investment Income

The control of investment income from insurance premiums has become a critical concern, as long as interest rates remain at high levels. In recent years, insurance companies began to give concessions in order to attract business via cash-flow underwriting. Throughout the insurance industry, the combined ratio of losses and expenses in relation to premiums is at an unprecedented high level. In the early 1980s, this ratio was frequently over 100 percent compared with historical averages closer to 70 to 90 percent. Many analysts believe that insurance companies can still be profitable when recording losses and expenses as high as 110 to 115 percent of their total premiums. Turning these calculations around, the high interest rates have resulted in unusually low premiums, i.e., the soft market occurring during the late 1970s and early 1980s. Where institutions have taken advantage of cash-flow underwriting, the savings help their cost-containment efforts.

Captives and Off-shore Placements

A captive is a limited purpose insurance company controlled by a single parent organization, a group or association engaged in a similar business. In the mid-1970s, captive insurance companies attracted widespread interest among health care institutions, to deal with the problem of scarce coverage and high insurance costs. (With off-shore domiciles in Bermuda and the Cayman Islands, the appeal of some captives was heightened beyond their purely financial advantages.) For many organizations, there were considerable advantages arising from the deductibility of premiums, shelter of investment income, control over the claims reserves and payments, and more direct access to the reinsurance markets. By the early 1980s, all of these advantages could usually be achieved through other methods that did not require the effort and financial commitment of setting up a captive. Therefore, the activity in captives has leveled off to a considerable extent, given the changes in market conditions.

For cost-containment efforts over the coming years, the appeal of captives will probably be quite selective. Most likely, it will primarily benefit multi-institutional organizations that want the long-run advantages of building a significant centralized fund for their insurable risks.

Pools

A pool is a group of organizations permitted by law to share a significant portion of their exposure for one or more areas of risk, without the need to establish a formal insurance company. In over 20 states, Workers' Compensation and/or liability pools can be formed. Most pools are designed to attract members of varying size but favor the small and medium-sized entities. There are often incentives to restrict access for those with poor claims experience and to attract those with good experience. The general attraction of pools is "economies of scale" whereby the smaller entities gain negotiating strength, breadth of coverage, improved services, and price reductions that were previously unavailable. Pools will be one of the most popular insurance mechanisms during the 1980s. The experience of Workers' Compensation safety groups and other pools indicates that they can offer positive results and tangible cost savings.

On the negative side, the lesser degree of regulation of pools can easily lead to abuses or inefficiency. There can be restrictions and penalties over how an entity leaves the pool or long delays before anticipated dividends are distributed.

PERIODIC REVIEW AND BIDS

Going beyond specific financing methods, it is appropriate to consider the more general topic of how to review an insurance program. The development of an insurance program is laborious. Proper design affects the total assets of the institution. A competent professional relationship is as important here as it is for other areas requiring critical judgment, such as law, accounting, and architecture.

A periodic review of the insurance program includes the systematic evaluation of the extent of coverage, the adequacy of services, and the appropriateness of costs. Going to the insurance market every three to five years will signal to all involved—insurance companies, brokers, those in administration, and trustees—that the institution is serious about its intention to receive the best value. (On the other hand, more frequent bidding will discourage the establishment of stable relationships, lessen the thoroughness of any review, and may not achieve any significant cost savings.) Here are a few thoughts about how a periodic review of the insurance/risk management program can contribute to cost-containment efforts.

An insurance review should address an institution's specific circumstances as follows:

- Specifications are important. Are the needs of the institution understood? Is the extent of coverage and services required explicitly described?
- Exposures must be determined. Has the institution identified and evaluated the areas where it is vulnerable to losses?
- Loss experience must be considered. Is there adequate information concerning the losses occurring in past years?

In addition to these basic topics, the decision to begin an evaluation and solicit bids for the insurance program should address further specific topics such as:

- Are the bidders qualified? Who will be included in the process and what criteria are particularly important in the choice of insurance advice?
- What markets should be selected? Must insurers meet criteria for size or financial strength? Must companies be admitted in the state(s) or can non-admitted and foreign companies be used?
- Policy language should be considered. Are there special requirements for the wording of insurance contracts to be acceptable?
- Adequate time is an important consideration. How much time is necessary to compile the critical information and develop the required proposals?
- Technical proposals must be reviewed. How will the selection be made among different proposals or various alternatives?
- Price and other financial terms should be considered. Are there requirements of the institution on method of payment? Are there deferred costs/benefits that will affect a choice of program?

The development of specifications and a thorough review of an insurance program are strenuous activities. At the very best, it requires close collaboration between the institution and some technical advisers, whether these latter are insurance brokers, attorneys, consultants, or board members with professional experience in this area. The thoroughness of the review will depend upon the adequacy of data and documentation available. It is important, therefore, to match the needs of the institution with the particular background of those doing the evaluation so as to assure the highest degree of professionalism.

Even when insurance is purchased from a direct writer, the institution may still seek advice from qualified risk management consultants. Consultants and brokers vary in the depth of their experience, size of their technical staffs, access to insurance markets, knowledge of current trends in the insurance market, negotiating strength, rapport with and understanding of the institution, and so on.

When brokers are involved, the selection should be limited so as to assure the level of professionalism and to avoid a free-for-all. A few ways to proceed in this direction are:

- Open bids, with no preselection of brokers, can be used. Any qualifying firm can respond to the formal specifications and obtain a quote from any acceptable insurance carrier. This approach minimizes the degree of professionalism and may discourage serious bidders who see little prospect of a long-term relationship.
- Broker qualification and competitive bids can be used. There is an initial selection of a small number of brokers (usually two to four). Each broker designates preferred insurance markets. This approach permits a measure of competition but may constrain the scope of alternatives to be considered if the institution requires all bids to be uniform.
- Broker selection is another strategy. There is competition among brokers to represent the institution. After designation of a single "broker of record," this firm negotiates with the entire insurance marketplace and develops a range of alternative proposals with recommendations for management considerations. This method encourages a systematic review while emphasizing the professionalism of the process.

Whatever process is used, emphasis should be on the development of long-term stable relationships around which the insurance program can evolve and improve. Emphasis on cost containment must consider the degree of professionalism and the extent of services under review, as discussed further in the next section.

ARRAY OF SERVICES

An effective risk management program must incorporate a wide array of services. Traditionally, whatever services were required were provided by an insurance company, including engineering inspections, education and safety programs, claims management, and legal defense. All were "bundled" within the total cost of an insurance policy premium. Some insurance companies emphasized their expertise and depth of service as a selling feature, as in the examples of boiler insurance, certain property insurers, and a few of the large multiline companies.

More recently, however, health care managers have questioned whether there may be advantages to "unbundle" risk management services. They now face the decision whether "to buy" professional advice from outside vendors or "to build" their own expertise in-house.

Along these lines, the Joint Commission on Accreditation of Hospitals (JCAH) standards and Medicare regulations have tended away from spelling out exactly what must be performed and have left the responsibility for defining the appropriate array of services to the institution itself.

A few areas of service are listed here to illustrate the potential for unbundling and the decision whether or not to seek out outside help. It is evident in these examples that unbundling can lead to pressures either toward spending more on desirable enhancements or toward cutting back on optional services. No generalizations are made about the net effect on cost containment.

Specific Areas of Service

Education

A wide variety of educational programs are available to institutions from outside sources, which reduces the need to "reinvent the wheel" in-house. On the other hand, the ongoing need to repeat educational programs for new staff and continuing education may offer cost savings from developing an in-house program. Whether purchased outside or developed in-house, a hospital can establish its own agenda for awareness and training programs that extend beyond those typically offered by insurance companies.

From an insurance viewpoint, education is an essential duty of an institution to provide adequate information, training, and supervision for the acts of its employees. Shortcuts may be assumed to increase the likelihood of losses caused through employee negligence or inattention.

Surveys and Inspections

In addition to accreditation surveys and regulatory reviews, expert and objective site evaluators are available to help reduce the exposures to loss. Some insurance companies even offer their staffs on a consulting basis. Such individuals are familiar with the state of the art elsewhere and can help identify personnel who may be equally thorough and who may have a better sense of what improvements are feasible. Whether there is more credibility for management to accept recommendations of an outside consultant or in-house personnel depends on the particular institution.

From an insurance viewpoint, key issues include the review of physical plant and equipment, as well as the evaluation of ongoing operations. More broadly, the institution should carry out a systematic analysis and evaluation of all significant exposures to accidental loss and liability. In most cases, the resulting recommendations will involve increased expenditures rather than cost savings. Presumably, there are long-term benefits through enhanced quality or reduced risks. Not surprisingly, the prospect of additional costs in this area may often meet resistance from some parts of management.

Organizational Bylaws, Standards, and Procedures

There is probably no more cumbersome job than to squeeze an ongoing organization into written form. The task is important, however, because such documents shape how an organization will function, and they govern its actions. To accomplish this job, outside help is often essential, especially because the scope of legal liability is constantly expanding. Poor drafting or inadequate scope can lead to problems later.

From an insurance viewpoint, the key issues are medical staff relationships, credentials and privileges, and the linkage to legal liability issues. Failure to address these issues could be very expensive.

Information Systems

Health care institutions rely on explicit written information. Adequate information is a key element in the resolution of risk management problems and the success of quality assurance programs. For example, an institution may not know of an adverse event and fail to take proper action, or there may exist a gap in the documentation of appropriate actions that did occur. In either case, a lost lawsuit can be equally expensive. Institutions cannot afford to "play ostrich" and keep themselves in the dark about the existence of adverse events.

Some large hospital systems and outside vendors have developed useful computerized information systems for risk management and quality assurance. By contrast, the information systems of insurance companies were designed for their needs and often will not offer the scope of an unbundled system. On the other hand, overly elaborate information systems for risk management programs can go beyond the point of cost effectiveness. The struggle to improve an information system and to justify the additional costs is probably a measure of management involvement in the risk management/quality assurance function, as much as it is a result of calculating costs vs. benefits.

Claims Management

The investigation, evaluation, negotiation, and settlement of claims have been unbundled already to whatever extent the financial risk has shifted from the insurer to the institution. Whoever pays the bills will manage the claims. On the other hand, a self-insured institution may have too few active claims each year to justify a high level of staff involvement or expertise in this critical area. In malpractice claims, for example, two to five new files per year might be expected for every 100 beds, and perhaps half of these may never become active claims. For active claims, specialized outside help is usually in order at some point in the process, whether during the investigation of the case, development of the defense, or negotiation of a cash settlement. Few people begrudge the level of expenditure for claims management services because it is easy to imagine how the results could deteriorate if insufficient efforts are made.

Legal

Virtually all health care institutions will seek outside legal advice and assistance for serious liability situations. Even when lawyers work within the institution, outside counsel will ordinarily be retained. One cost-containment trade-off may be in terms of legal posture—whether to defend every case rigorously or to seek a more compromising attitude when the source of litigation may stem from patient anger more than injuries due to negligence. In such a case, an effective ombudsman may serve to resolve the problem as well as to reduce the potential legal expenses required for an active defense.

One way to analyze unbundled services is to distinguish which services are targeted primarily prior and which are after an adverse event. Activities prior to an adverse event include engineering and safety surveys; education and awareness programs; the review of bylaws, contracts, standards, and procedures; and other efforts directed at loss prevention and hazard control. Activities after an adverse event include contingency plans for disasters and emergencies; incident reporting, investigation, and documentation; defense and settlement of claims; and other events comprising effective claims management.

Quality assurance and risk management programs differ in their relative degree of focus before and after the adverse event. In some institutions, the perception is that extensive loss prevention activities are the most cost-effective methods for the long run. Other institutions lean more toward rigorous claims management as their preferred strategy to place a lid on the outlay of cash. The viewpoint here is that an appropriate balance of activities both before and after events is essential to any strategy for building a cost-effective array of services.

WHO SHOULD BE THE RISK MANAGER?

Financing methods and services do not exist in a vacuum but must fit with the individuals involved in a risk management or quality assurance program. The job descriptions of hospital risk manager/quality assurance coordinator vary to fit the priorities of different institutions. By extension, the type of individual(s) who work on the risk management/quality assurance function will affect the extent of cost-containment efforts.

In some institutions, risk management and quality assurance persons report to an assistant administrator or the function may be an additional "hat" for the director of nursing, medical records, engineering, or security. In many cases, the director of finance is the senior administrative person supervising the risk management and/or quality assurance function. In a small number of hospitals, risk management is a responsibility of the medical staff, and the risk manager may be a physician or may report to a physician.

Given this variability in professional background and lines of reporting, it is useful to summarize different functional areas typically involved in the job description:

- The administrative function is to identify significant exposures to accidental losses and other adverse events; visit all parts of the organization to become familiar with new and changing exposures; and communicate with managers and employees about loss exposures, loss prevention, and the financial effects of losses.
- The financial function involves participation in the selection of appropriate financing methods to pay for accidental losses through insurance, self-insurance, or other programs and preparation of periodic budgets and financial reports of risk management activities. Records of accidents and losses and insurance reserves and recoveries must be compiled.
- The clinical function involves incorporating quality assurance and risk management programs into patient care services and coordinating efforts with the medical staff, other professionals and ancillary services.
- The legal function involves reviewing leases, contracts, and other sources of liability both inside and outside the organization and coordinating efforts with outside counsel regarding the level of duties imposed by law, regulation, and court decisions.
- The records and information management function is to maintain appropriate records on property and equipment; coordinate efforts with a patient record system; analyze historical loss frequency and severity; and prepare forecasts of future trends.
- The planning function involves planning and coordinating loss prevention and risk control activities and assisting in plans for emergencies and other contingency events.
- The general management function involves supervision of safety, security, and other areas of training and participation in appropriate staff meetings.

This list suggests the wide variety of tasks that may comprise the job description of risk manager/quality assurance coordinator.

Another approach to job description focuses in a more general fashion on the personality traits, psychological orientation, and habits found in an effective risk manager. From this viewpoint, important factors include the individual's degree of achievement needs (moderately high); degree of risk taking/risk aversion (someone who is more comfortable with intermediate probabilities that can be modified, rather than long-shots or certainties); and length of "time horizon" to carry out tasks (6 to 12 months rather than on a daily or weekly basis).

A third approach focuses more on level of authority and influence within the organization than on explicit job tasks or personality traits. Some consultants recommend a role for the risk manager with a wide scope of authority, reporting to the executive director, the board, or head of the medical staff. The implication is that the higher the position in the organization, the more likely the risk manager is to have successful results and to elicit change.

A contrary view is expressed by Stanley Skillicorn, a physician and risk manager in a California hospital.[1] Skillicorn prefers the reverse role with an apparently low level of authority in the organization. The risk manager should identify problems but is not responsible for solving them. In this scenario, the risk manager should refer problems and recommendations for action back to the appropriate department head or other line manager for solution.

A cost-containment perspective is an appropriate element in any of these job descriptions, regardless of the specific professional background or lines of reporting within the institution.

CONCLUSION

The purchase of insurance and related services involves sizable expenditures and opens up many possibilities to channel this cash flow to meet the goals of the institution.

Cost containment in the areas of insurance, risk management, and quality assurance requires a long-run perspective that takes account of institutional characteristics, the personalities of individuals involved, and the preferences for risk taking, as well as the calculation of how much cash is required in the short term.

Cost-containment efforts can be an important criterion in the choice of financing methods and selection of services that enable institutions to promote quality care and to avoid harm to patients and to themselves.

NOTE

1. S.A. Skillicorn, *Quality and Accountability: A New Era in American Hospitals* (San Francisco: Editorial Consultants, Inc., 1980).

Chapter 8

Quality and Competition

Donald W. Light, Ph.D.

The long-held assumption that professional control is necessary to ensure quality overlooks the role of competition. For a century, the medical profession largely escaped the competitive forces of the marketplace because the government, health administrators, and citizens entrusted it (and to a lesser degree other health professions) with monopolies and licensing arrangements in order to ensure high quality. The history of American medicine by Stevens,[1] which Starr has recently echoed and extended,[2] documents how the professional emphasis on "the best" has led to fee schedules, insurance policies, and a hospital-based delivery system that emphasizes the latest technological advances delivered primarily by physicians with an army of subordinates, all financed by insurance policies based on fees and costs.[3] This tale has been told so often and documented so well that it is surprising to read assertions like Paul Jellinek's that the medical sector could not be the source of escalating health costs in the past few decades.[4] The point here is that competition is throwing all these past institutional and professional arrangements into question, with far-reaching implications that only a few administrators and physicians realize.

While middle-level hospital administrators are concerned with implementing good quality assurance programs and running their units efficiently, senior administrators will need to take a functional, result-oriented view of how work is organized and carried out by physicians and other professional staff. Hospitals and medical centers will increasingly form alliances with large employers and/or unions to provide services at a reasonable cost. They must realize that this managerial, competitive approach to service differs profoundly from a professional one, with its emphasis on quality at all costs, state-of-art technology, and professional prerogatives rooted in social and cultural values.

The philosophy of competition rewards the hospital or provider that can do a competent job at the lowest price. This implies that standards of excellence are set *before* bids are taken, rather than striving for the best possible care at any price. As Blomqvist points out in his excellent little book, the best possible care can never be a standard of care for any health care system.[5] Developing criteria for quality before the competition begins also means that a given professional degree or license is less likely to be used than measures of process or outcome. The philosophy of competition also highlights the well-known conflict of interest of physicians benefiting in financial or other ways from their own recommendations about treatment.[3] In sum, the classic emphasis of American capitalism on competition is forcing us to reexamine the roles of professions in health care. It thus puts hospital administrators, insurers, corporations, and unions in growing conflict with the medical profession.

PUBLIC POLICY AND PROFESSIONAL QUALITY

A recent policy report from the National Center for Health Services Research systematically dismisses a number of arguments for exempting health services from a competitive approach; points out the ways in which more competition and consumer choice will solve major problems in health care services; and charges organized medicine with obstructing the health care market.[6] It concludes, in italics: *"Boycotting insurers, refusing to deal with competing organizations, and prohibiting providers who engage in certain competitive action from practicing in the profession are all among the anticompetitive practices with which provider groups have been charged."*[6a] It then turns to licensing, again in italics, *"Medical practice acts prohibit nonphysician professionals from practicing without the direction of a physician, even when appropriate and cost-effective. These acts prohibit a physician from providing services under the management of a nonphysician, creating barriers to the development of non-physician-owned HMOs."*[6b] Once heard from the socialist left, such statements are now coming from a conservative Republican administration.

Government programs are establishing the conditions for hospitals and other health care organizations to alter how work gets done. Fixed price contracts (whether like those for Medicaid services in Arizona, California, Illinois, New Jersey, and New York or whether in the form of a federal Diagnostic Related Group (DRG) system for Medicare) will reward those institutions and providers who offer services at an agreed-upon level of quality for the least cost. Initially, this new approach to health care financing has led to belt tightening, streamlining administration, and other activities within the traditional organization of services established over the two decades. Already, however, a second phase can be discerned in which the traditional, profession-oriented way of doing things will be challenged by the question: Can someone else with less training and a lower salary do just as good a job?

A series of court decisions since 1975 add another powerful tool for leaders of corporations, unions, hospitals, and states that want to see if adequate medical care can be provided at lower cost. Cases like *Virginia Academy of Clinical Psychologists v. Blue Shield of Virginia* (1981) find that there is sufficient physician control of Blue Shield to suggest a monopoly and to regard its refusal to pay for services of nonphysicians as restraint of trade. This is part of a larger pattern of cases against physicians and other professions for anticompetitive actions.[7] Since the purpose of antitrust law is to foster competition, it represents a different paradigm than a professional one. Moreover, the courts have confined their judgment to whether given acts restrict competition and not to whether those acts lead to "better" or "more appropriate" care. Their focus is on whether there are restrictions on who can enter the market and who can compete for price.

Accreditation and licensing are also under fire. Both the courts and the Federal Trade Commission have addressed them with the result that traditional professional control is being reduced. In a 1980 case, the Supreme Court ruled that a state licensing system must either show that its restraints are explicit state policy actively supervised by the state itself, or it would be subject to federal antitrust challenge.[8] Given the increasing interest among states to find less costly ways to provide health services, states may soon begin to reexamine the monopolies that licenses provide as a way of opening the health market to less costly providers.

The same kind of arguments apply to specialty certification and the control of specialists over beds or other resources. Such control can be and will be challenged as patients and competitors organize themselves. A major change in the American health care system is that consumers are becoming organized through unions that are given a set budget for health care, corporations that negotiate collectively for health services, and states that contract services for the poor and elderly. Thus, antitrust laws insist that professionals' ability to pursue their own interests be offset by competition in the marketplace. Quality of care is not to be entrusted exclusively to the medical profession, or any other profession, but to the marketplace.

QUALITY CARE AT LOWER COST

The central question, then, is to what degree and in what instances can medical care of good quality be delivered at a more competitive price than under current arrangements? There are many different marketplaces for medical care in which quality can be maintained or even improved at lower cost. Most of them do not involve the individual physician or patient buying services but rather concern the market decisions of large institutions or collective buyers. Various studies, for example, show that specialized units such as cardiac surgery improve their quality and significantly lower their costs per procedure when they perform the procedure often.[3] Not only does the proliferation of specialists and their workshops raise costs and lower quality as they each carry out fewer procedures on the average, but overall their larger number also increases the total number of procedures for the area and thus further increases costs. In comparative research between different regions of the United States and between the United States and Great Britain, more physicians in an area increase the number of procedures, with little or no measurable benefit to health.[3,9] Many more studies need to be done by hospital groups and governmental departments to identify how many physicians and workshops in a given region yield the best care at both the lowest average and lowest total cost.

A number of other studies indicate that quality can be maintained for less money by delegating or even substituting less expensive providers for more expensive ones.[10] For example, in a comparative analysis of five advanced countries, Roemer and Roemer reported that, outside of Canada and the United States, trained midwives play a major role in maternity care with no higher infant mortality or maternal mortality rates than here.[11] Obstetricians give all sorts of reasons why midwives cannot do their jobs well, but evidence abroad indicates they are doing well and that technical issues are not the problem. The difference is largely cultural and historical; midwives were well established in Europe long ago, and medicine came of age working with them. Roemer and Roemer report that "relationships between the doctor and midwife are usually very good. . . ."[11a] While midwives in the United States have been struggling to establish their legal and fiscal rights, with strong opposition from organized medicine, they may soon find strong allies among administrators, unions, and others who see them as able to maintain quality care at lower cost. As Roemer and Roemer conclude, "there is probably no better example of a function, now performed usually by doctors, that could be effectively delegated to other personnel."[11b]

While nurses have specialized in the United States, their domain of decision-making power has lagged behind their skills. In Norway, for example, nurse anesthetists handle 90 percent of all surgical operations under the supervision of an anesthesiologist.[11] Using functional criteria for quality has cut through professional prerogatives.

Most studies of what has been called "physician malutilization"[12] and substitutability concern primary care rather than hospital care, though they may suggest what questions need to be examined in the latter. A survey by the American Academy of Pediatrics in 1967 found that a large percent of office-based pediatricians were carrying out tasks that clearly did not require a medical degree.[13] Subsequent surveys of office-based internists and family physicians produced similar findings.[14,15] These and other reports suggested that many tasks done by physicians could be delegated to less elaborately trained and less expensive people. While delegation is a familiar and comfortable practice in medicine that is carried out extensively in hospitals, the interesting question is, "At what point does delegation become substitution?" The key answer has been, "When supervision by a physician is no longer done." However, even under supervision, a subordinate who carries out delegated work is, in effect, substituting for the physician. When this supervision becomes looser and more general, or even slides into a consulting relationship where the nonphysician takes the initiative when he or she thinks it necessary to have a physician's opinion, then substitution is even more complete.

Extensive research has been done on comparing the quality of care given by physicians' assistants and nurse practitioners when they substitute for physicians.[12,16,17,18,19,20,21,22,23,24,25,26,27] There are two major findings. First, on a wide number of measures, physicians' assistants and nurse practitioners provide comparable care to internists and family physicians in primary care. Whether diagnostic errors, treatment plans, prescription errors, referrals to specialists, or success of treatment are examined, there are no significant differences. As one review, echoing its predecessors, recently concluded, "In all cases, care rendered by physicians' assistants and nurse practitioners and the patient satisfaction and possibly compliance, [is] superior to that provided by physicians . . . it is notable that in the 15 years of their existence no events have suggested increased actuarial risk for the new health professional services."[12a]

No less a figure than Rogers is sufficiently persuaded by these studies to conclude that physicians' assistants and nurse practitioners are equal to physicians in the day-to-day care of patients.[28] Rogers wrote, "Obviously they must know their limits, when to refer, when to seek physician aid—but the studies show that they know this well."[28a] The educational implications are radical. For Rogers, they imply that "we now *know* that we can teach all of what we today regard as 'the facts' that are needed to *look* like we behave like a doctor in six months to a year."[28b] Rogers would therefore like to see the required curriculum in medical schools greatly reduced so that medical students can grow professionally and intellectually through their own initiative. But this is a luxury a competitive market may not be willing to afford. If the basics can be taught in a year, why not reduce medical school (which is so expensive to taxpayers and parents) to two or at most three years? It would reduce debt and discrimination against disadvantaged applicants. Why not license physicians' assistants as primary care clinicians? These suggestions are immediately rejected as politically unrealistic, but they are not unrealistic if those who foot the bill for medical care get serious about cost containment. As Roemer and Roemer conclude, "In general, a health care system should have health workers with the *least* elaborate training necessary to prepare them to perform a function *properly*."[11c]

The second finding shared by the body of comparative research is that non-physicians, especially nurse clinicians, are rated higher on subjective and psychological measures such as patient satisfaction and compliance than are physicians. To draw on the anthropological distinction between illness and disease, nurse practitioners attend to illness as well as disease. Since illness is the patient's experience with discomfort, attending to it effectively is bound to improve compliance and increase satisfaction. Studies have also found that nurse practitioners do more follow-up work on their patients than do physicians.[21] The economic implications of this finding are important. It is usually concluded that nurse practitioners are significantly less productive than physicians, taking from half again to twice as long with patients. The term *productive,* however, dismisses the caring function of medicine and its benefits for increased compliance as well as for satisfaction. A more accurate conclusion from these studies would be that in half to three quarters as much time as nurse practitioners, physicians take care of only the physiological and pharmacological aspects of patients' problems with little attention to their emotional feelings and concerns. If compliance is a measure of successful service (and consumer satisfaction the watchword of any service industry), nurse practitioners may have the better competitive approach. Certainly within the medical profession, family physicians are banking on the same approach to win over patients from other specialists. So far, however, competition apparently has not been real enough for the lower time cost of physicians' assistants and nurse practitioners to be passed on to patients. If they were, patients could choose between the quick, medical approach of physicians, a similar but cheaper approach by physicians' assistants, or the more comprehensive approach of nurse practitioners.

QUALITY HEALTH VS. QUALITY MEDICINE

An important dimension of the studies on nurse practitioners in primary care concerns the measures of quality to be used in assessing the cost effectiveness of services. Despite major changes in contemporary health care, quality is usually still measured by medical criteria. Implicit in these criteria is a model of health care that emphasizes the pathogen and not the person; the critical medical encounter and not the social ecology of the patient's life; acute intervention after normal functioning has broken down rather than prevention; and technical or chemical intervention rather than interpersonal care.[9] This disembodied view of scientific medicine holds that: (1) the specific functions of organs can be identified; (2) everyone's body functions about the same unless disturbed by injury or illness; (3) disease and the experience of disease do not vary much from culture to culture; (4) boundaries between self and body and between self and others are obvious and shared; and (5) bodies should be seen objectively. Extensive research spanning several decades, in fact, demonstrates that: (1) organs have shared and interacting functions so that only with great deliberation can they be separated analytically; (2) "normal" bodies function in widely differing ways so that the boundaries of injury and illness are not clear; (3) patterns of disease and especially experiences with disease vary markedly by ethnic culture, religion, sex, age, and social status; (4) the individual's relations with his or her body and with others are subtle and affect illness experiences even up to rates of death; and (5) only by disregarding the above can the artifact be created that our bodies are objectively separate from ourselves.

Thus, quality health implies rather different criteria than quality medicine, and this is the import of the higher ratings that nurse clinicians receive for follow-up care, patient satisfaction, and compliance. For some time, nurses have been taught a holistic, health-oriented approach to patient care, and consequently nurse practitioners have a notably different way of thinking than most physicians. The medical model of care, though dramatically successful in developing powerful tools for intervention, has been much less effective than most people realize. Careful analysis of mortality figures in Great Britain and the United States indicates that clinical medicine has accounted for only 10 to 25 percent of the decline during the past century.[29,30] A major reason for this modest contribution is that the infectious diseases that caused most of the deaths in the nineteenth century were already declining before miracle drugs became available, and the rate of decline did not increase markedly after their use. Since then, morbidity and mortality statistics show that quality medicine has been accomplishing less and less at more and more expense. The reasons are easy to understand. The killers that are left—heart disease, cancer, stroke, etc.—prove to be the most difficult to treat by medical intervention. The major causes of death today involve pollution, life habits, and social stress. High-technology medicine has little to say about these; health care has a great deal to say. Thus, in measuring quality, health leads to a rather different set of priorities and values than medicine. A comparison between health care providers and medical care providers is given in Table 8-1.

From a health point of view, every hospital admission is a sign of failure. Quality health would dictate wellness rounds or comprehensive care conferences at which the question would be asked, "What actions (or inactions) led to Ms. R. being hospitalized, and what can be done to minimize her chances of coming in again?"

CREATING THE CONDITIONS FOR COMPETITION

Once quality is clarified, from the patient's point of view, then the question is how favorable conditions can be created to allow those not currently dominant a chance to compete. To draw again on the studies comparing physicians to

Table 8-1 Comparison of Health Care and Medical Care Providers

Ranking of health care providers	*Ranking of medical care providers*
1. Self- and mutual-help groups	Hospital-based specialists
2. Nurse clinicians	Office-based specialists
3. Prepaid clinics oriented to prevention	General practitioners
4. Comprehensive or polyclinics	Comprehensive clinics
5. General practitioners	Providers oriented to prevention
6. Office-based specialists	Nurse clinicians
7. Hospital-based specialists	Self- and mutual-help groups

others in primary care, the more opportunity and autonomy given to nurse practitioners and physicians' assistants, the more they can do. This situation is similar to Japanese management, which brings out the potential in workers by encouraging participation and responsibility to their limits. Especially in hospitals with their heavily institutionalized hierarchies and detailed definitions of everyone's roles, there is a great deal of untapped energy and talent. For example, Mechanic and Aiken make a solid case for extending the range of tasks and degree of responsibility that nurses can take that will make physicians' lives easier and will improve medical care.[31]

But what of the power and vested interests of organized medicine? With a growing physician surplus and a decline in real income, organized medicine is not likely to take the cooperative attitude that Mechanic and Aiken urge but rather to think of ways in which physicians can expand into the domain of nursing. Already this is evident in the strategy of some medical schools to emphasize wellness, interpersonal skills, counseling, and other staples of the nursing curriculum. Organized medicine has successfully opposed the licensing of physicians' assistants in some states and the extension of limited licenses in others. Such anticompetitive tactics, of course, are not new. Therefore, it must be asked whether any of the changes contemplated here will occur. They will if powerful new groups such as hospital corporations, hospital administrators, state legislators, high state officials, large corporations, and unions are increasingly active in controlling medical costs and form various alliances to counter the past professional monopoly of medicine. The era of professional medicine is changing to an era of competitive and corporate medicine.

THE SOCIAL FOUNDATIONS OF PROFESSIONAL POWER

In order to gain perspective on the current organization of medicine and its underlying dynamics, it is helpful to understand what sociologists have found about the professions and how they work. Essentially, professions are occupations that succeed in claiming that they have knowledge or skills that can uniquely help clients solve problems. These skills and knowledge become a form of property for which rent (fees or salary) is collected. Title to this property is granted through licenses and other contractual arrangements. While others may have some of the same knowledge and skills, they do not have the right to use them as professionals, or they do so in a much more peripheral, weaker manner.[32]

Because a profession's knowledge and skills lie at the heart of its identity and economic life, it places great emphasis on them. Theory, specialization, and research receive the highest status. Yet these priorities can lead the profession away from addressing the needs of society and its citizens, which was the basis for its rights in the first place. This has certainly happened in medicine. Indeed it could be argued, as Stevens has, that the organization and financing of American medicine has been warped throughout the twentieth century by these priorities so that more and more energy and money goes to procedures that benefit people with fewer, more exotic disorders.[1] For this reason, professions periodically go through a phase when they reassert their commitment to treating the vast majority of technically uninteresting but demographically common problems. Community mental health, primary care, family medicine, and community law are some examples of these professional swings back to the sociological foundations of everyday practice. Moreover, during a swing towards specialization and research, a profession runs the danger that others will move in on the abandoned territory of primary care.

Thus, while skills initially are closely tied to tasks, the internal values and momentum of a profession lead it toward a separation of skills from tasks. This dynamic subject underlies the import of competition for quality and profession. To the extent that the skills can be codified and refined, they can also be taught to assistants and other groups, who then become the physician's competitors. On the other hand, the more general a profession's skills, the less defensible they are as unique. This is the central problem of family medicine as a "specialty."

Professional training usually involves considerable psychic investment and a large commitment of time and money. Professionals therefore come to identify with their skills as a measure of their personal worth, and this is why they resist attack from the outside as intensely as they do. Thus, becoming a professional is not only economic and strategic but also symbolic and personal. Professionals form subcultures that elaborate and further entrench these patterns.

Professions are also the products of social class and serve to perpetuate them. The history of different professions suggests that they served in the nineteenth century as a form of status transfer from the old status based on estates to a new status based on possessing technical knowledge.[32,33] This neo-Marxist view of professions as products of social class explains why, for example, medical schools have such a long curriculum at such great expense. In the nineteenth century, medical school graduates, if anything, did more harm than indigenous herbal healers,[34] and today in general practice they are apparently indistinguishable from physicians' assistants who have a short, inexpensive education. The prerequisites for training, the demand for years of discretionary time during which no income is earned, and the financial charges are essentially social class barriers that reserve this training for the children of affluent families. Granted that scholarship programs exist, the neo-Marxists argue, but they are token programs made by elite institutions. Conversely, few affluent children sign up to be physicians' assistants or even nurse practitioners. There is a sense of class-appropriate callings. If the neo-Marxists are right, then it might be expected that different health professions embody class values, expectations, and ambitions that do not directly stem from their body of expertise or training program.

An interesting case of status transfer is the history of Florence Nightingale and the creation of modern nursing in England. She essentially professionalized the charitable work in British workhouses that Victorian ladies had performed out of *noblesse oblige* with limited success.[35] Trained nurses were predominantly women because "the male more than the female was believed to be liable to usurp the functions of the doctor."[35a] This preserved the sexual division of labor between the master-actor and the mistress-helper, especially in primary care where nurses performed as well as general practitioners:

> The doctors feared that the nurses might become serious rivals and undercut the fees they charged for professional services. Nurses might flourish their certificates in front of patients and try to make out that they 'knew more than the doctor,' while the patients might be tempted to use the nurse as a substitute for the doctor as 'you can get a nurse for very little . . . while the doctor's fee is high.' Mrs. Fenwick [a director of district nursing] dismissed all this as 'ignorance of social relations and etiquette.' The suggestion that nurses would, if registered, compete with the doctors was 'very mischievous.'[35b]

Even the social nature of Fenwick's dismissal proves the point. Moreover, within nursing, class relations were retained from society at large in the form of the matron overseeing the less skilled nursing staff:

> Cure functions were seen as primarily male and upper class, and care functions predominantly lower class and/or female but, initially at least, carried out under the moral leadership of upper-class women. The social position occupied by the matron in the hospital power structure . . . bore a close relation to . . . an upper-middle-class woman in the Victorian home, had she married.[36] p. 32

A similar history has been documented for medicine and other professions, showing that the upper classes transferred their traditional status to professional coinage.[32,33,37] During the second half of the nineteenth century, when the professions took their modern forms, it was the upper class faction that solidified their position by controlling professional education and licensure.

This brief discourse on the social foundations of professional power serves to emphasize the forces both without and within the profession that will resist freely competitive approaches to providing services of quality at the best price. Both the social and psychic investment in professional work must be understood to deal effectively with it. A movement towards a "free" and rational market based on technical competence requires a cultural shift from a class-based professional paradigm to a health care culture that values competition based on measurable quality. At its root, economics is a branch of anthropology.

NOTES

1. R. Stevens, *American Medicine and the Public Interest* (New Haven, Conn.: Yale University Press, 1971).

2. P. Starr, *The Social Transformation of American Medicine* (New York: Basic Books, 1982).

3. A.E. Enthoven, *Health Plan: The Only Practical Solution to the Soaring Costs of Medical Care* (New York: Addison-Wesley Publishing Co., Inc., 1980).

4. P.S. Jellinek, "Yet Another Look at Medical Cost Inflation," *New England Journal of Medicine* 307 (1982):496–497.

5. A. Blomqvist, *The Health Care Business: International Evidence on Private versus Public Health Care Systems* (London, Ont.: The Fraser Institute, 1979), p. 6.

6. K.M. Langwell, *Research on Competition in the Financing and Delivery of Health Services: A Summary of Policy Issues* (Washington, D.C.: National Center for Health Services Research, 1982).

6a. Ibid., p. 13.

6b. Ibid., p. 14.

7. T.D. Overcast, B.D. Sales, and M.R. Pollard, "Applying Antitrust Laws to the Professions," *American Psychologist* 37 (1982):517–525.

8. California Retail Liquor Dealers Association v. Medical Aluminum, Inc. 445 U.S. 97, 105 (1980).

9. L.S. Levin and E.L. Idler, *The Hidden Health Care System: Mediating Structures and Medicine* (Boston: Ballinger, 1981).

10. J.B. Christianson and W. McClure, "Competition in the Delivery of Medical Care," *New England Journal of Medicine* 301 (1979):812–818.

11. M.I. Roemer and R. Roemer, *Health Manpower Policies under Five National Health Care Systems* (Washington, D.C.: Health Resources Administration, 1978), p. 81.

11a. Ibid., p. 2.

11b. Ibid., p. 19.

11c. Ibid., p. 7.

12. A. Yankauer, "The New Health Professionals: Three Examples," *Annual Review of Public Health* 3 (1982):249–276.

12a. Ibid., p. 256.

13. A. Yankauer, J.F. Connelly, and J.J. Feldman, "Pediatric Practice in the United States," *Pediatricians* 43 (1970):521–554.

14. F.A. Riddick et al., "Use of Allied Health Professionals in Internists' Offices," *Archives of Internal Medicine* 127 (1971):924–931.

15. B.H. Kehrer and M.D. Intriligator, "Task Delegation in Physician Office Practice," *Inquiry* 11 (1974):292–299.

16. M.W. Edmunds, "Evaluation of Nurse Practitioner Effectiveness: An Overview of the Literature," *Evaluation and Health Profession* 1 (1978):69–82.

17. S. Greenfield et al., "Efficiency and Cost of Primary Care by Nurses and Physician Assistants," *New England Journal of Medicine* 298 (1978):305–309.

18. D.M. Lawrence, "The Impact of Physicians' Assistants and Nurse Practitioners on Health Care Access, Costs and Quality: A Review of the Literature," *Health Medical Care Service Review* 1 (1978):1–12.

19. C.E. Lewis et al., "Activities, Events and Outcomes in Ambulatory Patient Care," *New England Journal of Medicine* 208 (1969):645–649.

20. R.W. Lubic, "Evaluation of an Out-of-Hospital Maternity Center for Low Risk Patients," in *Health Policy and Nursing Practice*. L.H. Aiken, ed. (New York: McGraw-Hill Book Co., 1981).

21. J.A. Ramsey, J.K. McKenzie, and D.G. Fish, "Physicians and Nurse Practitioners: Do They Provide Equivalent Health Care?" *American Journal of Public Health* 72 (1982):35–57.

22. J.C. Record, *Staffing Primary Care in 1990: Physician Replacement and Cost Savings* (New York: Springer, 1981).

23. J.W. Runyan Jr., "The Memphis Chronic Disease Program: Comparisons in Outcome and the Nurse's Extended Role," *Journal of the American Medical Association* 231 (1975):264–270.

24. D.L. Sackett et al., "The Burlington Randomized Trial of the Nurse Practitioner: Health Outcomes of Patients," *American Journal of Internal Medicine* 80 (1974):137–142.

25. C. Slone et al., "Effectiveness of Certified Nurse Midwives," *American Journal of Obstetrics-Gynecology* 124 (1976):177–182.

26. H.C. Sox Jr., "Quality of Patient Care by Nurse Practitioners and Physicians' Assistants: A Ten Year Perspective," *Archives of Internal Medicine* 91 (1979):459–468.

27. R.W. Wood et al., "Reproducibility of Clinical Data and Decisions in the Management of Upper Respiratory Illness," *Medical Care* 17 (1979):767–779.

28. D.E. Rogers, "Some Musings on Medical Education: Is It Going Astray?" *The Pharos* 45 (Spring 1982):11–14.

28a. Ibid., p. 13.

28b. Ibid., p. 14.

29. T. McKeown, *The Role of Medicine: Dream, Mirage or Nemesis?* (Princeton, N.J.: Princeton University Press, 1979).

30. J.E. McKinlay and S.B. McKinlay, "The Questionable Contribution of Medical Measures to the Decline of Mortality in the United States in the Twentieth Century," *Milbank Memorial Fund Quarterly (Health and Society)* 53 (1977):405–428.

31. D. Mechanic and L.H. Aiken, "A Cooperative Agenda for Medicine and Nursing," *New England Journal of Medicine* 307 (1982):747–750.

32. M.S. Larson, *The Rise of Professionalism* (Berkeley, Calif.: University of California Press, 1977).

33. D.W. Light, "The Development of Professional Schools in America" in *The Transformation of Higher Learning: 1840–1930*. K. Jarausch, ed. (Stuttgart: Klett-Verlag, 1983), pp. 40–49.

34. W.G. Rothstein, *American Physicians in the 19th Century: From Sects to Science* (Baltimore: Johns Hopkins University Press, 1972).

35. B. Abel-Smith, *A History of the Nursing Profession in Great Britain* (New York: Springer, 1960).

35a. Ibid., p. 52.

35b. Ibid., p. 35.

36. M. Carpenter, "The New Managerialism and Professionalism in Nursing" in *Health and the Division of Labor*, ed. M. Stacey (London, Eng.: Croom-Helm, 1977), pp. 14–40.

37. B.J. Bledstein, *The Culture of Professionalism* (New York: W.W. Norton, 1976).

Part III

Methodology and Concepts

Chapter 9

Health Care Evaluation and Planning

Gregory Parston, Ph.D.

LINKING EVALUATION AND PLANNING

Health program evaluation is a management tool. It is not the day-to-day delivery of health services. Rather, it is a mechanism that health institutions use to find ways of delivering services more effectively. When it is carefully designed and properly conducted, program evaluation can enable managers to clarify objectives, to measure performance, to identify options, to redirect programs, and to document successes and failures.[1] The intended results are assured quality and enhanced performance.

Other chapters discuss the general concerns and the specific issues of quality assurance and performance evaluation in hospitals. This chapter is not an attempt to reformulate those discussions but rather to look at the potential contributions of program evaluation, specifically, from the perspective of another management tool, long-term planning. According to Donabedian, who has contributed insightfully to the development of quality measurement and assessment of health care, "The purpose of quality monitoring is to exercise constant surveillance so that departures from standards can be detected early and corrected."[2] The argument posed here is that by extending the focus of program evaluation managers might be able to detect departures from standards *before* they occur and thus prevent lapses from desired levels of quality.

Planning, with its concern for the future commitment of resources, can provide opportunities to extend the focus of program evaluation in order to consider the implications of possible future performance. An example of how that has been done in planning health services for the elderly is presented and is cited to call for stronger links between planning and performance evaluation in hospitals.

Management Theory and Practice: Science and Art

The evolution of management theory during the twentieth century has been an attempt to establish the existence of systematic and rational relationships between events in human organizations. Many of the emerging theories of management have sought their proofs from scientific method. Phenomena have been observed, hypotheses have been advanced and tested, and principles have been deduced. Management research has advanced a body of modern management theory in which knowledge has been formulated and systematized to provide better understanding of management practice, as well as to guide that practice.

Although there is considerable disagreement among theorists about what constitutes management practice, Koontz and O'Donnell review several models of management systems and identify "five essential managerial functions: planning, organizing, staffing, directing and leading, and controlling."[3] Whether managers actually do these things and whether what managers do can be clearly identified as these functions remain questionable. Still, even though practice often trails theory, in practice, too, the scientific method finds its parallels. Observations are undertaken and performance is controlled through monitoring and evaluation activities; hypotheses of sorts are formulated and tested in planning; and organizations, staffing, and leadership are means by which principles of practice are deduced and implemented.

Certainly, the epistemological strengths of the scientific method have fostered its application and misapplication in many fields outside of the physical and biological sciences in which it evolved, including management. As a means to help explain the theoretical dynamics of human organizations, the scientific method also has influenced the ways in which those human dynamics work. Many warnings have been sounded about the appropriateness of a faithful reliance on scientific method in the "soft" or "inexact" social sciences, as well as about the political values that such reliance represents. Although it is not necessary to go into all of these concerns here, one warning merits recognition.

Rittle and Webber argue that the problems of social or policy planners are different from the problems in natural sciences. "The problems that scientists and engineers have usually focused upon are mostly 'tame' or 'benign' ones. . . . For each the mission is clear. It is clear, in turn, whether or not the problems have been solved."[4] "Wicked problems," on the other hand, do not enjoy this precision and clarity. They have no definitive formulation; there is no immediate or ultimate test of their solutions; and their explanations largely determine their resolutions. Unlike those tame problems that are most easily handled by the scientific method, there is no opportunity to learn without penalty by trial and error because every attempt counts significantly.

Although this distinction specifically concerns the problems of the public planner, it applies equally well to the problems of social organizations generally. This is particularly so when those social organizations provide an essentially public service, such as health care. The problems of health care managers are wicked problems. Scientific methods may help understand those problems, but their solutions lie more in the exercise of judgment than in the mechanics of experimentation. Management is as much art as science. When management practice bases its judgments more on contrived pseudoscientific models than on the artful realities that those models often distort, management fails.

Management practice can inform judgment, and the tools of practice can help managers to better understand the complexities of the problems they face before exercising judgment. Evaluation and planning are two of these tools. The first observes and assesses; the second hypothesizes and tests. By blending the usefulness of each, health service managers may be able to deal more systematically and make judgments more rationally within their institutional realities.

The Rift between Evaluation and Planning

What do program evaluation and planning have to do with each other? In theory, there is a significant connection, but in hospital management practice, there is much less of a link.

Management theory encourages the development of processes in which evaluation findings help set the agenda for planning and in which planning's achievements are monitored through evaluation. Evaluation and planning are ideally intertwined. Indeed, depending upon their professional interests, evaluation and planning theorists subsume each other's activity within their own sphere. Evaluation theorists Shortell and Richardson, for example, see the health program evaluation process as comprising a cycle with three basic phases: (1) assessment of program impact; (2) program planning; and (3) program implementation.[5] At the same time, Flexner and Berkowitz, advocates of the emerging and still indeterminate hospital strategic planning process, are certain enough of its jurisdiction to include evaluation as part of a similar three-phase cycle: (1) identification of problems; (2) descriptive and analytic studies; (3) strategic and tactical planning, implementation, and evaluation.[6]

Professional domains are unimportant here. What is important is that, in theory, evaluators and planners both recognize program evaluation as an initiator of planning and as a means to assess planning's success. Both recognize planning as a process that addresses the problems identified by evaluation and as a mechanism that establishes the standards against which evaluation is conducted. In most hospital management situations, though, things are not so tidy.

One sticking point in the management cycle is that the personnel who conduct program evaluation in hospitals are frequently not the same people who undertake planning in those institutions. (And it is just as seldom the case that those concerned with quality assurance have much to do with either program evaluators or planners.) This is not so much a result of different sets of requisite skills or of disciplinary competitions or contradictions. It is, in part, a matter of focus. Evaluators' concerns are the process and organizational details of individual existing programs; planners' concerns are the future structural composition and direction of the institution. Of course, individual programs will compose future institutional structures, and a future structure either supports or fails to support existing programs. Existing processes move directionally, and future direction of an institution is meant to guide existing processes. But even where this interface is recognized, there is likely to remain a practical interstice in the planning-implementation-evaluation cycle. A major reason for this management gap seems to be a consequence of the way in which planning and evaluation have changed in the hospital field.

Recent Moves Apart

Until the last decade or so, planning as a generic discipline has not enjoyed a good reputation in the United States. Associated with images of control and nondemocratic regimes by the red-baiters of the McCarthy era, organized planning was regarded—and often still is—as an interference in the affairs of a well-intentioned, pluralistic people. Of course, everyone plans anyway—from summer vacations to job moves—and so those who run our institutions, including hospitals, felt confident that they could plan institutional development without need for the professional planner. Insofar as planning has been undertaken as a discrete administrative activity in hospitals, it has been primarily facilities planning. Stimulated by Hill-Burton requirements, long-term master plans showing phased development of hospital buildings and medical center campuses became the *raison d'être* of hospital planning staffs. Planners were actually architects who produced reports and renderings of how their institutions would look in 20 years. Unfortunately, these master plans were often better used as accoutrements in executive offices than as aids in dealing with future uncertainties.

Influenced largely by the success of different forms of planning outside the health field—from the planned marketing strategies of corporate industries to the technical achievements of NASA programs—and partly in response to certificate-of-need legislation of the 1970s, planning in many hospitals is undergoing transformation. Strategic planning, with its emphasis on studying uncontrollable environmental factors and on analyzing market conditions, is emerging as the new style of hospital planning. Planners are sometimes still architects, but their planning tasks are beginning to shift from accommodating intended institutional changes to helping to manage the process of long-term institutional development. Establishment of mission statements, assessment of current market performance, programmatic design of institutional services, and development of internal consensus and external support are the jobs of strategic planners. These planners no longer report to engineering departments but to vice presidents for finance, to vice presidents for marketing, and, more appropriately, to chief executive officers.

At the same time, health program evaluation has developed as a discipline of its own. Larger federal government involvement in health care financing, establishment of peer review organizations, increasing technological capabilities, and economic crises have all contributed to the increased demand for evaluation for health services programs. Shortell and Richardson state, "The common thread running through is the emphasis on rationalizing the delivery of services . . . not only on whether the program worked (improved access, contained cost) but on *why* the effort was brought about."[5a] They go on to explain that while evaluation is a common activity in the daily work of administrators, planners, and providers, "what distinguishes program *evaluation* research from day-to-day evaluation decisions is the use of *scientific method* . . . to isolate causes of particular events or outcomes."[5b] So, while hospital planning has evolved toward a more corporate, more negotiatory model for dealing with future development, program evaluation has strengthened the quasi-scientific management armory required to administer existing health resources.

These stylistic and temporal differences have tended to move hospital planning away from the operational role of other management tools into a policy-oriented role. It has changed the question planners ask from "What do our programs need?" to "What programs should we have?" Along the way, somewhat surprisingly and quite unfortunately, responsibilities for answering the question "How well are our programs doing?" have been dispersed among quality assurance officers, program administrators, and planners such that there are many partial answers but seldom a comprehensive one. Hospital planners evaluate programs to determine the nature of their actual and potential contributions toward meeting long-term institutional and community goals. Program effectiveness and efficiency and quality of care, apparently divorced from the planners' corporate agenda, have become the objectives of those currently engaged in the provision of program services.

This rift between evaluation and planning is overstated here, but only to make the point. Although there are many hospital planners who actually research program quality and many program evaluators who actually plan long-term institutional changes, it appears more often to be the case that the regular work of hospital planning and health program evaluating are not integrated as management theory directs. Yet, clearly, the environmental conditions and future uncertainties with which hospital planning deals will influence the performance of hospital programs. Changes in institutional mission, in demographic patterns, in economic climate—changes that planning is meant to foresee—will affect the accessibility, continuity, and effectiveness of health service programs. So why can't evaluation programs be designed to enable evaluators to extend their analyses into the future environments that planners project? Why can't planning provide evaluators with information that will allow them to judge future performance and thus anticipate departures from standards before they occur? Why can't the gap between evaluation of existing programs and planning of future institutions be closed? In fact it can be, quite easily, if planning is willing to be more humble and program evaluation, less rigid.

Strategic Evaluation: The Ottawa-Carleton Case

There are not many well-documented examples of an ingrated planning and evaluation cycle at work in American hospital management. In truth, preoccupation with the ongoing development of strategic planning methods and the current changes in quality assurance and program evaluation requirements have left hospital administrators little opportunity to forge a practical integration of planning and evaluation, however desirable. But integration of planning and evaluation tools has been achieved elsewhere, and these achievements can be examined to guide similar developments in American hospital management.

One good example is a multi-institutional exercise that was undertaken in Ottawa, Ontario. Under the auspices of the Ottawa-Carleton Regional District Health Council, representatives from hospitals and agencies that provide health services for the elderly grouped together to evaluate performance of their existing programs, to determine needs for improvements in service, and to establish a means for ongoing evaluation and planning. One significant difference from community-wide planning in the United States is the level of direct involvement of local providers in both the planning work of the host agency and in the subsequent implementation of planned programs, an involvement that is fostered by Canada's very different method of publicly financing health care. Although the work in its present form is not directly transferable to individual hospital planning and evaluation practices in the U.S., it does offer lessons from which administrators of hospital services might draw some insight.

Strategic Planning and Evaluation Method

District health councils are local planning bodies in Ontario that have been established to advise the Provincial Minister of Health on organization and delivery of local health services. Councils are composed of 15 to 20 volunteers, including health providers, consumers, and elected officials, and are supported by small professional staffs. The councils have broad terms of reference, among which are mandates to identify and consider alternative methods of meeting community health needs, to encourage the development of a comprehensive range of health care programs, and to set funding priorities consistent with long-term goals.

The Ottawa-Carleton Regional District Health Council (OCRDHC) is the responsible agency for the Regional Municipality of Ottawa-Carleton, which comprises 11 municipalities in eastern Ontario, including the national capitol. Recently, the OCRDHC initiated a specially funded planning program intended to demonstrate that the agency could help plan effectively for the future development of community health services. The specific terms of reference of the Ottawa-Carleton planning program were interpreted to include the following objectives: (1) to develop a strategy for planning health services over the long term (comprising guidelines, procedures, and policies to assist and inform the council in its decision making); and (2) to employ the strategic guidelines, procedures, and policies to help establish short- and medium-term operational plans to strengthen and improve deliveries of health services.

In keeping with these objectives, OCRDHC's planning team began its work by developing a detailed methodology based on two interrelated premises that spell out the need to link long-term strategy with short-term performance.

First, health service planning is not a "once-and-for-all" approach that ends with the production of a master plan. Rather than trying to master the future, planning should be characterized by continuity and self-education. By undertaking incremental changes to the health care system and then evaluating the impacts of those changes, the council would learn more about how to develop a pattern of health services that would respond effectively to future community needs.

Second, it is impossible to formulate strategies for change that are sufficient to cope in advance with all possible occurrences. It is impossible to predict the future environment within which the development of health care will occur. The complexities of the health care system, imperfect knowledge of its operations, and uncertainties about future conditions require a planning approach that helps manage current resource commitment while retaining long-term flexibility.

Current concepts of long-range planning do not meet these requirements. Planners cannot predict the future events that will affect the long-term viability of actions taken today. As a result, those actions can inadvertently become the causes of inappropriate long-term momentum that is difficult and costly to reverse. What planning can do, though, is to anticipate a *range* of probable future events and then to evaluate how they are likely to affect the existing configuration of health care services. Equipped with those expectations, planners and providers can consider, "How will our services fare under different sets of future conditions? How does this action taken now help meet our objectives if these future conditions occur? Does another action allow more long-term flexibility? Does another action afford a more viable solution across a broader range of future conditions?"

This deliberation does not produce the single optimal decision or the master plan for a predicted future. Instead, it results in a list of alternative and variously desirable action sets to improve current performance. Choices can then be made between short-term performance and long-term viability; future risks of poor performance are identified; and short-term actions that are likely to be inappropriate to the future environment may then be avoided. Judgment, not science, becomes the key in program decision making.

Linking Action and Uncertainty

Consistent with the planning program's objectives, two types of planning were undertaken. The first led to alternative long-term strategies for health service development that were designed to identify possible future configurations of the region's health system. The second type of planning led to short-term action plans that were designed to improve or build on existing programs and that were to employ the long-term strategies as means to balance current needs for action against future viability. Because the OCRDHC had established gerontology as a high priority, health services for the elderly was the area for the first in a series of programmatic evaluations and short-term plans. To conduct that work, the OCRDHC convened a gerontology task force made up of providers of services for the elderly, who were to employ the planning method and develop a multi-institutional plan for gerontology services in the region.

The work that was undertaken in Ottawa-Carleton is described in detail elsewhere.[7] Briefly, the planning method comprised three streams of work, each stream containing a sequence of tasks relating respectively to development of goals, to measurement and evaluation of the existing health system, and to alternative projections of the future. With the integration of these three streams, changes to the health care system that were proposed to improve performance in the short-term were assessed within the context of alternative long-term futures.

The first stream, *Policies and Standards,* began with a study of the comparative performance of Ottawa-Carleton's health services with those elsewhere, with a survey of local pressures for modification to the health care system, and with the development of policy statements on desired performance of various sectors of the health care system. These inputs were structured into criteria for evaluation of existing programs and for subsequent assessment of alternative planning actions. In this stream of work, a number of evaluative measures were developed, including cost per unit of service, geographic distribution, language of services, total number of services available, accessibility to handicapped, referral patterns, waiting lists, and others. Of course, where provincial guidelines existed, standards were already in place; numbers of beds per thousand population was a common example. But as was more often the case, comparative standards from other provinces and countries were collected for use in subsequent evaluation.

The second stream, *Demand and Performance,* entailed the development of information on the operation of Ottawa-Carleton's health care services. A detailed inventory of all health care resources provided the baseline data that were then analyzed against the performance measures to describe the strengths and weaknesses of existing health care services. The gerontology task force found weaknesses in existing services that included areas of overprovision and underprovision, lack of coordinated referral, and difficulties in access to services for linguistic groups, among other findings. Information also was collected on impending changes to health care services (a new home nursing program about to open, for example) in order to develop an image of the probable shape and performance of the services at the time when planning recommendations would be implemented. But before using these evaluation findings and going on to plan changes to improve or strengthen performance of existing programs, the gerontology task force turned to the long-term planning work being done simultaneously by the OCRDHC planning team.

This work is best explained in the methodology's third stream, *Futures*. In this stream, various types of environmental uncertainties (for example demographic shifts and alteration of employment patterns) were condensed into a representative set of alternative future states within which the region's health services might find themselves operating. Employing a modified Delphi technique along with projection data from a number of official sources, the planning team constructed four representative futures. The futures varied in parameter but not in structure. Each future comprised demographic, economic, political, health care, and technological variables that could be expected to influence health service performance as measured by the evaluation criteria. Each future stood in for a range of conditions that were regarded as not improbable, as meaningfully different, and as relevant to the outcome of current program developments.

Once the alternative futures were developed, the products of the previous two streams were used to subject the Ottawa-Carleton health care system, as a whole, to an assessment within the conditions of each future. This work considered the performance of existing health care programs in light of each future's distinctive conditions. What were seen as potential future inadequacies depended on how existing services would measure up to desired performance in a particular set of future conditions, as well as on a variety of other factors, such as future pressures for change or comparisons with what may be happening elsewhere.

The performance criteria that were developed by the council and by the task force, the evaluative considerations of the health care system for each future, and the budgetary parameters of each future were brought together in order to generate alternative strategies for long-term alteration to the health care system. As a simplified example, given criteria about availability of services, the existing and future inadequacies in health services for the elderly, and a future in which funds for capital expansion are limited, a strategy for that future would include an increase in services provided through home care programs, an increase in day hospitals and mobile services, and decreases in more intensive chronic inpatient services. The configuration of the health care system in each future, then, represented the direction in which the impending health care system could be expected to evolve in response to the circumstances of that future. Each configuration was structured in terms of range, quality, and location of services. The resulting configurations, when taken together and like the futures within which they occur, represented a range of possible future developments of the health care system.

In one future, for example, long-stay institutional services would be increased significantly in response to expanded health insurance and would entail increased uses of health workers other than physicians as providers of community-based care. In another future, severe economic constraint and continued dominance of physicians' political influence in health care would limit growth of noninstitutional services. All future configurations shared common characteristics, such as at least moderate increases in day surgery services. However, where circumstances were unique to a particular future, they resulted in unique configurational characteristics.

This long-term multifuture, *strategic evaluation,* as the planning team called it, outlined the distinctive differences and similarities in the performance of existing programs, as well as what performance might be expected across the range of futures. It also identified those alterations to the health care system that could or should be pursued irrespective of future changes in health, economic, technological, and developmental environments.

With this information in hand, the gerontology task force proposed remedial actions to make up for current deficiencies and then examined those actions with respect to their impact on the performance of the future health system. The resulting analysis provided a detailed account of what services existed for the elderly in the region, of what improvements were required in order to meet council policies and task force criteria, and of alternative ways of achieving those improvements. The proposed actions then were assessed in terms of short-term performance and in terms of long-term viability. This is where the interactive nature of the planning and evaluation exercises is seen most clearly. The strategic evaluation presented an overview of how existing health services would perform and could evolve under various future conditions. It thus provided a basis for judging the long-term suitability of actions under consideration now, for making necessary trade offs between current performance and future flexibility, and for identifying risks of potential future failure.

The resulting products of operational planning were related to the three methodological streams. The first was a reconsideration of policy guidelines for gerontology services, which could be used in later planning and with which the council could respond to initiatives proposed by other agencies that have a mandate for planning health services in Ottawa-Carleton. The second was a short list of planning initiatives that the council and local providers could take or oversee. Increases in day care places for the elderly and the establishment of a geriatric assessment unit were examples. The third product included proposals that the council could promote for consideration by agencies that plan nonhealth resources in the region (such as the regional transport authority) as well as the identification of environmental variables (such as changes in ethnic composition of the population) that could affect future health service performance and that thus should be monitored by the council's planners.

Lessons for Hospital Evaluation and Planning

The Ottawa-Carleton methodology allows health service providers to evaluate current performances of their programs and to identify needs for remedial actions.

More importantly, it enables them to assess how well those programs would perform across a range of probable future circumstances. The assessment, to be sure, cannot be as rigorous or certain as the evaluation of current performance, but it nonetheless can provide useful information for judging the long-term appropriateness of short-term program changes.

The methodology poses a number of challenges to traditional concepts of long-term planning. It accepts uncertainty and the benefits of incremental change and so chooses to keep long-term options open rather than to set a determinate course now. While this reduces the demand for data that would be required to support the probability of a predicted future, it means that vigilant monitoring of environmental changes has to become an important task in continued planning work. Planners thus serve more as generators of information required to guide decision making than as technicians who provide answers for the problems facing health administrators. This does not mean that planners do not have a role in decision making. Indeed, the methodology stresses common understanding, deliberation, and informed judgment and thus encourages wider participation in decision making. It does mean that planners are no longer master craftsmen, and this is demonstrated best in the introduction to OCRDHC *Long-Term Strategic Evaluation:* "This is not a plan . . . [but] a tool for ongoing planning."[8]

No ultimate status is claimed for the Ottawa-Carleton methodology. Its development and application were influenced by economic, governmental, and organizational factors that, in other circumstances, would alter its composition and conduct. Many of the tasks that were undertaken (only some of which are described here) would not be entirely appropriate or adequate in planning for other organizations, particularly for individual hospitals. But the underlying philosophy and logic, the recognitions that predicted futures are more hazardous than helpful and that assessment of future performance can inform current decisions, provide important lessons for hospital program evaluation and planning.

Certainly, many of the factors that influence a health service program's structure, process, and outcome are among the environmental variables that hospital planning monitors. For example, credentials of attending health professionals will be influenced significantly by changes in the composition of the local health labor force. As another example, maintaining a ready access to service must take account of shifts in the linguistic characteristics of both users and providers. Information garnered through hospital planning's environmental and market research can provide important indicators of impending changes in program performance. These indicators, in turn, can provide a sense of desirable preventive actions, such as initiation of wider recruitment efforts or expansion of bilingual service programs, before program failure makes remedial actions necessary.

Linking the data bases of program evaluators and hospital planners is a required first step toward this type of preventive assessment. Obviously, many of the performance variables analyzed by evaluators are not related directly to the institutional and environmental variables studied by planners. But where they are, as in the examples above, the absence of common information can inexcusably undermine program quality, and it can also unnecessarily undermine the internal political support and understanding needed for long-term institutional development.

Construction of detailed alternative strategies for the long-term development of service programs is one way to identify the links between existing program performance and future institutional direction. Because these strategies are built within representative futures whose precise composition can never be known, studies of cause and effect between environmental change and program performance can be neither absolutely precise nor predictable. However, the investigation of where programs could go wrong and of how institutions would probably have to be altered as a result can enable hospital managers to act with more circumspection and with less surprise.

Managing hospital and health services is much more like planning for jungle survival than like planning for an expedition to the moon. Surprises can be frequent and deadly, and the certainty of future location is rare. Yet, it is certainly better to listen for the warnings of the beast that ends up never crossing our path than to fall prey to the undetected predator. Integrating program evaluation with planning can enable managers to hear those warnings and can help hospitals to survive and, indeed, to thrive. However, to accomplish that end, both evaluators and planners must be prepared to recognize the benefits of the others' management tools and the limitations of their own.

NOTES

1. J.S. Wholley, *Evaluation: Promise and Performance* (Washington, D.C.: The Urban Institute, 1979), p. 3.

2. A. Donabedian, "The Quality of Medical Care," *Science* 9 (1978):856–864.

3. H. Koontz and C. O'Donnell, *Management—A Systems and Contingency Analysis of Managerial Functions* (New York: McGraw-Hill Book Co., 1976), p. 125.

4. H.W.J. Rittel and M.M. Webber, "Dilemmas in a general theory of planning," in *Systems and Management Annual*, ed. R.L. Ackoff (New York: Petrocelli, 1974), pp. 219–223.

5. S.M. Shortell and W.C. Richardson, *Health Program Evaluation* (St. Louis: C.V. Mosby, 1978).

5a. Ibid., p. 7.

5b. Ibid., p. 7.

6. W.A. Flexner et al., *Strategic Planning in Health Care Management* (Rockville, Md.: Aspen Systems Corp., 1981), p. 114.

7. Ottawa-Carleton Regional District Health Council Planning Program, *Planning Health Services in Ottawa-Carleton* (Ottawa, 1978).

8. Ottawa-Carleton Regional District Health Council Planning Program, *Long-Term Strategic Evaluation of Health Services in Ottawa-Carleton* (Ottawa, 1979), p. 1.

Chapter 10

A Validation Theory for Quality Assessment*

William E. McAuliffe, Ph.D.

INTRODUCTION

A problem in the area of quality assessment is the absence of a conceptually adequate model for validation of assessments. Several years ago, two related essays by McAuliffe weighted the relative advantages of process and outcome approaches to measuring the quality of care.[1,2] Those analyses concluded that evidence on the validity of process measures was ambiguous and that there had been virtually no research on the validity of outcome measures. The essays argued that a major reason for the sorry state of evidence on quality assessments was the limitations of the "medical-effectiveness" validation model that dominated the field. Although offering no obvious way to evaluate outcome assessments, the medical-effectiveness model estimated the validity of process measures by examining their correlation with outcomes. However, since the size of process-outcome correlations depends on the strengths and weaknesses of both process and outcome measures, the logic of the model requires some basis for assuming high outcome validity. A review of existing evidence, pertinent to the validity of outcome-based assessments of quality, suggested many reasons for believing that the validity of outcome-based assessments could not be assumed to be high.[2] Despite this fundamental difficulty in interpretation, researchers have continued to depend upon the study of process-outcome correlations as virtually the only method of evaluating the validity of quality assessments.

The main purpose of this chapter is to present an alternative to the medical-effectiveness model. This alternative, the psychometric model, offers a broader conception of validity and provides methods for evaluating outcome assessments and methods other than process-outcome correlations for evaluating process and

*Work on this chapter was performed as part of the Kaiser Research Program in Health Policy and Management, Harvard University School of Public Health. Support for the program comes from the Henry J. Kaiser Family Foundation.

157

structural assessments of quality. The model also explains how studies of process-outcome correlations can be designed and interpreted more effectively. The model derives from an overall theory of health measurement described in the next section.

The chapter serves as a guide to validation methodology for hospital administrators, quality assurance committees and practitioners. The first sections explain validity's role in the measurement process. The remaining sections present a brief description and evaluation of the range of approaches to validation. The discussion provides a framework for what is being done in the field, corrects common misconceptions, and suggests new strategies.

A THEORY OF HEALTH MANAGEMENT

Central to this theory of measurement is a metaphysical conception of two worlds: one of ideas or qualities and the other of things.[3,4] *Concepts* or qualities of varying levels of abstraction (e.g., health status, people, institutions, quality of care, and athletic ability) populate the idea world. Concrete *objects* (e.g., patients, students, hospitals, case records, and track stars) inhabit the world of things. To bridge these two worlds satisfactorily, some established procedure must be followed, and it is for this bridging operation that the theory uses the term *measurement*. (It is common in physical sciences to employ a much more restricted definition of measurement that includes only ratio and interval level measurement, but for social and medical sciences that definition would be too restrictive.)

The basic elements of measurement are revealed when a determination is made of the sex (concept) of a person (object) by implicitly checking his or her characteristics against the characteristics of males and females. A determination if a person is male or female is the value produced by this elementary measurement process. Similarly, a person's athletic ability can be judged impressionistically by observing him or her at play. Athletic ability can be assessed precisely by recording the individual's performance, by using sophisticated timing instruments, or just by using a tape measure in a set of carefully selected events, as in a decathlon. Thus, *measurement* is a process or procedure (including use of instruments) applied to objects (things or events) to determine symbolic values that are assumed to represent a particular quality or concept.

How well those values (measurements) actually reflect the categories or gradations of the concept is the question of *validity*. The connection between measure or concept is known as an *epistemic assumption*, emphasizing that the connection is ultimately no more than an assumption or hypothesis, although it may be studied by logical analysis or empirical research, just as any hypothesis. Such an effort is termed *validation*.

MEASURING QUALITY OF CARE

The skepticism of many physicians toward measures of quality of care should not be unexpected, since many persons are uncomfortable with the idea of measuring highly abstract concepts. *Intelligence* and *quality of life* are classic examples of other concepts whose measurement evokes reactions of disbelief. The roots of this doubt about assessing quality of care are not entirely clear, but at least a few of them can be identified.

In the first place, the concept *quality of care* could itself be problematic, either because it has received little intellectual attention and is therefore poorly developed or because it has meant different things to different observers. The many definitions of *quality of health care* show that its meaning varies, but only somewhat. It is neither as vague as *quality of life*, nor does it have as many different interpretations as *intelligence*.[5,6] At this time, another sophisticated theoretical analysis of the concept *quality of care* might prove to be helpful, but minor differences in definitions frequently have little bearing on how a concept is measured. For example, the concepts *health status* and *opiate addiction* have many theoretical definitions each. Yet, despite these conceptual differences, the measures used in most studies are essentially the same. Health status indexes include mortality, morbidity, and functional status, and opiate addiction is almost always measured by the presence of withdrawal sickness. Some further refinement of the concept *quality of care* may be useful, but what is more clearly missing is experience in working with measures of the concept. Quality of care should be better grasped when scientists have greater knowledge of its variations and relationships with other phenomena (its causes, consequences, and correlates) and when providers have had firsthand experience in judging and being judged by quality measures.

In part, these problems of belief also stem from certain paradoxes of abstraction and the measurement of abstractions. As an example, suppose a baseball fan was interested in evaluating the "quality of play" of the Baltimore Orioles last season. Quality of play subsumes many relatively concrete dimensions, including hitting, fielding, pitching, base running, scoring, and winning. Each of these, such as hitting, subsumes still more concrete aspects, such as team batting average, total bases, strikeouts, walks, runs, etc. In general, any variable subsumed by a concept is eligible as one of its indicators. Practically speaking, no component or collection of components can be expected to capture it all. Even a grand composite index would still miss some of the intangibles that do not get into the record books. This difficulty is as true for measuring the Orioles' play as it is for measuring the economy, the job performance of managers,[7] or the quality of medical care. As a result, highly abstract concepts seem unmeasurable (intuitively something is always lacking), and for the same reason, they seem hard to define precisely. Yet, a highly abstract measure designed to cover as much as possible, such as *quality of play,* unavoidably includes so much that its meaning is difficult to grasp.

However, a key implication of the two-world model is that all concepts, no matter how concrete, are still abstractions that can only be inferred when a measurement process is applied to objects. Although concepts do vary in how closely they are linked to phenomena, the relationship between concepts and their measures differs only by degree, and there is nothing formally different in the way various concepts are measured.

Sometimes a seemingly qualitative distinction is drawn between concrete concepts, called *observables,* and more abstract concepts, termed *hypothetical constructs.* Heroin use and heroin addiction illustrate the difference. Addiction is more abstract than use in that addiction is inferred from a wider range of phenomena, including heroin use, physiological symptoms, subjective states, and so on. But, again, both addiction and use are abstractions that are measured in fundamentally the same way. In this model, there can be no direct measures of a concept; all measures require inferences. Consequently, contrary to the claims of some authors, outcome measures are not direct indicators of the quality of care, and they, like other measures, must have their validity demonstrated.

In principle, measurement of quality of care could attain sufficient refinement so as to command the same kind of respect given to many physical measures. If a highly abstract concept cannot be measured satisfactorily, it is because, as formulated, it embodies faulty theoretical propositions about nature; but that conclusion can be determined only after study and analysis. Burwen and Campbell tried to measure the construct, "general attitude towards authority figures," but found only attitudes towards specific authority figures.[8] So far, studies employing measures of quality of care suggest that the concept is a defensible one.[2]

OPERATIONALIZING VALIDITY IN QUALITY ASSESSMENT

This section discusses operationalization of the concept of measurement validity. An *operational definition* of a concept specifies the conditions of measurement for a particular context. The previous paragraphs defined validity in a theory of measurement; the next step is to spell out how that definition applies specifically when assessing the quality of medical care. First, however, it is necessary to examine critically the currently popular operational definition that equates validity with medical effectiveness and correlation with outcomes. Then, an alternative operational definition of validity will be presented.

A Critique of the Medical-Effectiveness Model

In the quality assessment literature, the validity of a criterion has usually referred to its effectiveness in making a patient well. For example, Sanazaro and Williamson stated, "The validity of any criteria of clinical performance is determined by the extent to which such performance is causally related to patient outcomes."[9] This medical-effectiveness model of validity is, in most cases, employed only in connection with the validation of structural and process criteria, but Barro,[10] for one, extended the range of its applicability beyond types of criteria to methods of observation, namely, the direct-observation approach employed by Peterson[11] and by Clute.[12]

Medical effectiveness is an inadequate validation model because medical effectiveness is not equivalent to measurement validity. The recordings of observations that a medically effective procedure was performed could be invalid, because the recordings may have been falsified, and so, in fact, the procedure was never performed. The measurements of effective procedures could also be highly unreliable (and therefore, largely invalid) because of carelessness in keeping medical records, because of errors made by medical record abstractors, or because medical audit reviewers could not agree on a case's adequacy. Finally, it is even conceivable, theoretically, that the recording of an ineffective procedure could be a somewhat valid measure of quality if it was substantially correlated with good provider performance. This situation could happen, if the element of care was new and was mistakenly thought to be efficacious and had been adopted by only the most advanced physicians. It could also occur if the procedure required expensive equipment, available only in large teaching hospitals where care was excellent. (Of course, when developing measures for a regulatory program, the evaluator wants measures that are not only validity indicators but also useful guidelines for changing behavior. Consequently, ineffective procedures would not be criteria for quality assurance.)

Another major problem with the medical-efficacy approach is that it offers no guidance for evaluating the validity of outcome measures themselves which cannot be taken for granted.[2]

Quality of Medicine versus Quality of Care

Part of the attraction of the medical-efficacy model, to many physicians, is their understandable interest in simultaneously promoting both the quality of medicine and the quality of care. However, dual goals would be beyond the scope of quality assurance programs. What quality assurance is designed to do and should be concerned with is the optimum, or at least, acceptable application of existing medical technology. If, in the process, something is learned about the nature of medical technology, all the better, but active pursuit of medical technological advances is truly beyond the scope of a quality assurance program and, undoubtedly, is also beyond the capability of many providers participating in a quality assurance program. It is the job of medical research to improve the quality of medical knowledge by discovering new medical procedures and by investigating the medical efficacy of existing procedures. It is the job of quality assurance to make sure that procedures based on the best medical technology have been employed and that they were employed appropriately and skillfully.

An Alternative to the Medical-Effectiveness Model of Validity

This section presents the psychometric model of validity that derives from the measurement theory described above. As explained earlier, the belief that the records produced by certain structured observations or procedures bridge the gap between concept and object is an epistemic assumption, and validity is the degree to which this assumption is correct.

In this measurement theory, each concept can have many indicators. For example, the concept of quality of care is connected with many phenomena, i.e., factors that produce it, factors that result from it, and factors that constitute it or that simply correlate with it. Any one of the causes (structural inputs), constituents (process) or correlates, or effects (outcomes) can serve as the objects for valid measures of quality. Many writers have stated that there must be a causal connection between a valid indicator and what it is trying to measure.[13,14] (Also, see the quotation from Sanazaro and Williamson above.[9]) However, that view would be overly restrictive because a stable correlation, whether causal or not, is sufficient for measurement. For example, a score on a test of medical knowledge could be a measure of quality of care (even though the test score and quality performance are only correlated) because both measures have the same cause. It is certainly true that causal relations may be more desirable because they are more useful from the perspective of policy making or regulation, but this is distinct from the question of measurement validity. In fact, evaluators often feel uncomfortable with measures that are not constituents conceptually and refer to them, not as measures, but as *proxies*. Few evaluators would be satisfied with a measure of heroin use that did not involve some direct indication of actual use, either the individual's statement or some observation of use. Yet, correlates of use that might be employed as proxies would include the use of other drugs; circumstantial evidence, such as having friends who use the drug; or anything that is a cause or consequence of heroin use. The same dissatisfaction evaluators would feel regarding these measures should also apply in the case of quality of care measures based on structures or outcome.

In this measurement theory, not only can each concept have many measures, but it is also true that each of those measures can be an indicator for many other concepts simultaneously (e.g., death can serve as a measure of health status on the one hand and quality of care on the other). In theory[15] and in practice, none of the many measures of a concept is perfectly valid, which would mean being *pure* (reflecting only that concept), *complete* (encompassing all the concept's relevant aspects), and *representative* (having the right mix of aspects). Since no measures are perfect, validity is not an all-or-nothing quality, but one that varies along a continuum.

For the purpose of formalizing this theory, facilitating operationalization, and establishing continuity between single items and composite measures, points made in the last paragraph can be expressed statistically in terms of the components of the variance of a set of measurements:[16]

$$\sigma_x^2 = \sigma_v^2 + \sigma_{se}^2 + \sigma_{re}^2.$$

This theoretical equation expresses the proposition that the differences between the values x_i of a set of measurements (a single item or a composite index), as measured by their total variance, σ_x^2, is made up of three components. One, σ_v^2, is the variance of the measurements due to or associated with the concept being studied or simply the *valid variance*. The remainder of the total variance is due to other concepts and is divided somewhat arbitrarily into two *error* components: systematic error, σ_{se}^2, and random error σ_{re}^2.

The validity of a measure is then defined as the proportion of the total variance that is valid, that is:

$$\text{Validity} = \frac{\sigma_v^2}{\sigma_x^2}$$

Readers with statistical training will recognize that this variance ratio is algebraically equal to the squared correlation coefficient, P_{xc}^2, between the concept, c, and the measure, X. It is a hypothetical correlation, called the *validity coefficient*, which is the most commonly used index of validity. Although this theoretical correlation between measure and concept can never be estimated directly, it may be approximated in empirical validity studies by substituting in place of the concept another measure already possessing accepted validity. Also, in order to describe the direction of the relationship, either positive or negative, an estimate of ρ_{xc} rather than its square is usually reported.

Systematic measurement error is the stable variance associated with concepts or factors other than the concept being measured. Should the same measure, X_i, be used as an indicator for one of these other concepts instead, then the parts of the total variance that are regarded as valid variance and systematic-error variance would naturally change. After accounting for the valid variance and systemic-error variance, the rest of the variance is *unreliable,* that is, it is thought to be due to random effects of other factors. Reliability of a measure is defined as the proportion of its variance that is free of random error, that is, the stable variance including valid variance and systematic-error variance.

Readers familiar with multiple regression may understand this model more easily by viewing measurement as observations being explained by a theoretical regression analysis with many concepts as independent variables. The validity of the measurements would then be the proportion of variance explained by the concept being measured; systematic-error variance would be the additional variance explained by the other concepts in the regression; random-error variance would be the residual variance unexplained by any of the concepts in the regression; and the measure's reliability would be the total variance explained by the regression equation.

One important implication of the psychometric model is that a measure's validity is an ingredient of its reliability.[17] Therefore, measures with low reliability must have low validity. For example, if implicit quality assessments correlate only .50 across physician reviewers, only half the assessment variance is reliable, and therefore no more than half the total variance can be valid. Consequently, increasing reliability (say, by using the combined judgments of more than one reviewer or by providing explicit criteria to increase inter-judge agreement) is an obvious first step towards attempting to increase validity. Furthermore, the level of aggregation affects reliability (e.g., conclusions about a hospital based on evaluations of 50 cases are more reliable than conclusions about a physician based on evaluation of one such case). Greater reliability in turn permits greater validity. Consequently, even though most of the reported validity estimates of quality assessments have been rather modest, those estimates focus on judgments of individual cases. Greater validity would be anticipated when the same assessments are aggregated for the purpose of quality regulation at the hospital level, e.g., for hospital certification.

Thus, the advantages of this model of validity over the medical-effectiveness model is that it does not have causal assumptions; does not confuse the advancement of medical science with the purpose of quality assurance; relates reliability to validity; and, as the next section shows, provides several means for estimating the validity of all types of measures, including outcome-based measures.

METHODS FOR ESTIMATING THE DEGREE OF VALIDITY

Measurement specialists have devised several strategies (methods) to estimate the validity of quality assessments. Although more than one strategy can sometimes be employed so that the results can be somewhat independent of a particular validation strategy, the choice of method usually depends on the type of measurement problem. In quality assessment, there are two broad validation questions, and all but one of the commonly used strategies should be useful for investigating them. The measurement questions are: (1) Is it really possible to measure something as abstract and intangible as the quality of medical care? and (2) Are practical methods of assessing quality, e.g., patient questionnaires or criteria applied by medical records technicians, sufficiently valid to be useful in a national quality assurance program? Although studies often seem to want to address both questions simultaneously, the methods for dealing with each type of question differ. Therefore, to avoid confusion, investigators should consider the questions one at a time. The next sections of this chapter will present validation strategies most useful for these purposes. Question two is addressed first for ease of exposition.

Concurrent Validity

Concurrent validation is typically employed when an acceptable measure (traditionally called the *criterion* by measurement experts) already exists but is not practical—usually in terms of expense—for the problem at hand. A cheaper measure is constructed, and the evaluator wants to know whether it retains sufficient validity to be useful. In some instances the newer measure will eventually prove to be more valid than the present criterion, but in the beginning a new measure is judged by its correlation with an established measure. A classic example of this strategy is the concurrent validation of questionnaire measures of psychopathology by comparing them with psychiatrists' ratings.

Researchers have already used concurrent validation in several ways on problems of quality assessment. Two studies examined the validity of quality assessments by nonphysicians. Novick et al. compared audits by physicians with quality ratings by nonphysicians for 48 cases of anemia and found that correlations ranged between .31 and .46 across five broad categories of care (e.g., diagnosis, treatment).[18] In a second study, Richardson compared a surgeon with two nurses in their use of explicit criteria in medical audits; the surgeon's ratings correlated .86 and .83 with those of the nurses.[19] In another example of concurrent validation, Brook compared physicians' assessments based on explicit criteria with assessments based on "implicit" criteria: the assessments correlated .48 for 296 cases.[20] Finally, Zuckerman et al. compared pediatric outpatient medical records with tape recordings of the doctor-patient interactions.[21] Although Zuckerman et al. themselves did not give the cases independent quality ratings based on the two types of data, to do so would have provided an opportunity to estimate the concurrent validity of medical-record-based quality assessments.

These examples illustrate that the established measure of criterion does not necessarily possess high validity in an absolute sense, and therefore a modest correlation with the criterion does not necessarily mean that the new measure has low validity. An empirical correlation from a concurrent validity study can be expected to be a good estimate of the theoretical validity coefficient only insofar as the criterion is itself highly valid. Practical considerations however often require that a criterion be employed that is merely the most accepted measure available (e.g., psychiatrists' ratings) while recognizing this criterion's limitations (e.g., low reliability). Methodologically, it is obviously highly desirable in validation studies to spare no reasonable expense to refine the criterion as much as possible (e.g., combine the ratings of a panel of psychiatrists).

This last point gives insight into the current situation regarding validity research in the quality assessment field. To date, almost all quality assessment studies have sought to develop a practical assessment technique that could be used in a national program of quality regulation. Consequently, designers have assumed that the method would have to employ or build upon existing hospital data, personnel, and resources—despite obvious adverse effects on validity (e.g., medical record data is known to be faulty). Since no one would claim that these assessment methods, including outcome approaches, represent medical science's all-out attempt to measure quality of care, it should be obvious that today's validation research focuses on question number two above, namely, whether these practical methods of assessment have sufficient validity to be useful and which one is most cost valid.

Concurrent validation would be a validation strategy well suited for these purposes if there existed a method of quality assessment that could serve as a criterion. Some experts have treated outcome assessments as if they were suitable criterion measurements, thus supposedly making process-outcome comparisons instances of concurrent validation. However, there is little reason for regarding any existing outcome measure as a highly valid criterion for they too have been developed as inexpensive, practical measures.[2] The author has suggested that, while no true criterion measure currently exists, one could be developed especially for validation studies with relatively little technical difficulty.[1] Since expense would be much less decisive in a small validation study, high validity of criterion quality assessments could be assured rather easily by performing comprehensive assessments based on tape recordings or direct observations, coupled with special attention to coding accuracy. The study by Zuckerman et al. described above employed this principle.[21] In the author's view, creating a criterion for use in concurrent validation research would resolve many of the validity problems presently facing the field.

Predictive Validity

Another criterion-oriented strategy of validation, known as *predictive validity*, may be relevant to some of the measurement issues in quality assessment. Predictive validity is useful when an adequate measure (the criterion) is already available but measurements are needed that can be obtained earlier in the time stream. Classic examples are measures designed to assess how students would perform in a school or on a job if admitted or hired. Predictive validation is thus useful when timeliness is being traded for loss in validity; the question is how much validity can be retained.

Convergent Validity

A current major obstacle to using criterion-based approaches for validity quality assessments is that the existence of a criterion presupposes the answer to the first question regarding whether quality of care can be measured at all. Critics would want to know how the validity of the criterion could be estimated. Convergent validation and the next two validation strategies presented below— content and construct validation—do not presuppose the existence of a criterion and are thereby suitable for validating a criterion candidate. It is important to keep in mind, however, that all validation depends ultimately on inference or assumption. The principle underlying these three validation methods is to examine the consistency of a network of assumptions with empirical findings.

Convergent validity depends upon the correlations among two or more alternative measures of a concept. The different measures are assumed to be valid to some degree, but in contrast with concurrent validation no one measure is singled out initially as obviously superior. Examples of convergent validation are common in the quality literature, even if not so named. Brook's pioneering study examined correlations of alternative process measures with each other, outcome measures with each other, and process measures with outcome measures.[20] (See also McAuliffe.[1]) Other studies have also correlated structural measures with each other, with process measures, and with outcome measures. (See Scott et al.[22] and Palmer and Reilly.[23]) According to the logic of convergent validity, a strong positive correlation between two contending measures lends credence to the claims of validity for each, although it is possible that they correlate for irrelevant reasons, such as from a common form of systematic-error variance. The absence of a correlation or a low correlation is harder to interpret, since a correlation's size may reflect several substantive and statistical factors.[2] Either one or both of the measures may be faulty; they may simply measure different aspects of the same concept; or there may be one of a variety of statistical problems (e.g., a lack of variance in one measure) that are artifacts of the validation study design or analysis. Despite these serious obstacles to interpretation, convergent validation studies, especially studies of process-outcome correlations, continue to be very popular, almost to the exclusion of any other validation approach.

A Critique of the Process-Outcome Correlation Strategy

After reviewing numerous attempts to evaluate the validity of quality assessments by process-outcome correlation, the author has concluded that, as currently designed and analyzed, studies of process-outcome correlations will almost always fail to find strong correlations and that the current approach should be substantially modified and relied upon less heavily. The next paragraphs present the basis for this view, first by describing key elements of the process-outcome approach and then by critically analyzing the problems apparent in each element.

While every process-outcome study has its own unique features (see McAuliffe[1] for a review), most have a fairly standard design: (1) sampling—cases are a series of approximately 50 or more selected from hospital outpatient records according to diagnosis, with any cases having special management complications excluded, presumably because the assessment criteria would not apply to those cases; (2) content of process measures—process assessments are based on a list of explicit process criteria covering diagnosis, treatment, and follow-up; (3) outcome measurement—the outcome criteria include the patient's mortality, physiological evidence of morbidity, functional status, subjective symptoms, and, sometimes, patient satisfaction; and (4) statistical analysis—validity is estimated by a simple correlation between a sum of the process criteria complied with and a sum of the outcome criteria met. Each of these design features can be criticized.

Sampling cases by diagnosis rather than by presenting complaint systematically excludes cases that could demonstrate the value of diagnostic criteria, often by far the largest category of process criteria. Since subjects who failed to receive proper treatment because of misdiagnosis are absent, any variation in compliance with diagnostic criteria can have nothing in the outcome score with which to correlate because all cases have confirmed positive diagnoses. Similarly, excluding cases with special management problems (e.g., co-morbidity, pregnancy, etc.) makes irrelevant those diagnostic criteria specifically included in the medical process to identify such problems.

Diagnostic process criteria of this last type raise even more serious sampling and design problems. Although a relevant diagnostic criterion should be performed for every patient, its performance can impact only the outcomes of the statistically small number of special cases that the criterion is designed to identify. Consequently, for a study to find a substantial correlation between compliance with the criterion and patient outcome, the sample would have to include *only* subjects with the characteristic in question. For example, suppose an evaluator wanted to assess the validity of a process criterion requiring physicians to ask patients whether or not they were pregnant (the diagnostic procedure) in order to avoid undesirable side effects of drug treatment on the fetus (the relevant outcome). To validate this criterion by a process-outcome correlation, the evaluator would have to study only pregnant women with the disease; observe variations in diagnostic compliance; and then relate variations with the outcomes of the *babies*, not the mothers. It should be obvious that the usual process-outcome study, which often contains none of the crucial features of this special design, could hardly reflect the validity of this criterion. More importantly, no single validation study could generally evaluate more than one or a few such diagnostic criteria from a set. Consequently, these special patients and the criteria for identifying them would ordinarily have to be validated in a series of separate process-outcome studies or in a very large study, or otherwise should be excluded from the usual process-outcome study. A single process-outcome study could validate a series of these criteria under the following conditions: (1) the sample would have to be large or carefully stratified to contain adequate numbers of each type of special patient (independently of the care performed); and (2) the scoring of the process assessment or statistical analysis would have to adjust each time for the correlational relevance of every criterion for a particular patient.

In general, the effects of a diagnostic process are only indirectly and incompletely felt by the usual diagnosis-specific therapeutic outcome because of the way cases are selected; because the impact of diagnostic compliance depends on compliance with therapeutic process criteria (proper treatment, instruction, and follow-up) and on patient compliance; and because some errors (e.g., treatment of misdiagnosed patients with antibiotics) rarely have major effects on diagnosis-specific therapeutic outcomes. It seems possible, therefore, that it is usually a mistake to include any diagnostic criteria in a process assessment in the usual process-outcome study. Instead, all diagnostic criteria would have to be validated against carefully considered diagnostic outcomes in appropriately designed studies with proper samples. It is noteworthy that the concurrent-validation approach described earlier would not require separate studies to validate diagnostic criteria.

Elsewhere, the author has discussed in detail the many problems concerning the validity of the individual outcome measures and composites employed in the usual process-outcome study.[1,2] Therefore, a brief summary will suffice here. The validity of outcome measures has not been established and cannot be assumed because they are often incomplete (they fail to measure all relevant effects), impure (they reflect effects of variables other than the quality of care), and unbalanced. Also, appropriate matching of process and outcome content is essential if sizable correlations are to result. Unless serious attempts are made to refine obviously deficient process and outcome measures, the results of process-outcome correlations will always be disappointing and difficult to interpret.

Patient compliance is one factor whose influence on outcomes is usually not considered in studies of process-outcome correlations. Even if a process assessment included only therapeutic and follow-up criteria, low patient compliance could profoundly lower the correlation between process and outcome. Two solutions—unfortunately, not employed in most studies—would be either to study only compliant patients or to adjust for compliance statistically, say, by interactive terms with treatment and with follow-up as part of a multiple regression analysis.

Timing of outcome measurement can profoundly affect the validity of outcome measures of quality. Measurement of outcome should be guided by medical knowledge of when the effects of the process of care are most clearly and fully evident, but practical considerations have often resulted in measurements that are too early (e.g., at discharge) or too late in the causal sequence.

As illustrated by the discussion of patient compliance, zero-order correlations between simple process and outcome scores will often not reflect the potential validity of quality assessments. Medical processes that involve conditional relationships, such as between diagnosis, treatment, and follow-up, have to be considered in the scoring of process assessments, in analysis of the relationship between process and outcome, or in the study design. For example, directing a patient to return for follow-up can only affect a patient's disease outcome if the original course of treatment is ineffective; the patient returns as directed; and the subsequent treatment is effective. If these complexities are not taken into account in the scoring of the process measure, in the data analysis, or in the research design (e.g., validating the follow-up criterion on only compliant and diseased patients), then a resulting lowered process-outcome correlation might mistakenly lead to the conclusion that quality of care cannot be measured with sufficient validity.

A final point about process-outcome correlations is that they seem to presuppose that a choice must be made between the two types of measures rather than a combination of the two. It is unlikely that a truly satisfactory assessment of quality could depend on only one type of measure, and a composite would likely be more valid. Consequently, the ultimate relevance of validity estimates based on process-outcome correlations can be questioned.

Content Validity

Content validity offers a radically different approach to the problem of validity. Compared to the other strategies, content validity depends more upon qualitative judgment and does not, by itself, yield a quantitative estimate of the degree of validity. In place of a quantitative estimate, it indicates why a measure appears to be deficient and thereby suggests how it might be improved. Consequently, content validation is a strategy most appropriate to use when constructing a measure of a concept that has never been measured before or constructing a criterion measure against which others may be judged.

Content validation has two steps: (1) specifying the measure's substantive domain based on an analysis of the concept; and (2) constructing measures of each aspect of the domain and combining them in an appropriately balanced manner. The method assumes that a measure will have adequate validity if its domain is appropriately specified and each aspect is validly measured and weighted.

Specifying the substantive domain of quality is the essential job performed by hospital quality assurance committees when they select process or outcome criteria for an assessment. Deciding upon the substantive domain is properly a medical issue to be based on medical knowledge gained through research, clinical experience, and analysis. Disagreements over substantive content are problems for quality assurance specialists and committees, not for validation researchers.

The second step in content validity includes construction of a measure for each part of the substantive domain, developing scoring rules, and deciding how the data will be collected, processed, and analyzed. Statistical techniques may be used at this step to adjust out the effects of unwanted factors (e.g., the effects of patient mix on outcomes), to weigh different components empirically, or to decide on the measurement validity of each of the components.

Unfortunately, this second step has received relatively little attention in the construction of quality measures, due probably to the implicit constraints of cost.

The importance of this step, however, becomes apparent when it is realized that even when there are no arguments about substance, the validity of a measure can be almost completely undetermined by low-quality data. In general, when the components are identified correctly, the more valid the component measures and the rules for combining them, the greater faith can be placed in the validity of the overall measure. Thus, adequate content validity requires both correct specification and measurement of the concept's domain.

For problems of quality assessment, especially the problem of whether quality can be measured at all and how a criterion could be constructed, content validation's great advantage over other approaches (such as convergent validity) is that content validation suggests ideas for how the measure might be improved. For example, if the content validity of an existing measure of quality of care was challenged because it failed to measure the psychosocial aspects of care or because medical skill was poorly represented in the medical record data upon which the measure depended, the evaluator would have a fairly clear idea of how those challenges might be met and tested. Once the process of construction is completed to everyone's satisfaction so that there appears to be adequate content validity, the next method, construct validation, can be used for an external, empirical confirmation of the overall measure's validity.

Construct Validation

If content validation evaluates validity on the basis of how a measure is put together, construct validation evaluates validity on the basis of how a measure performs. Proposed by Cronbach and Meehl, the construct validity of a measure is judged by whether or not the measure behaves as it should.[24] The measure's behavior is predicted by theories in which the concept being measured plays a role. These predictions are then tested empirically using the measure in question and measures of the other concepts contained in the theory. For example, the construct validity of a quality assessment would be evaluated by whether or not it behaved as quality of care should. Knowledgeable persons in medicine generally believe that the quality of medical care is better in large teaching hospitals than in small community hospitals, that specialists deliver better care in their areas of specialization than do nonspecialists, that programs designed to improve quality are effective, and so on.[13] A valid measure of quality of care, when applied to actual situations, should confirm these hypotheses. If not, the validity of the measure of quality must be questioned, as long as the soundness of the hypotheses and the validity of the other measures are not in question. Construct validation also encourages continued evaluation of a measure's performance in a wide network of theoretical research contexts, e.g., as part of prospective experiments of training designed to improve quality, observational studies in actual treatment situations, econometric studies of the effect of cost containment on quality, and so on.

The value of the construct validity approach can be appreciated when the results of certain previous studies of outcome measures are considered. Studies have occasionally found negative correlations between process and outcome measures or between structural measures (teaching versus community hospitals) and patient outcomes.[13,25]

These results were troublesome because they were contrary to theory (common sense). The construct validation strategy produces an urge to look for a plausible explanation. Since it seems unlikely that better care truly harms patients, it must be considered which of the measures, process or outcome, is most likely to be negatively related to quality of care. Although process measures may be far from perfect, it is hard to see how they could be negatively related to quality. By contrast, disease outcomes could easily be negatively related to quality if the sickest patients receive the best care but still have relatively poor outcomes. The analysis suggests that outcome measures must be corrected statistically to adjust for disease severity, patient's physical status, etc. The subsequent performance of an adjusted measure, in a variety of situations, if it were consistent with theoretical expectations, would then argue for its greater construct validity (see Roemer et al.[13] for example).

CONCLUSIONS

This chapter's main purpose has been to adapt psychometric validation theory to quality assessments and other health care measurements. The limitations of the current approach, called the medical-effectiveness model, were described in detail. In the author's view, adherence to the medical-effectiveness model and its emphasis on studying process-outcome correlations has stagnated the field's research on validity and will probably continue to produce discouraging results.

The chapter argued that adoption of psychometric theory (see Nunnally[17]) would be advantageous because it is broader in conception than the medical-effectiveness model, systematically incorporates other work already performed in the field, and suggests a range of validation methods for addressing the main questions presently facing the field. The chapter pointed out that outcome measures could be validated by all of the methods described, including concurrent, content, convergent, and construct validation. By contrast, the medical-effectiveness model offers no means of validating outcome measures. The psychometric model also helps keep distinct quality assessment and basic medical research.

Application of psychometric theory to quality assessment suggests a program of basic measurement research. The need to validate low-cost assessment methods and lingering doubts about whether quality of care can be measured at all suggest the great value of work on constructing a criterion—a measure against which less costly measures could be judged and one that could perform credibly in construct-validity studies. This program would provide a sound research foundation for the entire field of quality assessment.

For the consumer of validation results, the chapter has attempted to provide a background for interpreting recent validation studies and for understanding the need for additional research. The chapter devoted special attention to process-outcome studies, which have been widely misinterpreted. Alternative approaches, which avoid many of the problems inherent in the process-outcome approach, were described. For a comprehensive assessment of the validity of quality assessments, see review articles.[1,2,26,27]

NOTES

1. W.E. McAuliffe, "Studies of Process-Outcome Correlations in Medical Care Evaluation: A Critique," *Medical Care* 16 (1978):907–930.

2. W.E. McAuliffe, "Measuring the Quality of Medical Care: Process versus Outcome," *Milbank Memorial Fund Quarterly* 5 (1979):118–152.

3. J.R. Royce, "Factors as Theoretical Constructs," *American Psychologist* 18 (1963):522–528.

4. L.J. Cronbach, "Test-Validation," in *Educational Measurement*, 2nd ed., ed. R.L. Thorndike (Washington, D.C.: American Council on Education, 1971), pp. 443–507.

5. A.R. Jensen, "How Much Can We Boost I.Q. and Scholastic Achievement?" in *Environment, Heredity, and Intelligence*. Harvard Educational Review Reprint Series no. 2 (Cambridge, Mass.: 1969), pp. 1–123.

6. R.L. Hamblin et al., "Compensatory Education: A New Perspective," *University of Toledo Law Review* 2 (1970):459–499.

7. L.R. James, "Criterion Models and Construct Validity for Criteria," *Psychological Bulletin* 80 (1973):75–83.

8. L.S. Burwen and D.T. Campbell, "The Generality of Attitudes toward Authority and Nonauthority Figures," *Journal of Abnormal and Social Psychology* 54 (1957):24–31.

9. P.J. Sanazaro and J.W. Williamson, "Physician Performance and Its Effects on Patients: A Classification Based on Reports by Internists, Surgeons, Pediatricians, and Obstetricians," *Medical Care* 8 (1970):303.

10. A.R. Barro, "Survey and Evaluation of Approaches to Physician Performance and Measurement," *Journal of Medical Education* 48 (suppl. 1973):1051–1093.

11. O.L. Peterson, "An Analytical Study of North Carolina General Practice: 1953–54," *Journal of Medical Education* 31, Dec., Part 2 (1956):1–165.

12. K.F. Clute, *The General Practitioner: A Study of Medical Education and Practice in Ontario and Nova Scotia* (Toronto: University of Toronto Press, 1963).

13. M.I. Roemer et al., "A Proposed Hospital Quality Index: Hospital Death Rates Adjusted for Case Severity," *Health Services Research* 3 (1968):90–118.

14. C.G. Osborne and H.G. Thompson, "Criteria for Evaluation of Ambulatory Child Health Care by Chart Audit: Development and Testing of a Methodology," *Pediatrics* vol. 56, 1975 (No. 4, suppl.), pp. 625–692.

15. L.V. Jones, "The Nature of Measurement," in *Educational Measurement*, 2nd ed., ed. R.L. Thorndike (Washington, D.C.: American Council on Education, 1971), pp. 335–355.

16. F.N. Kerlinger, *Foundations of Behavioral Research: Educational and Psychological Inquiry* (New York: Holt, Rinehart, and Winston, 1965).

17. J.C. Nunnally, *Psychometric Theory*. Rev. ed. (New York: McGraw-Hill Book Co., 1978).

18. L.F. Novick et al., "Assessment of Ambulatory Care: Application of the Tracer Methodology," *Medical Care* 14 (1976):1–12.

19. F.M. Richardson, "Methodological Development of a System of Medical Audit," *Medical Care* 10 (1972):451–462.

20. R.H. Brook, *Quality of Care Assessment: A Comparison of Five Methods of Peer Review,* Publication No. HRA-74-3100 (Washington, D.C.: Department of Health, Education and Welfare, 1974).

21. A.E. Zuckerman et al., "Validating the Content of Pediatric Outpatient Medical Records by Means of Tape-Recording Doctor-Patient Encounters," *Pediatrics* 56 (1975):407–411.

22. W.R. Scott et al., "Hospital Structure and Postoperative Mortality and Morbidity," in *Organizational Research in Hospitals,* eds. S.M. Shortell and M. Brown (Chicago: Inquiry Book, Blue Cross Association, 1976), pp. 72–89.

23. H.R. Palmer and M.C. Reilly, "Individual and Institutional Variables which May Serve as Indicators of Quality of Medical Care," *Medical Care* 17 (1979):693–717.

24. L.J. Cronbach and P.E. Meehl, "Construct Validity in Psychological Tests," *Psychological Bulletin* 52 (1955):281–302.

25. M.E. Goss and J.I. Reed, "Evaluating the Quality of Hospital Care through Severity-Adjusted Death Rates: Some Pitfalls," *Medical Care* 12 (1974):202–213.

26. A. Donabedian, "The Quality of Medical Care," *Science* 200 (1978):856–864.

27. R.H. Palmer, "Quality Assessment," in *Assuring Quality in Medical Care: The State of the Art,* ed. R. Greene (Cambridge, Mass.: Ballinger, 1976), pp. 11–136.

Chapter 11

Legal Counsel and Risk Management

David J. Slawkowski, J.D.

A BRIEF HISTORY

Over the past eight years, the operations of health care providers have come to embrace many different concepts and functions that were previously unrecognized. Some of the most widespread and divergent of such functions have developed into the related fields of quality assurance and risk management. Up until the notorious malpractice crisis that struck many states and caused many gray hairs in physicians and administrators in the early 1970s, virtually every hospital and other institution had the benefit of relatively low-cost, fixed-rate professional liability insurance. Most such insurance policies carried with them a number of incidental services, such as fire and safety surveys, consultations, auditing services, and other loss control functions, in addition to the more traditional insurance service, such as the review of accident reports, the investigation and settlement of potential claims, and the retention and direction of defense counsel. This separation of what has come to be known as *loss control* or *risk management* from the organization being serviced led to an attitude in the institutions that such functions were not a concern to administration and could safely be left to outsiders. As long as insurance was available at reasonable cost there was little incentive to change.

Developments in law and medicine forced a rapid change in this complacency. The abolition of charitable immunity, beginning in the late 1950s and continuing into the 1960s made charitable institutions that had previously been immune from suit plump targets for lawsuits. The development of legal theories seeking to place responsibility for the acts of negligent physicians on deep-pocketed corporations increased exposure. The erosion of the deep reluctance of physicians to testify on behalf of patients and the evolution of the traveling "hired gun" to testify as plaintiff's expert made verdicts in favor of patients more likely Changes in the pattern of medical practice that replaced the kindly "family" doctor who cared for a patient for life with board-certified subspecialists who rarely made house calls or conversed understandably or sympathetically with their patients made laymen with poor results more interested in a lawsuit. A general increase in the amounts of awards and settlements in all litigation complicated an increasingly deteriorating situation.

In the face of such pressures, insurance carriers could do nothing but increase rates or cease offering professional liability insurance. Both were done. Many companies left the market, and the premium demanded by others become prohibitive. With premiums approaching or exceeding 100 percent for primary insurance coverage, many hospitals began to explore available alternatives such as quota share insurance, captive insurers, self-insurance trusts, or risk pooling groups to provide for losses. But the passage of the liability insurer also meant the cessation of its ancillary services to claim management. Uncomfortable as it was at first, administrators suddenly found themselves in the unaccustomed position of safety inspector and claims adjustor.

RISK MANAGEMENT

Faced with these new functions, many hospitals elected upon centralizing the duties in a single job description, one popular title for which has become the risk manager. Despite the prevalence of the term or similarities of function, there seem to be as many different definitions of the risk manager's function, training, and *modus operandi* as there are institutions with risk managers. Based upon the observations of an outside spectator, most risk managers tend to be: (1) individuals with previous university or vocational training in safety management; (2) nurses or other health professionals who have moved into administration; (3) administrators or financial officers who have historically dealt with outside insurors and attorneys at their institutions; and (4) insurance claim executives who have experience in professional liability work. Individuals from differing backgrounds invariably bring their own insights and limitations to the position of risk manager. There may yet be no adequate definition of the professional risk manager. Once again, observation from the interested outsider seems to indicate functions within two broad categories: (1) loss prevention; and (2) loss control or claim management. Loss prevention includes functions formerly performed by insurors, such as safety inspections, seminars, employee education, and statistical analysis of the sources of potential claims. Loss prevention functions can also include less traditional practices, some of which are discussed below. Loss control functions are all those steps necessary to identify, investigate, evaluate, and dispose of claims. Virtually all of these functions are new to hospitals. These include the review of incident reports to identify injuries, interviews of witnesses, negotiation of settlements, and assistance in trial preparation.

Risk managers from different types of backgrounds obviously bring their own individual strengths and weaknesses to their jobs and may even define the duties differently. Thus a manager trained in safety engineering may provide superb inspections of the premises but be totally unaware of potential problems arising in policy and procedure manuals. A former nurse may understand the dangers inherent in the operating room but have no idea of how to negotiate a settlement. Such comparisons are endless and readily apparent. Further complicating an already murky situation are innumerable outside contractors who offer services to institutions. Captive insurance companies may offer some necessary services to their assureds, but they are rarely as complete as those offered by traditional carriers. The personnel providing loss services in captives vary widely in training and experience themselves. Many insurance agents and brokers offer claim management contracts at widely varying costs. Again, generalizations about the types and qualities of such services are impossible. Many consulting services have sprung up overnight, and they use the expertise of many different types of personnel, including physicians. Unfortunately, the only prerequisite to offering such services as a risk management expert seems to be the hanging of a shingle. The only rule to be observed among the purchasers of such services is *caveat emptor*.

OUTSIDE COUNSEL IN RISK MANAGEMENT

Since no two risk management programs or risk managers are alike, it is impossible to suggest a general program for the use of outside legal counsel. There are, however, a number of common areas where an attorney can be of considerable assistance in both the design and operation of the loss prevention and loss control functions. As with the other types of outside suppliers discussed above, the principle of *caveat emptor* must apply. The field of health care law is beginning to be recognized as a subspecialty of law, but there is no guarantee of competence or experience. There are few law school courses specializing in health care issues and even fewer schools with a genuine program in which students can concentrate on a health-related program. It must therefore be considered what type of outside counsel is best equipped to assist the newly-coined risk manager in his or her important functions.

At present, and for years to come, the only attorneys with a true specialty (although bar associations do not recognize any such concept) will be those who have spent a significant amount of time practicing medical professional liability law. A limited or occasional practice in the field is not enough. It is well recognized among most attorneys, although not by most hospitals, that medical malpractice litigation is not for the tyro. For example, in Chicago, probably 60 percent of all malpractice lawsuits are filed by about a dozen plaintiff's attorneys. Probably 85 percent of all malpractice defense work is handled by a half dozen defense firms. Although there are a number of other attorneys who handle malpractice claims, the best and most consistent results come from the "regulars."

It should also be noted that the selection of outside counsel to work with risk management in the loss prevention and loss control field does *not* mean the automatic selection of the institution's corporate attorney. Familiarity with the corporate structure, bylaws, and institutional politics can be helpful, but it is not essential to the institution's goals in the field.

Having thus identified the type of attorneys who will not be helpful, how should one be chosen? Perhaps the same type of thought process attorneys use can be instructive. In drafting contracts and instruments and in formulating negotiations or correspondence of all types, an attorney considers and plans for the worst possible result—litigation. What will a contract look like in court if there is a breach? How can a testator's intention be made most clear to a probate judge if there is a will contest? What will a jury think about a particular conversation or letter if there is a lawsuit in which it becomes evidence? If all the loss prevention and loss control efforts are for nought and claim is filed, who will be able to obtain the best result? A malpractice specialist with considerable experience in handling the types of claims faced by institutions should be the logical choice. The type of attorney with the knowledge and experience to take a claim to trial and verdict is the logical choice to participate in the full scope of risk management functions. A lawyer who can comfortably handle a trial in which claims of negligence are based upon policy and procedure manuals or Joint Commission on Hospital Accreditations (JCAH) standards is well suited to amending an institution's manuals or ensuring JCAH compliance to prevent future litigation. The lawyer must ensure that claims are more defensible and ultimately less expensive. Such a lawyer will be recognized by the number and types of cases he or she has handled and his or her ability to speak intelligently about concrete problems found by institutions. In selecting an attorney, a person who can give concrete answers to these general questions as they relate to specific hospitals will be the attorney of choice.

The Lawyer in Loss Prevention

Although most institutions are well aware of some of the uses of attorneys in the claims management process, fewer are aware that outside counsel can be useful in the realm of loss prevention as well. The attorneys are therefore underutilized in this field, and many opportunities to prevent or lessen the impact of claims are missed.

A major area where outside litigation counsel can be of assistance is in the review and evaluation of internal working documents (such as rules and regulations of the institution), of the medical staff, and of policy and procedure manuals. Such a review cannot, of course, be addressed to the mechanics of medical or nursing care. Many such documents, however, contain an excess of flowery or philosophical language of uncertain legal effect. For example, an institution might include language in a policy manual that "it is the policy of this hospital to strive to provide the best medical care available.'' Such language is encouraged by many hospital accreditation agencies and associations. But in states where the law allows the standard of care by which an institution is measured to be shown by its own internal documents, such language may result in subjecting the institution to a much higher standard of care. Courts could hold that such a hospital was required to provide the *best* care, rather than reasonable care, thus having a significant effect on individual claims and on the hospital's entire exposure. Many other examples can be found by a quick review of an institution's manuals. Allowing outside counsel to review and make suggestions to change offending language can cost the institution a small amount in fees but could result in savings of tens or hundreds of thousands of dollars in litigation. For example, the language quoted above might be amended to simply state, ''provide the best care obtainable consistent with the requirements and resources available.'' Such a change should be favorable to necessary accrediting agencies yet be fluid enough so as not to set an unobtainably high standard of care.

Another fertile field for the use of outside counsel is in the review of internal working procedures in order to present them in the best light in view of possible future litigation. The entire concept of quality assurance in the form mandated by the JCAH is of concern to all institutions. What the JCAH has not addressed is the effect its mandated procedures have on individual institutions who find themselves in court. While a quality assurance program provides for the beneficial effect of identifying and correcting potential hazards, in so doing it may expose the institution to increased liability in individual cases. For example, the actions of the quality assurance committee may identify that a particular piece of equipment or a particular staff physician or employee might be a risk to patients. If, for example, evaluation shows that a particular surgeon has had a higher than average complication rate in a particular type of surgery, corrective action might be instituted. If a particular patient who has suffered complications seeks legal redress, a distinct danger exists that deliberations of a quality assurance committee (or morbidity committee, medical care evaluation committee, or tissue committee) might be discoverable, or even admissible in the event of a trial, to show prior knowledge of a dangerous condition and failure to act to correct it. This rather simplistic approach, which is favored by many patients' attorneys, ignores administrative realities in terms of the length of time required to identify and correct such problems, especially in view of due process rights to be guaranteed to staff physicians. Perhaps even more important, when institutions and the committees devoted to improving patient care are subjected to this type of outside interference, a real possibility exists for a so-called ''chilling effect.'' Free and open discussion of problems and how to correct them will not occur if members of these types of committees may be hauled into court to testify or if their memoranda or reports are to be rifled by attorneys of disgruntled patients.

Some states recognize such dangers and have provided safeguards, such as the Illinois Medical Studies Act,[1] that provide protection for such committees.

Legislation of this type is not universal, and local rules must be consulted. Even in Illinois, the seemingly express language of this statute is much disfavored by both plaintiffs' attorneys and judges, and extreme care must be taken to remain under the literal wording of the Act to have any opportunity of successfully claiming the privilege.

Institutions would be well served to consult counsel familiar with whatever statutes or court legal protection might be available to protect the sanctity of its quality assurance program from judicial examination. An audit of such procedures by outside counsel could be most helpful in preventing or minimizing interference.

It may even be possible to aggressively use such protection as might be available to shield the actions of the risk manager from discovery. No generalizations can be made because of the wide variety in local law and the functions of the risk management, but the possibility can be explored.

Other areas of loss prevention can also be suggested. Some consideration should be given to types of litigation that are not within the strict confines of professional liability but where the expertise of counsel might be of significant help in preventing or containing a lawsuit. A very significant area in which much litigation seems likely is in the area of staff privileges. With the new thrust toward quality assurance and increased public pressure and internal policing of the medical profession, it seems inevitable that institutions will more often find themselves in the position of measuring the skills of practitioners and being forced to take disciplinary action. The perils of such actions are well known, and it sometimes seems that virtually any such actions result in litigation. While it is somewhat outside the common concept of risk management, common sense would seem to militate that the same problems apply. A thorough review of the staff privilege and discipline requirements to ensure that they are understandable, workable, and legally sufficient can prevent significant litigation costs in the future. Furthermore, when disciplinary action is contemplated, it seems prudent to act as though a lawsuit will be filed. Calling in trial counsel to advise on the procedures from their very inception in order to memorialize the process in a light more favorable to a judge's review can be invaluable.

These examples of the participation of outside counsel in law are not meant to be exhaustive. Consideration of an institution's individual circumstances will readily show areas where additional protection might be obtained by the thorough legal checkup.

The Attorney in Claim Management

The use of outside counsel in claim management is more familiar to health care providers, because they have long been accustomed to working with defense attorneys in the defense of actual lawsuits and occasionally in the preparation of claims for litigation. At the risk of being repetitious, it should again be stressed that each institution will have different needs based upon the strengths and weaknesses of its own staff. The depth of participation of outside counsel is defined by the goal that is to be achieved, which is to ensure that the institution has a thorough understanding of each individual claim, including both the likelihood that there is liability and the extent of exposure. This goal also encompasses the need to obtain this information as quickly as possible, have it as accurate as possible, and have it as up to date as possible as new facts are developed through investigation and litigation. Losses are inevitable. Surprises are not. It is upon just such a thorough understanding of each individual claim that an institution's entire insurance or self-insurance program turns.

Experience teaches that the prompt participation of outside counsel can lead to effective results. This participation can take numerous forms. Some institutions have found it very helpful to rely on the attorney's experience in recognizing potential claims and to have counsel review all incident reports. (Where the in-house reviewer has such experience, as from insurance industry experience, this depth of participation is obviously unnecessary.) One helpful and less expensive alternative has been for the attorney to work closely with the risk manager or other in-house reviewer on a temporary basis to share and impart a feeling for the type of claims that are asserted in the jurisdiction. Outside counsel should have a wide breadth of experience in all types of institutional litigation and will often be able to spot potential claims that are likely of assertion even though the individual institution may have had no experience with such a claim. Once potential claims are identified, the attorney can be of considerable further assistance as discussed below.

Before moving on to the area of claim investigation, however, one important alternative method of early identification of potential claims bears mentioning. As has been intimated, professional liability claims are most often brought by a relatively few attorneys. In larger jurisdictions, such as Chicago, the most serious cases are almost always brought by one of a relative handful of plaintiffs' attorneys. The mere expression of interest by one of these attorneys in a patient's hospital chart should be sufficient to set alarm bells ringing, whether or not an incident report was made. A request to inspect or copy a chart by an attorney prominent in the field of professional liability litigation should trigger an immediate investigation into the circumstances. Often a review of the chart will disclose that a less than desirable result was obtained, and the thrust of further investigation immediately becomes clear. In other cases, it may appear that the reason for a chart review is an auto accident, industrial injury, or other cause for hospitalization, rather than any potential problem in the treatment itself. Nonetheless, the chart should be carefully checked in order to determine whether there were any real or apparent shortcomings in treatment that might lead an experienced plaintiff's attorney to conclude that a malpractice action might also exist. Outside counsel should be well aware of attorneys practicing in the professional liability area, and the attorney's experience should be sought in developing a list of such attorneys in order to "red flag" any chart requests.

Once a potential claim has been identified, it is again appropriate to define the depth of participation of counsel by the exigencies of the case. Since attorneys generally charge by the hour, the extensive use of counsel can be expensive. It is therefore imperative to make the necessary expenditure only in those cases where the potential benefit outweighs the cost. In cases where there is less exposure, attorneys still can be of use in developing a working protocol by which the hospital or other institution can generally operate. Some examples follow.

In true disaster losses, such as an intra-operative anesthesia incident resulting in death or severe injury to a patient, the participation of counsel can be well justified. Under certain circumstances, depending upon the patient's age, marital status, social background, and income, a lawsuit may be virtually inevitable. Under these facts, an immediate phone call (perhaps even while the patient is still in the recovery room if the incident is immediately identified) can be of tremendous help. Defense counsel may have the rare and extremely desirable opportunity to identify and interview witnesses while their recollections are still fresh. It may even be possible to identify, inspect, and preserve documentary evidence, such as notes that have been scrawled on scraps of paper, disposable equipment and supplies, or other vital pieces of physical evidence upon which the successful defense of a claim might turn. Such evidence is seldom available when a substantial time lag exists before defense counsel is engaged. Prompt contact with defense counsel can also instill in the institution's personnel an immediate realization of the gravity of the circumstances and prevent the type of offhand, thoughtless remarks to the patient or family that might later be construed as admissions. Experience also teaches that, since nurses and physicians (particularly house staff) are so geographically mobile, the immediate interview may be the only opportunity to contact witnesses. Nothing can be more frustrating to defense counsel than to be called in to defend a case only to find that the only knowledgeable witnesses have dispersed to the far corners of the country or even of the world.

The impact upon the institution in such a case can be very significant. As has been stated, prompt investigation and participation by defense counsel can ultimately make the difference between a substantial verdict in favor of a plaintiff and winning a case. Perhaps even more significantly, prompt investigation may show that liability does indeed exist. It may be possible to conclude that a settlement should be offered, and such a matter might even be put to rest before the patient or family contacts an attorney. Since a claimant need not share any settlement with an attorney by means of a contingent fee and need not wait the one to five or more years necessary to resolve a lawsuit, it is quite likely that a settlement can be effected at a substantial discount. Thus, even when liability exists, proper use of an attorney can result in substantial savings.

Other cases, because of less severe injury and smaller potential damages, will not warrant this type of intensive preparation. Nonetheless, when it appears that litigation is in the offing, the attorney can be used to help plan and direct an investigation. Since counsel will ultimately be charged with conducting a defense, it is reasonable to obtain his or her suggestions in order to best develop the facts that will be necessary later. The attorney should be used to identify what facts will be at issue in the case and therefore what witnesses will be necessary. After potential witnesses have been identified, they may be contacted and interviewed, and statements may be taken in order to preserve their recollection for later testimony. Once these points have been identified and cataloged by the attorney, the actual legwork involved can be delegated to an outside investigator or even to the institution's own personnel.

It will be important to the facility to keep in contact with outside counsel even after the initial investigation has been performed. His or her experience and training in evaluating the facts that are developed will be important in ensuring that there are no hidden aspects involved in the case. Thus, interviews with witnesses and reviews of records and policy or procedure manuals can result in significant changes in the case that must not be overlooked. Once again, practices must be tailored to the needs if the particular institution. For example, a risk manager with training and practice as a nurse may be well aware that an elderly patient who has suffered a fall and a fracture can go on to develop pneumonia and perhaps even expire. Individuals from a claim or financial background might be unaware of such danger and might feel that the dealth of a patient following an in-house fall might serve only to reduce damages rather than exacerbate them. Review by an outsider can serve as a fail-safe mechanism to ensure that most information developed through the investigation is properly evaluated.

The Lawyer as Negotiator

Reference has previously been made to the possibility that certain claims might be advantageously settled prior to a suit being filed. If the patient has not retained an attorney it would not be ethical for the institution's counsel to negotiate directly with the claimant. Nonetheless, outside counsel can be used very profitably in evaluating the worth of a claim and in suggesting the size of an offer to be made. Counsel's experience will be especially important in calculating what discount would be available in settling a case before suit is filed.

Although some cases are settled before the patient retains an attorney, more, if not most claims, will be initially asserted by a lawyer. The same considerations as to early settlement will apply. When the decision is made to compromise a claim before suit, the use of outside counsel as negotiator is virtually a necessity (except where the risk manager is an experienced claims adjustor). Attorneys are well known for their many antics, and the institution will be well served by having a negotiator as well versed in negotiating techniques as its opponent.

CONCLUSION

The filing of a lawsuit brings the institution to the point where defense counsel is inevitable and where the relationship between attorney and client is well known. The absence of the insuror or intermediary does not have as much effect, and the attorney-client roles are familiar. The relationship need not be further discussed here.

Prior to suit, there are, unfortunately, no clear answers as to what an institution should delegate to outside counsel or keep within its own walls. While some suggestions have been made as to areas where the use of such an attorney might be helpful or profitable, all of the foregoing can be summarized into questions involving four principles:

1. What does the institution need?
2. What are the institution's own strengths or weaknesses in a risk management program?
3. Can the use of an outside expert be cost effective?
4. Where can the outside counsel bring experience and expertise to strengthen the program?

The answers to these questions, which will involve considerable thought and imagination, will dictate how each institution should use outside counsel.

NOTE

1. Illinois Medical Studies Act, Section 8-2101 Code of Civil Procedures of Illinois, et seq.

Chapter 12

Diagnosis Related Reimbursement

Sankey V. Williams, M.D.

The increased attention that has been devoted to hospital cost has led to better understanding of the relationship between resource consumption and hospital output. One consequence has been the development of new measures of the relationship. They are potentially so powerful that already they are being used for new reimbursement programs and new internal control mechanisms. They may help contain costs, improve efficiency, lead to better budgeting and planning, and alter the relationships among hospital power groups. They are known generically as case-mix measures.[1]

The most highly developed and studied of the case-mix measures is the Diagnosis Related Group (DRG) system that was developed at Yale around 1975 and reformulated in 1981.[2] The DRG system is being used in experimental programs to reimburse hospitals in Georgia, New York, and Maryland, but it is the social experiment in New Jersey that has captured the most interest because of its size and its early start.[3] Based on preliminary results from these experiments, the Health Care Financing Administration has proposed using the DRG system to pay hospitals for most Medicare patients.[4]

THE CLASSIFICATION SYSTEM

DRGs are categories in a classification system for inpatients. Each patient can be placed in one, and ideally only one, category based on the patient's primary and secondary diagnoses, surgical procedures, age, and complications. Information from the hospital abstract is used to assign patients to categories.

Creation of the classification system involved identifying which combinations of patient characteristics should be used to define categories. The categories had to meet two requirements. They had to define patients who required similar amounts of hospital resources during the admission, and they had to be compatible with existing classification systems that grouped patients together if they had similar illnesses. The requirement for similar resource consumption meant that patients who were in the same category could be combined for the purposes of reimbursement, budgeting, planning, and other management functions that depended on resource allocation. The requirement for compatibility with existing classifications meant that the categories would recognize clinical characteristics, which were accepted as important measures of resource consumption. It also meant that existing information in the medical record could be used for category assignment and that the system would be understood better by the people who would have to use it.

The patient's length of stay was chosen as the measure of resource consumption because it was easily measured and because it correlated closely with the cost of stay. The patient's primary and secondary diagnoses, the surgical procedures that were performed during the admission, the patient's age, and any comorbid conditions or complications arising during the admission were chosen to describe patients for the analysis.

Major Diagnostic Categories

The analysis that was used to create the reformulated DRG categories began by using the clinical judgment of a representative sample of national experts to identify 23 major diagnostic categories.[2] Each major diagnostic category contained all patients whose primary diagnoses involved the same organ system or a similar pathophysiologic process. Examples include "No. 5 Diseases and Disorders of the Circulatory System" and "No. 18 Infectious and Parasitic Diseases (Systemic)."

Diagnosis Related Groups

The next step of the analysis required the examination of actual data from representative admissions. A sample of 400,000 records was chosen randomly from 1.4 million discharges during the last half of 1979. The records came from 332 of the 2,100 hospitals from throughout the country that provide data to the Commission on Professional and Hospital Activities (CPHA). The 332 hospitals were similar to all 2,100 hospitals with respect to bed size, regional distribution, location with respect to a metropolitan area, and teaching status.

Using these 400,000 records, each major diagnostic category was divided into DRG categories with the help of a computer program.[5] For each major diagnostic category, the program used a statistical technique, automatic interaction detection (AID), to help identify which single patient characteristic best accounted for variation in the length of stay and thus which characteristic best grouped patients together who had similar lengths of stay. For 18 of the 23 major diagnostic categories, the best patient characteristic was the presence and type of surgical procedure, which was then used to define temporary subgroups.

Next, the computer program was used to examine each subgroup to help identify which single remaining patient characteristic best grouped patients who had similar lengths of stay together within the subgroup. For many subgroups, this was the primary diagnosis, which was then used to define still smaller temporary groups within the subgroup. The search for other useful patient characteristics continued as long as groups with more similar lengths of stay could be identified or until predetermined limits were reached. When the groups suggested by the statistical analysis were not compatible with clinical experience, the judgment of a panel of experts was used to choose alternative groups. The end result was a set of terminal categories for each major diagnostic category.

These terminal categories became the DRG categories. Each DRG thus was defined by a combination of patient characteristics that identified a group of patients with similar clinical problems, all of whom had similar lengths of stay. For example, DRG 121, in major diagnostic category No. 5 Diseases of the Circulatory System, included patients without an operation who had an acute heart attack and who survived the admission despite complications. DRG 122 included patients who differed from those in DRG 121 only because they were free of complications. DRG 111 in the same major diagnostic category included patients who underwent surgery for a major vascular reconstruction and who were at least 70 years old or had complications or a comorbid condition. In all, 467 DRGs were identified.

THE REIMBURSEMENT PROGRAM

The purpose of the reimbursement program is to replace the traditional method of hospital payment, which does not provide incentives for efficiency, with a new method that encourages efficiency. The basic idea is to pay the hospital a standard amount for each patient in each DRG regardless of the cost of the admission. Efficient hospitals are allowed to retain the difference between revenues and cost, and inefficient hospitals must absorb the difference. The new method is a prospective reimbursement program because, each year, the hospital knows in advance what it will receive for each patient and, based on its projected case mix, what its overall revenues will be.

For the program to work, every hospital must report information in a uniform way. Patient characteristics are reported using the ICD-9-CM system.[6] Information on the cost of each admission is reported using a standard hospital accounting system developed by the state department of health. Information on patient characteristics and cost are merged and reported together.

In a series of calculations, this information is used to determine the different reimbursement rates for the different DRGs.[3] There are two stages to the calculations. The first calculates the amount to be paid for the variable costs of providing direct patient care The second calculates the amount to be paid for fixed costs, such as the costs of administration, utilities, and depreciation on buildings and equipment. Hospitals are divided into major teaching, minor teaching, and nonteaching groups, and the groups are considered separately in calculating reimbursement rates to recognize the additional costs of training health care personnel.

Variable Costs

In the first stage of the calculations, information on variable costs from every hospital in the three groups is used to calculate a statewide average cost for patients in each DRG during the base year. Differences in regional labor rates are recognized in these calculations by adjusting each hospital's costs according to its regional labor rate. Using information only from the hospital, the hospital's average cost for patients in each DRG also is calculated.

Several categories of patients are excluded from these calculations: those who leave the hospital against medical advice, those who die during the admission, and those who are admitted and discharged on the same day. Also excluded are other patients who have unusually short or long stays regardless of the reason. The definition of an unusually short or long stay is different for different DRGs, and "trim points" have been established to identify these patients.

For variable costs, each hospital's set of reimbursement rates for the different DRGs is calculated by combining the average cost for each DRG in the hospital's labor market with the hospital's average cost for the same DRG. The relative proportions of the two costs that are used to determine the reimbursement rate for a DRG depend on the differences in cost among patients for that DRG. When the differences are small, more of the labor market average cost is used to determine the reimbursement rate. When the differences are large, more of the hospital's average cost is used to determine the reimbursement rate because large differences in hospital cost may mean that different hospitals are treating different types of patients in that DRG.

The reimbursement rates for variable costs that are calculated in the base year are adjusted in the year of payment to account for price inflation of the hospital's inputs. The adjustment factor is calculated from components of the consumer price index, the producer price index, and the employment cost index. (Adjustments are not made for the increased costs that result from increases in the number of hospital personnel or for changes in services.)

The hospital's total reimbursement for variable costs in a given year is calculated by multiplying the number of expected cases for each DRG times the hospital's reimbursement rate for the DRG and then adding the resulting values for all DRGs together. Reimbursement for patients whose admissions fell outside the trim points or were otherwise not included in the calculations is determined by a system of controlled charges.

Fixed Costs

The hospital's reimbursement for fixed cost is calculated separately. For indirect patient-care services that are defined as fixed costs, such as maintenance and administration, the hospital is allowed either actual cost or 110 percent of the median cost of all hospitals after adjusting for the number of admissions, whichever is lower. (If actual cost is less than 90 percent of median cost, the hospital retains one-half of the difference.) The hospital's fixed costs also include the capital costs resulting from leasing expenses, long-term debt, major movable equipment, and property taxes. Allowances are made for working capital. Special allowances are made for uncompensated care, outpatient costs, and some other costs.

Overall Reimbursement

The hospital's overall reimbursement is calculated by adding the total reimbursement for variable costs to the total reimbursement for fixed costs. Using projections, this calculation can be done at the beginning of the payment year so the hospital has a prospective budget, although reconciliation is made at the end of the year if there are discrepancies between the projected and actual inflation rates, number of patients, or other measures.

The overall reimbursement provides two types of incentives. One is the prospective determination of reimbursement, which sets limits within which management must operate. The other is contained in the reimbursement rate for variable costs, which encourages the hospital to manage each admission as efficiently as possible because there is an opportunity for retaining and a risk of losing the difference between reimbursement and cost for each admission.

Billing Rates

To recover its overall costs, the hospital must bill each patient or the third party payer for both the variable and fixed costs. The hospital's billing rate for each DRG is determined by combining the DRG reimbursement rate for variable costs with the hospital's total reimbursement for direct costs. The reimbursement rate for variable cost in each DRG is increased by a constant factor (the fixed costs divided by the total fixed and variable costs) that allows the hospital to recover all its fixed costs. The result is a standard biling rate for each DRG.

Because different third party payers have different contracts with the patient and the hospital, different adjustments must be made to the standard billing rate for different third party payers. These adjustments are complex and depend on provisions for covered services, shared coverage, responsibility for uncompensated care, and negotiated payer differentials.

ANTICIPATED EFFECTS

The effects of using the DRG classification system for a reimbursement program in New Jersey are being evaluated by several different groups, including the Health Care Financing Administration, the Health Research and Educational

Trust of New Jersey, the National Center for Health Services Research, and many others. Definitive answers to the most basic questions about effectiveness are not yet available. Nevertheless, it is the perception of many who are involved that there is enough evidence of probable effectiveness to proceed.

Cost Containment

The single most important question is whether the reimbursement program will control hospital costs. Little is known for certain about this question other than the observation that the increases in hospital costs in New Jersey have been smaller than national averages during the program. Comparable differences existed before the program, however, and it is uncertain to what extent the special features of the DRG reimbursement program can be credited with this apparent effect.[7]

Improved Management Information

More certain, but not much better documented, is the likelihood that the system will help hospital administrators improve internal control by providing improved and timely management information.[8] Hospital administrators who are familiar with the system describe substantial improvements in information and management controls just in meeting the reporting needs of the system.[9] Additional improvements are anticipated as they receive periodic reports that describe their hospital's activity in detail fine enough to identify departmental and even physician differences in patient cost after adjusting for case mix.[7]

Relations between Administrators and Physicians

The reimbursement program puts considerable pressure on administrators to limit costs, which they can do in two general ways. One is to limit the unit cost of the hospital's inputs by limiting increases in employee salaries and the prices paid for drugs, equipment, and other supplies. The other is to limit the number and change the mix of inputs that are used in patient care, but these decisions are under the direct control of the hospital's physicians. Therefore, administrators must influence physicians' patient-management decisions if they are to respond most effectively to the incentives in the reimbursement program. Whether this can be done and how it might be done are issues that are being addressed. Early reports suggest that the attempt is being made and that there are some successes.[7,9] The results will have important implications for how the quality of hospital care is monitored. It may even affect how the hospital is governed and how physicians are paid.[10]

Medical Records

Because the hospital's reimbursement depends on information in the medical record, the quality of that information has become more important than it was previously. In the past, few problems were caused when a patient's age was mistakenly coded as 69 when it was actually 70, but under the new reimbursement program this mistake alone might cause the patient to be assigned to the wrong DRG category and thus for the hospital to receive the wrong reimbursement rate. The new importance of the medical record has made it necessary for hospitals to improve data collection and monitoring procedures, which has been costly in some cases and has given added importance and prominence to medical records departments in all cases.[3,9]

Utilization Review

The purpose of utilization review has changed under the reimbursement program.[3] Previously, utilization review was used to control unnecessarily prolonged stays, but this function is now provided by the incentives in the fixed reimbursement rate for each admission. In the new program, utilization review should be used to monitor for unnecessarily shortened stays that might be induced by the reimbursement incentive. Utilization review should also be used to identify stays that were prolonged inappropriately so the patient's admission would cross an upper trim point and thus qualify for reimbursement outside the program, which means greater hospital revenues.

PROBLEMS

Enough practical and research experience has been gained to identify important problems. Some of the problems result from application of the reimbursement program, but some result from the classification system itself.

Errors in the Discharge Abstract

Because patients are assigned to a DRG category based solely on information contained in the hospital abstract, the system is subject to classification errors that result directly from errors in the abstract.[3] Most studies have found many errors in the abstract. A study of national samples of patients discharged in 1974 reported misclassification errors of 22 to 40 percent.[11] A similar study of patients discharged in 1977 failed to show any significant improvement.[12] A study of 3,000 Medicare patients in one Chicago hospital compared concurrent with retrospective abstracting and found that the two approaches led to the same DRG assignment in only one-third of the cases.[13] A detailed audit, published in 1978, of 50 randomly selected patients in each of 50 New Jersey hospitals found that 20 percent were misclassified.[14] Another study of 2,774 patients discharged from 56 New Jersey hospitals in 1977 found that 17 percent were assigned to the wrong DRG.[15] Nevertheless, it is likely that improved surveillance by the state and third party payers (which now recognize that how much they pay depends on DRG assignment) and by each hospital (which now recognizes that how much it receives also depends on DRG assignment) will result in improved abstract data.

DRG Creep

Because assignment of patients to DRG category depends on information from the medical record, it is possible for systematic errors to influence reimbursement rates. This might occur, for example, if the hospital exerted less effort to detect errors that increased reimbursement than it exerted to detect errors that decreased reimbursement. The result would be a "creep" upward in the distribution of DRG categories with high reimbursement rates.[16] This was a much greater potential problem in the original than in the reformulated DRG classification system because there were considerable discretion in the original system for patient assignment to a DRG category depending on which diagnoses were considered primary and which secondary.

Severity of Illness within DRG Category

Studies of the original DRG classification system have found that, despite the efforts to group patients with similar illnesses together, differences remain that can be explained by differences in the severity or stage of the illnesses.[17] When the classification system was reformulated, considerable effort was expended to reduce this problem. How successful these efforts were is now being studied.

Reproducibility

Reseachers from Blue Cross of Western Pennsylvania were unable to recreate the original DRG classification system when they used data from different patients. They concluded that there were inherent flaws in the DRG approach that precluded its widespread use.[18] The controversy that followed failed to resolve the issue.[19,20,21] The most likely explanation of the failure is that inadequate information was provided by the formulators of the original DRG system on how clinical judgment was combined with statistical considerations in creating the system, which has raised questions about the adequacy of those judgments. This deficiency was addressed directly when the DRG system was reformulated.

In the reformulated DRG system, extensive effort was made to ensure that clinical judgments were the consensus of a representative sample of national experts.

Outliers

Because some patients' lengths of stay are too short or too long and thus fall outside the trim points for the DRG category, these patients are treated as outliers in the classification system. In the reimbursement program, their bills and those of other outliers are based on controlled charges. As many as 30 percent of all admissions are treated as outliers, and this percentage is even higher in some hospitals with fewer admissions.[3] This means that many of the hospital's admissions are not included in the reimbursement program, thereby weakening the program's incentives.

Small Sample Sizes

In a small hospital, in any given year, there may be too few patients in some of the 467 DRG categories. With small numbers, the hospital may admit patients who, by chance, are unusually sick and who require more than the average amount of care. Because the hospital's reimbursement for these patients is based on the average patient, the hospital could receive less than is required to provide care for these patients. Obviously, the hospital could also receive more than is required if the patients who are admitted are by chance less ill than the average. Because these effects occur at random, in any year the increase in one DRG will likely offset the decrease in another DRG, and year-to-year changes will offset each other.

Cost Allocation

Traditionally, many hospital costs have been allocated to patients when indirect measures were used that do not reflect the value of the resources used to provide care. When costs are allocated by multiplying the patient's charges by the hospital's ratio of costs to charges, which is done by almost all hospitals, the allocated cost does not reflect the actual cost because the hospital does not uniformly charge for services in proportion to their cost. Because the DRG classification system uses the length of stay as the dependent variable, attention has not been focused on this problem. Cost allocation still can be a problem, however, because the reimbursement program is based on cost even if the classification system is not. One study has shown that patients in some DRGs are assigned more than the actual cost of their care with the traditional method of cost accounting and, therefore, that the traditional method prevents the DRG system from providing accurate information either for the reimbursement program or for management purposes.[22]

OTHER DRG REIMBURSEMENT PROGRAMS

Within limits, New Jersey's reimbursement program pays the hospital for each admission regardless of the length of stay. The DRG classification system is used to adjust the amount paid for different patients to account for differences in the types of patients admitted.

Other states also are using the DRG classification system to adjust what the hospital is paid for different patients. In these other programs, however, the hospital is paid an adjusted amount for each day of the admission and not for the admission itself. Both types of reimbursement programs provide incentives for more efficient care because they provide the hospital with a prospective budget, and both types of programs adjust payment to recognize differences in the hospital's case mix.

Because one type of reimbursement program pays for the admission and the other type pays for the days of care, however, there are differences in the incentives. An extreme example can be used to illustrate these differences. Assume that one hospital with 467 beds admitted one patient in each DRG category on the first day of the year and did not discharge any of the patients until the last day of the year, when all 467 patients were discharged together. If the hospital were paid for the number of admissions in each category, as is done in New Jersey, it would be paid much less than if it were paid for the number of days in each category, as is done in other states. Both types of reimbursement programs have features that would not permit the extreme differences that are suggested in this example. The existence of trim points in New Jersey's program means that all these patients would fall outside that state's reimbursement program, and effective utilization review in the other state's programs means that the full cost of care would not be reimbursed. Nevertheless, there are more restricted conditions in which the differences in incentives do apply. Under these conditions, New Jersey's reimbursement program, which focuses on admissions, provides more powerful incentives for efficient care than other reimbursement programs, which focus on the days of care.

Three other states are using reimbursement programs that are based on the DRG classification system to pay hospitals.[3] Still another program has been proposed to pay all hospitals for Medicare patients.[4] All but one of these programs focus on the days of care. In Maryland, where the focus is on admissions, the hospital can select one of several case-mix classification systems for its reimbursement program. Although patients are billed for controlled charges, at the end of the year actual revenues are compared with projected revenues, which are guaranteed, and any discrepancies are adjusted. In New York, the DRG classification system has been modified to include additional categories that are defined by the patient's age and other variables. The revised system has been used to develop four sets of per diem rates to correspond to four types of hospitals that are defined by teaching status and geographic location. In Georgia, hospitals are divided into 11 peer groups based on their case mix as defined by the DRG classification system and other variables. Different overall cost ceilings are established for different peer groups, and reimbursement for Medicaid patients depends on each hospital's performance in relation to its peer group's ceiling. Proposals for Medicare patients include the identification of hospital peer groups and the use of an index based on a modification of the DRG classification system.

OTHER CASE-MIX CLASSIFICATION SYSTEMS

The DRG system is only one of several case-mix classification systems, which are at different stages of development.[1] One of the oldest is the Professional Activity Study (PAS) List A, which was developed by the Commission on Professional and Hospital Activities. PAS List A has been used for some time to characterize national hospital activity in yearly publications. PAS List A has so many different categories, however, that it has not been used in reimbursement programs because of the problem of small sample sizes in many hospitals.

The Disease Staging system was developed using only the clinical judgment of a panel of experts to identify patients who were in different stages of their illnesses. Unlike the DRG system, statistical techniques were not used to identify patients with similar lengths of stay or similar costs. Both the DRG and the Disease Staging systems account for roughly equal amounts of overall variation in charges.[23] Because of the differences in development, however, it is possible that the Disease Staging system accounts for different characteristics than the DRG system and that some combination of the two might further improve both.

The Patient Severity Index is the most recent of these case-mix systems.[24] It differs from the others because there are only four categories in the index. The goal has been to identify patient characteristics that are independent of diagnosis and other traditional patient characteristics yet that identify patients who are more or less severely ill. The Patient Severity Index is also being studied as a way of modifying the DRG system to further account for the severity of illness.

NOTES

1. J.D. Bentley and P.W. Butler, "Measurement of Case Mix," *Topics Health Care Finance,* Summer, vol. 8, 1982 no. 4, pp. 1–12.

2. R.B. Fetter, *The New ICD-9-CM Diagnosis Related Group (DRG) Classification Scheme: User's Manual,* vol. 1 (New Haven, Conn.: School in Organization and Management, Yale University, 1981).

3. P.L. Grimaldi and J.A. Micheletti, *DRGs: A Practitioner's Guide* (Chicago: Pluribus Press, 1982).

4. J.K. Iglehart, "The New Era of Prospective Payment for Hospitals," *New England Journal of Medicine* 307 (1982):1288–1292.

5. R. Mills et al., "AUTOGRP: An Interactive Computer System for the Analysis of Health Care Data," *Medical Care* 14 (1976):603–615.

6. *ICD-9-CM International Classification of Diseases, 9th Revision, Clinical Modifications.* Ann Arbor, Mich.: Commission on Professional and Hospital Activities, 1978.

7. J.K. Iglehart, "New Jersey's Experiment with DRG-based Hospital Reimbursement," *New England Journal of Medicine* 307 (1982):1655–1660.

8. J.D. Thompson et al., "Planning, Budgeting and Controlling—One Look at the Future: Case-mix Cost Accounting," *Health Service Research* 14 (1979):111–125.

9. D.A. Bradley and P.S. Cooper, "Perspectives on the DRG Experiment: the Administrators' Reactions (Interviews)," *Interchange* (The National Health Care Management Center, University of Pennsylvania) 1 (Summer 1981):7–12.

10. H. Schwartz, "Can the U.S. Make Hospital Costs Go Down?" *Wall Street Journal*, November 2, 1982, p. 28.

11. L.K. Demlo et al., "Reliability of Information Abstracted from Patients' Medical Records," *Medical Care* 16 (1978):995–1005.

12. L.K. Demlo and P.M. Campbell, "Improving Hospital Discharge Data: Lessons from the National Discharge Survey," *Medical Care* 19 (1981):1038–1040.

13. C. Barnard and T. Esmond, "DRG-based Reimbursement: The Use of Concurrent and Retrospective Clinical Data," *Medical Care* 19 (1981):1071–1082.

14. New Jersey State Department of Health, *Reliability of New Jersey Hospital Discharge Abstracts,* DHEW-HRA Contract no. 230-76-0681, December 1978.

15. R.F. Corn, "The Sensitivity of Prospective Hospital Reimbursement to Errors in Patient Data," *Inquiry* 18 (Winter 1981):351–360.

16. D.W. Simborg, "DRG Creep: A New Hospital-acquired Disease," *New England Journal of Medicine* 304 (1981):1602–1604.

17. S.B. Horn and D.N. Schumacher, "Comparing Classification Methods: Measurement of Variations in Charges, Length of Stay, and Mortality," *Medical Care* 20 (1982):489–500.

18. W.W. Young et al., "Assessment of the AUTOGRP Patient Classification System," *Medical Care* 18 (1980):228–244.

19. J.M. Cameron and R.A. Knauf, "DRGs: An Assessment of the Assessment," *Medical Care* 19 (1981):243–245.

20. W.W. Young et al., "Response to Dr. Cameron and Dr. Knauf," *Medical Care* 19 (1981):245–248.

21. W.W. Young et al., "The Measurement of Case Mix," *Medical Care* 20 (1982):501–512.

22. S.V. Williams et al., "Improved Cost Allocation in Case-Mix Accounting," *Medical Care* 20 (1982):450–459.

23. R.P. Ament et al., "Three Case-Type Classifications: Suitability for Use in Reimbursing Hospitals," *Medical Care* 20 (1982):460–467.

24. S.D. Horn, "Measuring Severity of Illness: Comparisons across Institutions," *American Journal of Public Health* 73 (1983):25–31.

Part IV

Quality Assurance Strategies

Chapter 13

Information Management in Quality Assurance

Jesus J. Peña, M.P.A., J.D.; Richard Quan, M.B.A., J.D.; and Joseph N. Cintron, M.H.A.

The Joint Commission on Accreditation of Hospitals (JCAH) has developed a working definition of the term *quality assurance* as follows: "A system to evaluate and monitor the quality of patient care and the quality of facility management."[1] The goal of quality assurance is to improve the quality of patient care and the performance of all health professionals involved in the delivery of health services. This is an integral part of the mission and hospital function at almost every hospital.

The quality assurance process involves the following five steps:

1. problem identification;
2. problem assessment;
3. implementation of corrective action;
4. follow-up; and
5. report of findings.

The effectiveness of a quality assurance program is measured and evaluated by comparing the quality of care delivered to the objectives and standards that are previously set. These standards must be reasonably quantifiable and measurable to eliminate bias and subjective results.

The information needs of a quality assurance program require the coordination of many components of the health care delivery system. As a result, quality assurance programs in health care institutions have become dependent on data from many sources within the hospital. These data sources include (but are not limited to) medical records,[1] utilization review, Professional Standards Review Organization (PSRO), incident reports, infection reports, and activity summaries. Since every data source has its value, it's up to the administrator to decide what data source is best, not only for the internal management of the hospital but also for external parties who review the institutions, such as JCAH; federal, state and local regulatory agencies; and third party reimbursors. In order to coordinate and manage this large volume of data relating to the quality assurance function, many hospitals have adopted the computer to meet this need. At the present time, the application of information systems and computer technology to quality assurance presents the administrator with an excellent opportunity to develop a system that will link clinical and administrative information for planning and control purposes.

ROLE OF EVALUATION IN QUALITY ASSURANCE

There are generally three accepted approaches to the measurement of the quality of patient care in the hospital environment: structural, procedural, and performance.[2] An experienced administrator should be familiar with these three approaches in order to set up an information management system in quality assurance.

The structural approach involves the analysis of the material and social instrumentalities that are needed to provide development of medical bylaws that reflect the institution's needs, the proper credentialing mechanism, and the environmental factors used by the JCAH in relation to space, equipment, age of the facilities, and other environmental characteristics of the hospital.

The procedural approach to quality assurance is based on an analysis of the process of the delivery of care. This approach closely interrelates with the structural approach.

Most institutions use a mix of direct evaluation of practices and a retrospective review of medical records, cost analysis reports, and regulatory agencies' recommendations. The new technology available through the use of computers has made possible the integration of direct evaluation and retrospective review and even the projection of events through the use of forecasting techniques. The primary role of the administrator in the procedural approach is to develop the internal controls that are going to be used as a standard of measurement.

The third approach is the performance approach—how the institution performs in relation to the standards developed for similar institutions. What is the length of stay in comparison with the standards of utilization review, morbidity, and mortality in relation to the community served? The administrator is the ideal person to refine the relationship between these indicators and the quality of care provided at the institution, as well as evaluating and incorporating the external variables that affect the quality of care delivery at the institution.

The three approaches, when combined, should produce the basis for the quality assurance program.[3] In addition, the evaluation of the results should be used for cost control and financial management purposes. For instance, by comparing pre-operative and post-operative diagnoses, a system can be established for quality assurance in the operating room and some unnecessary costs can be determined. If the number of repeat X-rays is over the standard, determination can be made as to whether this is due to the training of the technician, film quality, poor processing, or outdated film or chemicals. In any case, a proper evaluation of the circumstances will improve the quality of care and eliminate unnecessary costs.

Computerized Information Systems and Quality Assurance

Four years ago, a leading U.S. management consultant stated that "the most significant management development of the 20th century—the computer—is not being used effectively by hospital management in their greatest hour of need."[4]

Unfortunately, this statement still holds true for many hospitals, especially the small ones with less than 100 beds. Dorenfest found that only 50 percent of these small hospitals with less than 100 beds used computers in their operations in 1980. (See Table 13-1 on page 204.)

Because of the large amount of capital investment, time, and training involved in the hospital's decision to use computers in their operation, most of the hospitals chose to computerize the financial management areas such as billing, payrolls, and financial reporting. The financial benefits are more visible and the return on the computer investment can be calculated more easily than in other areas of the hospital. The returns on the use of computer systems continued to improve as the costs of the hardware declined due to rapid advances in computer technology.

During the last few years, the success of computerized billing has led to a reevaluation of the attitude of hospital directors and administrators toward a more extensive use of computers, especially in the areas of information management and quality assurance. The computer's attributes of timeliness, speed, accuracy, data access, and reliability are now being recognized by hospital personnel in the labor-intensive hospital environment. Hospitals that use computer systems have noted increased productivity, cost savings, and increased revenues as a direct economic benefit. For example, the reduction or elimination of handwritten, manual forms frees valuable staff time for better patient care and management with a resultant increased productivity. Cost savings are achieved through personnel reductions since many clerical functions are eliminated. In addition, the elimination of manual forms reduces paper costs. With more timely and accurate information provided by the computer, previously "lost" charges and claims can be "recaptured" and thus increase revenues for the hospital.

There are many noneconomic benefits to the use of computerized information systems. The National Center for Health Services Research has documented improvement in response time for communications and increased availability of nursing staff time for direct patient care in hospitals that used computerized information systems.[5]

Computer applications are becoming the norm in the medical industry. They can be generally classified according to the functional departments in hospital administration: patient management; outpatient-E.R.; billing and accounts receivable; medical records and utilization review (PSRO), payroll-personnel management; accounts payable; general ledger; pharmacy; inventory management; fixed assets accounting; preventive maintenance; radiology; risk management monitoring; and dietary systems. Information management in quality assurance includes all of the nonfinancial computer applications mentioned above. The common denominator of these systems from the quality assurance point of view is that they simplify the logistics of tracking patients through the hospital and enhance decision-making ability with clinical and management information in usable report format.

A computerized patient management system provides an efficient means of centralizing information for patients undergoing treatment at the facility. Admissions for inpatient care, billing and accounts receivable, outpatient services, medical records, and PSRO reporting are maintained by the computer system. On-line data entry, file maintenance, editing, or correcting information on file can be readily achieved using the computer terminal.

A computerized medical records and utilization review (PSRO) system provides a patient tracking and charting system with the capability of abstracting and indexing the information. Detailed and summary reports can be produced for all phases of the patient/hospital/physician activity. For example, a computerized medical records system can maintain a profile for each patient stay; provide a location file for medical records; search medical records files for historical information; assign medical record numbers automatically; accumulate data from outpatient and inpatient activities; provide on-line access to chart location; provide automatic notification of admission/discharge/transfer activity; remind doctors of incomplete charts; produce periodic indexes for diseases, physicians, procedures, and infection control. A utilization review system can provide a review worksheet upon admission; identify patients requiring interim bills; produce patient activity worksheets; provide periodic activity summaries; select inpatients prior to expected discharge for extension review; and provide attending physician summary and activity listings.

Rogers and Haring conducted a study of 241 patients whose records were computerized and 238 control patients whose records were kept manually.[6] Their findings indicated that patients with computerized records and the proper automated utilization review spent fewer days in the hospital and received more complete referrals for consultation. In general, their records reflect a higher detection of new problems than those of the patients under the manual system.

A computerized outpatient-E.R. system can trace the patient's visit to the hospital from registration through billing. The most efficient systems can use on-line processing of patient information. These systems can assign patient account numbers; update the historical file with current information for each visit; retain a permanent file on each patient; reprint registration forms on demand; provide the patient with a preliminary bill at time of discharge; provide current billing information; and generate periodic statistical reports.

A pharmacy system provides control of medication purchasing, inventory, receiving, and distributing functions. The system provides management with drug utilization analysis, narcotic control, and reporting of pharmacy charges. In addition, auxiliary messages or cautionary statements can be entered to assist nursing personnel in the proper administration of drugs.

Risk Management and Quality Assurance

In a previous chapter, it was pointed out that risk management is the newest addition to quality assurance and is a factor that is increasingly considered by the JCAH, insurance companies, unions, and the hospital staff. As hospital staff and the general public become more aware of the alarming number of incidents happening daily in all hospitals and the costly implication of some incidents, more institutions across the country will work toward the creation of programs on loss prevention and examination of problem areas. The same situation has been a source of concern to the JCAH, insurance companies, and unions.

Most risk management programs have been developed with two goals in mind: (1) to prevent harm to patients, visitors, and staff; and (2) to minimize financial loss to a facility. The effective risk management programs tend to emphasize harm prevention and are incorporated into an overall facility-wide quality assurance program. A comprehensive quality assurance/risk management system is designed to gather and evaluate important information on all undesirable events or trends and to use professional time and resources efficiently with minimal duplication. A QA/RM system includes all clinical and administrative functions that seek to identify or solve problems related to the quality of patient care, such as medical and other professional staff activity reviews, cost-containment programs, standards compliance activities, and risk management. There is no doubt that quality assurance and risk management share: (1) the commitment to eliminate or reduce problems in patient care; (2) harm and loss prevention; and (3) analyses of related data. As a result, a great number of hospitals have developed combined QA/RM programs that focus on this new dimension of the health care industry.

Because each of the quality assurance and risk management functions produce and use the same or similar information, this area is an ideal candidate for a computerized system. Each function can feed and draw information from a central data base.

A typical computerized risk management program includes the recording and coding of data for each incident. For example, the incident might include data identifying the patient; the specific place, date and time of the incident; how many people (patients and/or staff) were involved and their roles (i.e., aggressor, victim, etc.); and the general cause of the incident. Usually over 30 types of incidents are recorded by the hospital staff. The incidents range from animal bites or insect stings to incorrect medication, assaults, and suicides.

Table 13-1 Sample Hospitals Classified by Computer Use

Bed Size	Total	Using Computers 1979		Using Computers 1980		Not Yet Using Computers December, 1980	
		Number	% of Total	Number	% of Total	Number	% of Total
Under 100	42	16	38.1%	21	50.0%	21	50.0%
100–199	58	53	91.4%	55	94.8%	3	5.2%
200–299	45	43	95.6%	43	95.6%	2	4.4%
300–399	33	32	97.0%	32	97.0%	1	3.0%
400–499	25	25	100.0%	25	100.0%	0	0
500—Over	47	47	100.0%	47	100.0%	0	0
Total	250	216	86.4%	223	89.2%	27	10.8%

Source: Copyright 1980 by Sheldon I. Dorenfest & Associates, Ltd. Not to be reproduced without permission.

An initial report on incidents for a given period of time will generally include a breakdown of types of incidents by service unit. Comparing a series of these figures can give an accurate indication of trends in various types of incidents over time. Once the relevant issues and problems are identified, more detailed reports can be generated that focus on specific types of incidents. Corrective action can then be taken.

Trends on the Horizon

The latest developments in information system technology, in conjunction with the availability of computer hardware at extremely low cost and the introduction of specific software packages designed to meet hospital needs, offer the potential for hospitals to use such technology to improve the quality of care at reasonable cost. The current computer systems have the attributes of modularity, integration with other systems, flexibility, relative ease of use and operation, reliability, and confidentiality. These systems are highly cost effective in the hospital environment.

Indications are that information systems are now used more extensively as an aid to quality assurance in hospitals, especially those with medium to large capacities. More hospitals have the capability to integrate the patient management and financial data from computerized information files, and the results have been better use of data at a lower cost and higher performance.

The availability of computer services based on distributed data processing systems and time-shared large off-site computers offers the small hospitals, those with 150 beds or less, the chance to establish a quality assurance system to satisfy their needs. The trend, however, is for individual departments within a hospital to acquire their own "turn-key" micro- or minicomputers capable of "networking" or communicating with other computer systems. Networking of systems allows the rapid sharing and exchanging of localized information, pooling of resources, and greater accessing to centralized files.

Daniel S. Schechter, publisher of the *Journal of the American Hospital Association*, recently stated that:

> Many would argue that no single area of technology has been more pervasive in its impact on society than that encompassing the use of computers to store and analyze vast quantities of data. The so-called information explosion owes both its birth and its continued intensity to the computer phenomenon.
>
> Successful management of hospitals in a time of rapidly changing environmental conditions necessitates timely acquisition and application of information on all aspects of a hospital's internal operations and on its relationship to other providers and to its community. Although hospitals have long been involved with computer technology, the arrival of mini- or microcomputerization has extended the use of

data processing well beyond the traditional applications in accounting and financial management. The "buzz" term now is management information systems, and hospitals are responding enthusiastically to the need to accumulate and analyze data on operations.[7]

With the ever-growing use of automated hospital information systems, the hospital administrator must recognize the need for the right people to coordinate or direct an effective quality assurance program. What is needed in the modern health care facility are people with the proper training in information systems analysis and design and program evaluation. In addition, any program in quality assessment should take into consideration risk management as an integral part of the quality assurance program. The administrative staff as well as the trustees of the health care facility should raise their level of awareness and understanding about the role of the computer in the hospital environment through continuing education and management seminars. In addition, education and training programs in using and operating the computer should be made available to all staff members. With the full support and commitment of the administrators and staff to automated hospital systems, the quality of care provided will improve significantly.

NOTES

1. The Joint Commission on Accreditation of Hospitals, *Accreditation Manual For Hospitals* (Chicago: Joint Commission on Accreditation of Hospitals, 1982), p. 152.

2. A. Donabedian, "The Quality of Medical Care," in *Quality Assurance in Hospitals*, ed. N.O. Graham (New York: Aspen, 1980), pp. 15–20.

3. A. Ricklin, *Quality Assurance*. Paper presented at the conference on Program Evaluation: A Tool for Health Care Administrators, Hofstra University, Hempstead, N.Y., July 17–18, 1981.

4. J. Navarro, "Future of Hospitals." Paper presented at the First Latin-American Health Exposition, Panama, September 15, 1981.

5. "Demonstration and Evaluation of a Total Hospital Information System," NCHSR Research Summary Series, DHEW Publication No. (HRA) 77-3188 (Washington, D.C.: U.S. Government Printing Office, 1977), p. 7.

6. J.L. Rogers and O.M. Haring, "The Impact of a Computerized Medical Records Summary System on Incidence and Length of Hospitalization," *Medical Care* 17, no. 6 (1979):618–630.

7. D.S. Schechter, Editorial, *Hospitals* 15 (1981):14.

Chapter 14

Quality Assurance and the Patient Record

Christine T. Kovner, R.N., M.S.N.

The patient record provides documentation of the care given and the patient's response to that care. Although much of the literature refers to the medical record, the author prefers the term *patient record* because it reflects the reality that the record is about a patient and many health providers contribute information to the record. This chapter will focus on the patient record used in hospitals and will discuss the relationship of the patient record to the hospital's quality assurance program. The advantages and disadvantages of using the patient record in evaluation will be discussed. Some suggestions for improving patient records used in quality assurance programs will be made.

Quality assurance and the patient record are so interrelated that it is hard to determine which should come first, the design of the patient record or the design of the quality assurance program.

WHY HAVE PATIENT RECORDS?

There are several reasons that health care providers maintain records of patient care. The American Hospital Accreditation identifies three as follows:

1. a means of communication among practitioners caring for the patient;
2. a source of data for present and future research; and
3. a record of how the patient responded in the past guides future treatment.[1]

In addition to the above reasons, the record serves as written documentation of care given, which can be useful in the event of legal action. When both the nurse's and the physician's progress notes indicate, through objective and subjective notation, that a patient's casted leg was evaluated four times per day during hospitalization, and the leg was found to have good color and circulation, it is more difficult for the patient or his attorney to convince a jury that his leg was injured by physician and/or nurse neglect.

207

Many hospitals maintain patient records because records are required by the Joint Commission on Accreditation of Hospitals. Finally, the patient record serves as a source of valuable data for the quality assurance program. This chapter will focus on the use of the patient record in quality assurance programs.

SOME OBSERVATIONS OF QUALITY ASSURANCE PROGRAMS

The quality of health care can be conceptualized in many ways. It can mean structure, process, or outcome or some combination of the three. In Chapter 10, McAuliffe discusses the pros and cons of using process or outcome when measuring quality. Whatever conceptualization the organization chooses to use (and it is important that the organization identify what conceptualization of quality it is using), some system for implementing the quality assurance program will have to be developed.

A variety of quality assurance models are described elsewhere in this book; however, quality assurance programs typically follow a model similar to that shown in Exhibit 14-1.

The exact process used for a quality assurance program varies from hospital to hospital and often varies by service within a hospital. The Joint Commission on the Accreditation of Hospitals recommends that the record be standardized for the entire hospital.[2] This facilitates the staff's ability to document care. Although this offers autonomy for each hospital and service, it makes comparisons among hospitals almost impossible. The requirements of the quality assurance program should influence the nature of the patient record, although often the organization and structure of the record influences the quality assurance program. Remember that a hospital can be held legally accountable to its own standards and expectations, both for the quality of care expected and the specified requirements regarding the patient record.

TYPES OF PATIENT CARE RECORDS

Currently there are two common types of patient care records in use in hospitals in the United States. The unit record is a chronological record of all hospital, emergency room, and outpatient care. The unit record may have integrated progress notes where nurses, physicians, and other health care providers enter their notes in the same section in chronological order. The unit record can also be organized by specialty with separate progress notes for physicians, nurses, and other providers.

Exhibit 14-1 Quality Assurance Model

General Model	Example
1. Values are identified. (This step is not always explicit.)	1. The philosophy of the organization specifies that patients will actively participate in their care.
2. Problems and/or areas of interest are identified. (These can be identified by any staff member.)	2. The quality assurance committee decides to evaluate patient participation in care.
3. Criteria are established. (At this point it could be decided to use implicit criteria and evaluate structure, process, or outcome, or some combination, partly depending on the identified problems.)	3. The quality assurance committee meets to determine what the criteria will be. Perhaps they review journal articles, survey physicians and nurses, and see what other hospitals do.
4. Standards are developed. (Again this can be implicit.)	4. The committee decides to audit hysterectomy patients; the expectation is that 90 percent of patients will participate in making decisions about their care. A tool found in the literature will be used.
5. Data are collected.	5. Concurrent patient records are audited for all hysterectomy patients operated on in June 1982.
6. Action is taken to remedy situations if deficient. Praise is given if successful.	6. An audit finds that 75 percent of patients have actively participated in their care. The committee reports this to staff and administration. The committee decides to repeat data collection on patients who had hernia surgery. The in-service department schedules a session on patient participation in care.

The other common type of patient record is the problem-oriented record (POR).[3] When using the POR, the staff identifies patient problems. Notes are then written with specific reference to patient problems with the record no longer precisely chronological, but chronological for each identified problem. The POR can be organized by specialty and is often referred to as the problem-oriented medical record (POMR). Medical problems and other health provider-identified problems are identified and noted in separate sections. The POR can also be integrated in relation to a single patient problem list. All providers must then make progress notes with reference to each problem. When using the unit record, separate note sheets are usually kept in chronological order for laboratory results, temperature, pulse and respiration, weight and other "objective" measures. The POR system requires the notation of some of these objective measures on the POR progress notes, though some separate note sheets are also included.

THE RELATIONSHIP OF THE RECORD TO QUALITY

There are many indicators of the quality of care provided. These indicators are (or should be) operationally defined by the hospital. Such definitions will relate to how the institution conceptualizes quality care. Once the concept is clarified, there are many sources of data to use to evaluate the care provided and received. Providers and consumer patients can be interviewed and/or observed. An end result of care, such as mortality rates, can be examined. However, the patient care record is by far the most common source of data about what the providers do for the patient and how that patient responds.

The major reason to use the patient record as a source of data for quality assurance is that the record is a readily accessible source of data. Other reasons for using a written record include its use as a base for sampling a health problem; for verification of diagnosis in the record with data recorded (such as lab reports); for review of data; to find missed diagnoses; and as a source of information on outcomes before discharge.[4]

There are many disadvantages or limitations in the use of data as usually recorded in the patient record in quality assurance. Williamson lists seven, as follows:

- No check is possible on the quality of recorded data;
- A substantial percentage of relevant hospital data are not recorded;
- Pertinent preadmission ambulatory care data are not recorded;
- Focus on organic pathology often precludes recording of psychosocial factors, patient understanding, and compliance information;
- Missed diagnoses go unrecognized, especially for patients who are not admitted and thus have no charts;
- Health outcomes are usually not recorded except as "improved," "not improved," or "worse" at discharge; and
- Post discharge follow-up data are not obtained.[4]

The above are subjective statements based on Williamson's long experience in the evaluation field.

There are few studies that empirically test whether the record is an accurate representation of the care provided. Starfield et al. report on a study of primary care providers.[5] They compared medical records with independent observations for information on coordination of care. The authors conclude that overall there was congruency between the record and observation in 70 to 85 percent of the interactions with patients. In the researchers' view, when the information was important, there was a higher level of congruency—95 percent for distinctly identified problems, 96 percent for major drugs, 94 percent for abnormal tests, and 83 percent for problems in the text of the progress notes. The researchers conclude that the findings of the study support using the record to evaluate the recognition by practitioners of important information relevant to patient treatment.

In a similar study by Romm and Putnam, medical records were compared with verbatim transcripts of ambulatory care visits of patients and physicians.[6] The information in the record was broken down into information units, such as chief complaint, diagnosis, and tests, and 59 percent of the units present in either the record or the recording were found in the written record. For the chief complaint, there were 92 percent of the units present and for the medical history 29 percent present. A particularly interesting finding in this study is that the record had *more* complete information than the recording about therapies and tests. In the recording, the physicians told patients they were prescribing drugs or ordering tests, whereas in the record the specific drugs and/or tests were mentioned. While there has been an assumption that more care is provided than the record indicates, it may be that in some cases less care is provided than is indicated.

Both of these studies support the position that not all that goes on in an encounter between patient and provider is recorded. It should be noted that both studies were conducted in ambulatory care settings, and the results may not be directly applicable to an inpatient setting. To what extent should organizations insist that the data even more accurately reflect actual practice before using it for an evaluation study? The costs of increasing the accuracy of recorded data may be too high to justify certain levels of accuracy. Accuracy can be increased by allowing more time to chart, a personnel expense. Accuracy can also be increased by audio recording all interactions and preparing a written record from the recording.

Related to accurate recordkeeping is a physician encounter that the author experienced. While seeing a rather prominent university faculty obstetrician to determine if she was pregnant, the author was pleased at the detail with which he commented on her health status. He made such comments as "breasts engorged," and "vaginal bluish color." As is typical in gynecological examinations, there was a woman in white present. After happily hearing the physician state that he was quite sure that she was pregnant, the author commented at her pleasure in having such an informative exam. The obstetrician said that as he examines a patient his secretary (the woman in white) writes down what he is saying on the patient's chart. Following the visit, he reviews the secretary's notes and signs the chart. Although somewhat expensive, as it requires two people, it seems to be an accurate way of recording patient data. (And it also keeps the patient informed!)

The mentioned empirical studies compare what is written on the record to what is either audio recorded or observed. How does what is recorded compare to what actually happened? How reliable is information abstracted from a patient record? Demilo et al. report on two particularly well designed and implemented studies of information abstracted from medical records.[7] Participants in the study were drawn from a controlled stratified national sample of nonfederal short-term hospitals. The purpose of the study was to assess the reliability of abstracted patient record information. Independent reabstracting of records was conducted, and results were compared to the original abstract. When discrepancies were found, the records were reviewed to find reasons for the discrepancies. Both studies found data on admission and discharge dates and sex to be quite reliable. However, reabstracting agreed with the original abstracting in only 57.2 and 65.2 percent of the cases for diagnosis. For procedures, reliabilities were 78.9 percent and 73.2 percent. Reliability varied with the particular diagnosis. In one study for the diagnosis of cataract, there was agreement of 97.3 percent, while for the diagnosis of cerebrovascular accident there was only 41.5 percent agreement.

The authors propose that discrepancies are often large enough to "preclude the use of such data for detailed research and evaluation. . . ."[7a] When using abstracted data, it is important therefore for the investigator to verify that observed changes are "real" rather than a result of increased reliability.

The above empirical data suggest that the patient record should not be the sole source of data for a quality assurance program. However, given the availability of the record, it will most likely continue to be one important source of data for quality assurance programs.

IMPROVING THE RECORD AS A SOURCE OF DATA

When viewing the patient care record as a data source, it is important to look at the retrievability of data because it can be difficult, expensive, and, as the previous study mentioned, unreliable to abstract data. Several potential problems can occur. Handwriting is often illegible. Abbreviations are used that are not familiar to chart reviewers. Information about a particular problem is often found in several sections of the chart. Information is missing or is not dated clearly. The dilemma for the evaluator is whether missing or illegible information means the action was not taken or observed or merely not recorded or not understandably reported.

Careful organization of the record can enhance recording. The use of checklists and charts can make recording easier to write down and read and therefore more likely to occur and be used. Health care providers can be encouraged to write legibly perhaps by reminding them that "if it can't be read, it didn't happen." Typewritten transcripts can be used. Abbreviations can be standardized. The

American Hospital Association suggests a list of acceptable abbreviations that, if accepted by all institutions, could help standardize abbreviations across institutions.[1] Each institution must decide how nonrecorded information will be handled. Legal implications for each jurisdiction should be kept in mind.

Though no clear figures are available, the cost of a quality assurance program can be great. Clearly the cost of professionals' time is more expensive than nonprofessionals. In the interest of cost saving, some of the data retrieval for a quality assurance program can be done by nonprofessionals. The ability of nonprofessionals to do this will depend to some extent on the organization and legibility of the patient record. It will depend on the clarity of the quality assurance guidelines that state which information is needed. Those designing both the record and quality assurance programs should keep in mind who will be extracting the data. It may be worth the initial costs of modifying a record for the long-term personnel savings of data collection by nonprofessionals.

For example, if an outcome audit is to be performed, it may be worthwhile to have a section of the chart where patient goals achieved are noted. Using a traditional progress note, the fact that the patient is afebrile may be noted on the physician's progress notes and in nurse's notes that are buried in a narrative in the middle of the chart. Information on temperature may also be found on the temperature, pulse, and respiration sheets. One solution would be to have clear audit directions for finding this information. An example is shown below.

Example of Audit Directions for Finding Information

Criteria	Standard	Chart Location
patient afebrile 48 hours post surgery	100%	TPR Sheet Nurse's notes up to 48 hours post-op*

Another option for the organization concerned with outcomes is to have a section of the chart for patient goals (outcomes) such as that shown below.

Patient Outcomes

Patient name_____	Goal Met		Date Achieved
Afebrile 48 hours post surgery	yes	no	10/6/8—
Ambulatory without assistance	yes	no	10/8/8—

In addition to assisting in data extraction, listing goals achieved gives the staff a sense of accomplishment and reminds them of areas in which further effort may be required.

---

*If a patient has no fever following surgery, this may never appear in the nurse's progress notes, but would have to appear in TPR Sheet. However, if the patient has a fever, this would be in the nurse's notes.

In some ways, the problem-oriented record organizes goal achievement with the use of a problem list. Resolution of problems is usually achievement of goals (or favorable outcomes). Whether an organization uses the POR or unit system depends on the needs and political climate in an institution. Quality assurance staff should note which system is in use and work with medical records personnel and others to devise appropriate audit directions.

DESIGNING APPROPRIATE QUALITY ASSURANCE PROGRAMS

In addition to his recommendations to devise appropriate records and to enforce standards, Donabedian suggests allowing for discussion of findings with the caregivers.[8] This last point is perhaps the most important. For the quality assurance program to function effectively, staff must be able to offer explanations and suggestions for change. There may be compelling reasons why standards of care were not met.

For example, a sample of patient records of diabetics in community hospital A was audited. Low adherence to agreed-upon quality assurance standards was found in June. This was in the recorded references to patient teaching by both physicians and nurses. Small group discussion with staff later revealed that a health educator was hired at the beginning of June. There was confusion among staff about the educator's role and responsibility for both the actual patient education and recording of educational efforts. Clarification of the role and responsibility of the health educator with both the educator and the staff involved brought charting and presumably patient education to a satisfactory level the following month. Had the quality assurance staff merely referred the problem of low adherence to patient education standards to the in-service department, staff in the in-service department might have prepared extensive programs on how to teach patients. The how-to was apparently not the problem in this case, but rather the problem was a confusion in whether the health educator, nurses, or physicians would perform the teaching.

Any quality assurance program should also provide information about the findings to the staff being evaluated. It is important for the staff to be able to discuss findings perhaps in small group sessions or in one-to-one discussions, where staff may be in a non-threatening environment.

Organizational Relationships

The activities of the patient record (medical record) department and the quality assurance program should be coordinated because of the close interrelationship of their activities. At the very least, a member of the quality assurance team should participate in patient record committee(s), so that changes in the patient record can be viewed in relation to the quality assurance program. Patient record personnel can make a contribution to quality assurance programs. Their expertise in data retrieval, analysis, and tabulation can aid the quality assurance program.

Computerized Records

A technological innovation that is influencing the relationship between the patient care record and quality assurance is computerization. The use of the computer for recordkeeping is becoming more common. A packaged program for recordkeeping can be purchased or rented, or a system can be designed for or by a particular hospital.

The use of the computerized record offers the opportunity, or some would say the constraint, of standardizing the data accumulated about patients. Manual data accumulation, such as a typical progress note, offers an array of choices limited only by the imagination and pen of the health provider. Computerization limits the choices to those options programmed into the system. Common problems such as abbreviations and illegible handwriting are eliminated, and data retrieval has the potential to become easier. There is also the opportunity to program the computer to retrieve data to compare relationships of preselected variables that can be useful for both research and quality assurance.

Inherent in this is clarification of roles and responsibilities of health providers. Romeo,[9] in a review of several computer systems for nursing documentation, offers the observation that "Computers have forced nurses to define their functions with clarity and precision."[9a] The same can be said for physicians and other providers. She describes the computer system used at the Clinical Center, the research hospital of the National Institutes of Health. In use there is the Technicon medical information system where all services ordered by physicians, most clinical findings, and observations are recorded on the computer. Romeo stresses the importance of a model of practice being a prerequisite for computer use.

Does computerization improve the evaluation (audit) phase of a quality assurance program? Because the use of computers is still limited, it is probably too early to tell. McNeill, in describing another computer system, problem-oriented medical information system (PROMIS), concludes that the system assists with the audit process.[10] In a study about the problem-oriented medical record, Stratman et al. compared the usefulness for audit purposes of manual problem-oriented medical records and PROMIS, a computerized system.[11] In a study of 69 matched pairs of patient records, a randomly selected sample of residents in internal medicine was asked which record (manual system or PROMIS) best enabled them to assume responsibility for care of the patient. The authors concluded that ". . . users of PROMIS did not create records with any more thorough, reliable or analytically sound information than that contained in a comparative sample of manual records."[11a] It is not clear from the author's analysis whether the information needed to assume responsibility for care is the same as that required for an audit for quality. In addition, in the above study the manual records were typed to appear the same as the computerized records. In reality, one of the advantages of the computerized system for audit is the legibility of the data and the standardization of abbreviations.

One of the obvious dangers in computerization of records is the potential for breach of confidentiality in the use of the record. With a manual record, more careful control of access to the record can be easily maintained. With computerization, access to patient records is more difficult to control. For example, a physician who wants to see a patient's manual record has to go to the unit where the record is, while with computerization the physician has access to the record from any cathode ray terminal (CRT or computer terminal). Although it is probably true that no one would stop a physician from looking at a patient's record in any unit, many physicians would be reluctant to go to a unit and take a chart of a patient under the care of another physician. If viewing a record can be done without anyone seeing the physician doing it, in the privacy of the medical records office, the temptation may be greater. By the use of codes, hospitals maintain security about who can and cannot get information from the CRT. Computer misuse is a well-known phenomenon. By breaking the code, those people who want access to the data can probably obtain it. In addition, because physicians can usually enter orders from any CRT, it is tempting for the busy intern or even attending physician to enter all orders from a central location and not even visit with the patient or have the information interaction that occurs when physicians are on units. Both of these have implications for quality of care and should be monitored carefully.

The Joint Commission on Patient Records and Quality Assurance

The Joint Commission on the Accreditation of Hospitals is specific in its requirement for a quality assurance program.[1] It states "There shall be evidence of a well defined, organized program designed to enhance patient care through the ongoing objective assessment of important aspects of patient care and the correction of identified problems."[2a] The manual also states "The effectiveness of a hospital's quality assurance program shall be emphasized in determining a hospital's accreditation status."[2b]

The sources of data for the quality assurance program may come from many places, but the medical record remains an important source of data according to JCAH. The review may be prospective, concurrent or retrospective.

The *Accreditation Manual for Hospitals* is also quite specific in its requirements for medical record services (i.e., patient records).[2] For example, Standard I is "An adequate medical record shall be maintained for every individual who is evaluated or treated as an inpatient, ambulatory care patient, or emergency patient, or who receives patient services in a hospital-administered home care program."[2c] The interpretation of this standard includes specification of the purposes of the record. Other standards and their interpretations are quite specific in the content required and the timeliness of including data. Requirements for organization of the chart are not specified. In addition to quality assurance and medical record services requirements, JCAH requires an effective utilization review program, demonstrating "appropriate allocation of its resources."[2d]

A record system consistent with JCAH guidelines is desirable both to gain or maintain hospital accreditation and as a way to defend against malpractice suits. Nonadherence to a nationally recognized norm (JCAH guidelines) can be used by plaintiffs as an argument when suing a hospital.

SUMMARY

This chapter has discussed the relationship of quality assurance and the patient record. The advantages and limitations of the patient record as a source of data for evaluation was discussed. Advantages of the use of computerized records have been mentioned, though empirical evidence does not necessarily support the premise that the computerized record is more accurate than the manual record as a source of data for evaluation.

Although knowledge in the field of quality assurance is continuously expanding, in the next ten years the patient record is likely to continue to be a major source of data for evaluation. Until the record becomes less widely used as a data source, more empirical information is needed about the validity and reliability of data in the record along with ways to improve the record as an accurate data source.

The best defense to charges of poor quality care is a good offense consisting of patient records that are planned with quality assurance in mind and quality assurance programs that are based on realistic and planned use of patient records.

NOTES

1. American Hospital Accreditation, *Medical Records Departments in Hospitals* (Chicago: American Hospital Association, 1972), p. 1.

2. The Joint Commission on Accreditation of Hospitals, *Accreditation Manual for Hospitals* (Chicago: Joint Commission on Accreditation of Hospitals, 1982), p. 83.

2a. Ibid., p. 151.

2b. Ibid., p. 154.

2c. Ibid., p. 83.

2d. Ibid., p. 193.

3. L. Weed, *Medical Records, Medical Education, and Patient Care: The Problem Oriented Record as a Basic Tool* (Cleveland: Case Western Reserve University, 1969).

4. J. Williamson, *Assessing and Improving Health Care Outcomes* (Cambridge, Mass.: Ballinger, 1978), p. 88.

5. B. Starfield et al., "Concordance between Medical Records and Observations Regarding Information on Coordination of Care," *Medical Care* 17 (1979):758–766.

6. F. Romm and S. Putnam, "The Validity of the Medical Record," *Medical Care* 19 (1981):310–315.

7. L. Demilo et al., "Reliability of Information Abstracted from Patients' Medical Records," *Medical Care* 16 (1978):995–1005.

7a. Ibid., p. 1003.

8. A. Donabedian, "Some Issues in Evaluating the Quality of Nursing Care," *American Journal of Public Health* 59 (1969):1833–1836.

9. C. Romeo, "Nursing Documentation: A Model for a Computerized Data Base," *Advances in Nursing Science* 4 (1982):43–56.

9a. Ibid., p. 56.

10. D. McNeill, "Developing the Complete Computer-Based Information System," in *Computers in Nursing*, ed. R. Zielstorff (Wakefield, Mass.: Nursing Resources, 1980).

11. W. Stratman et al., "The Utility for Audit of Manual and Computerized Problem-Oriented Medical Record System," *Health Services Research* 17 (1982):5–26.

11a. Ibid., p. 25.

Chapter 15

The Role of Nursing in Quality Assurance

Marianne D. Araujo, R.N., M.S.N. and Joanne T. Jurkovic, R.N., M.S.

The role of nursing service in quality assurance, risk management, and program evaluation is as significant as the impact of direct nursing care on total patient care. At Mercy Hospital and Medical Center, Chicago, nursing service plays an active role in determining its own policies and procedures that establish evaluative criteria and in addressing issues of risk management. Inferred in this statement is the evaluation of nursing decisions, based on broad standards set by various accrediting organizations.

Often, the theory of evaluation has been a roadblock in looking at standards in a pragmatic way. The process for evaluating practice as it affects patient care is just beginning to evolve. At Mercy, the authors have developed mechanisms through which nursing management is able to look objectively at practice, the environment, and managerial functions that have implications for patient care. The chapter will discuss quality assurance, risk management, and program evaluation and their practical application to nursing service within the total hospital delivery system.

PRACTICAL APPLICATION OF THE STUDY PROCESS TO QUALITY ASSURANCE

The Division of Nursing quality assurance program at Mercy is based upon the premise that the quality assurance process is a major stimulus for growth and not merely an activity to be pursued in the quest for accreditation. This premise of growth has allowed nurses directly involved in patient care to determine the criteria by which nursing practice is to be defined and measured within the framework of the nursing care delivery system.

Also important to the success of the quality assurance system was the selection of the quality assurance chairman. In reviewing the requirements for this position, the authors determined that the primary consideration was a recognition by nursing staff of the chairman's high level of nursing care. This, as well as a commitment to the use of group processes and participative management skills, seemed to be necessary traits.

In the past eight years, nursing quality assurance activities have evolved from a centralized system of peer review involving representatives from nursing units to a decentralized concurrent review system designed to meet each unit's specific needs. Further determination was made that the intent of the study process would be to evaluate the practice of nursing within the system, as opposed to evaluating the practice of an individual nurse. Strong support was articulated for the unit supervisor to maintain responsibility for individual nurse review. The following discussion will present the practical application of the major components of the study process: topic selection, tool design, data collection, data analysis, corrective action, and reevaluation.

Topic Selection

As noted above, the quality assurance program was begun as a centralized, concurrent peer review system with a single audit conducted simultaneously on all nursing units. Nursing staff responded to this system with the feeling that much of the audit was nonapplicable, while identified problems were not being evaluated. In response to those concerns, each nursing unit has a nursing quality assurance representative who plays an important part in decentralizing the quality assurance study process. This person no longer serves only to represent her or his unit on the committee but also to lead the quality assurance activities of the unit. Since each unit focuses on a different aspect of nursing care, the staff develops its own study tool. This tool is designed after selecting the topic for audit (e.g., pain assessment), based on input from either external or internal sources.

External sources are defined as data from hospital and/or nursing committees, information from other departments, and input from consumers. Internal sources are also used to determine the specific aspect of care to be reviewed. Such sources include previous study results, unit goals and objectives, discussions in staff meetings, or suggestions from staff members and/or the supervisor.

Following the topic selection, the rationale for selection and topic source are documented by the unit quality assurance representative and his or her unit peers. Specific items to be measured are then identified, and questions are stated to reflect quality nursing care as it relates to the particular practice issue. Standards of care, as articulated by the Division of Nursing, are the determinants of the level of care expected. The quality assurance representative seeks input from peers, nursing management and/or nursing clinicians in the field, to further validate the standards to be studied. A review of current literature, policies, and procedures is done when appropriate. Once the questions have been refined through this process, they are placed as criteria into the study format. (See Exhibits 15-1 and 15-2.)

Exhibit 15-1 Nursing Care Quality Review Instrument—Pain Assessment

8th FLOOR

PAIN ASSESSMENT

Revised May, 1982

Patient Section: (This section of the Instrument is completed on a specific number of patients at random.)

Date: _____   Reviewing Team: _____   Department: _____

Hospital #: _____   Room #: _____   Age: _____

Diagnosis:

Exhibit 15-1 continued

8TH FLOOR PAIN ASSESSMENT

Page 1

	MET-1 N/M-2 N/A-3		COMMENTS
	Direction: Select a patient whose diagnosis would indicate the patient may have complaints of pain. Review the chart for the above information.		
	Assessment of Pain		
	Check the Nursing Interview Guide and/or Progress Notes for assessment of pain. Does the note indicate the following:		
1.	Location of the Pain?		
2.	Type of pain (e.g. sharp, dull, aching, burning, throbbing, etc.)?		
3.	Duration of pain (e.g. constant, periodic, brief, etc.)?		
	When the patient is admitted with pain is the following documented on the Interview Guide:		
4.	Duration of pain (e.g. week, 2 days, 1 hour, etc.)?		
5.	Factors associated with pain (e.g. none, eating, walking, lifting, etc.?)		
6.	Relief measures taken (e.g. over the counter drugs, alcohol, heat, rest, elevation, etc.)?		
7.	Does the pain effect ADL (eating, sleeping activity, etc.)?		
8.	If ADL's are effected, how is the patient coping (e.g. assisted by others, stopped eating, reduced activity, neglected personal hygiene, etc.)?		
9.	When a problem is identified with ADL's, is it on the Care Plan?		
10.	Are interventions listed on the Care Plan consistent with the initial assessment (e.g., when heat helps, is there heat in the Plan)?		

Exhibit 15-1 continued

8TH FLOOR PAIN ASSESSMENT

Page 2

	MET-1 / N/M-2 / N/A-3		COMMENTS
		Review Progress Notes for entries regarding pain management	
11.		Is documentation in the Progress Notes of the intervention (e.g., Tylenol #3 given, heat applied)?	
12.		Is there documentation in the Progress Notes of the patient's response to the intervention (e.g., relief obtained, heat causing increased discomfort, etc.)?	
13.		When the interventions do not relieve the pain, are other interventions instituted (check Progress Notes for documentation)?	
14.		If ADL's are effected by pain, does the Care Plan identify the problem and appropriate interventions?	
15.		Looking at the Medication Profile, is there a pattern of pain medication administration (can Auditor assess when pain meds given appropriately, e.g., q4° after surgery)?	
16.		When PRN pain medication is administered, is there documentation of pain in the Progress Notes and evaluation of the intervention?	
17.		When PRN pain medication is changed, is reason for change documented?	
18.		Does the Progress Note document tolerance to new medication?	
19.		When a problem with pain management is identified, does the Care Plan contain appropriate interventions (e.g., too dependant on meds, not getting relief, patient afraid of medication)?	
20.		Does the Progress Note reflect and evaluate these interventions?	

Exhibit 15-1 continued

8TH FLOOR PAIN ASSESSMENT

Page 3

	MET-1 N/M-2 N/A-3	COMMENTS
	Patient Interview	
	Check to see if patient is fairly comfortable and able to be interviewed.	
21.	Does the patient feel his pain is being managed well by the Nursing staff ("Do you feel the nurses help you in managing your pain")? _____	
22.	Is the patient's perception of what helps to manage his pain reflected on the Care Plan (Ask patient what helps him tolerate the pain. Check the Care Plan. Document Patient's perception and the Care Plan entry when not met)? _____	

Exhibit 15-2 Nursing Care Quality Review Instrument—Sterile Technique/Nurse Interview

OPERATING ROOM

MAINTENANCE OF STERILE TECHNIQUE/NURSE INTERVIEW

April, 1982

Patient Section: (This section of the Instrument is completed on a specific number of patients at random.)

Reviewing Team: _____   Department: _____

Date: _____

Hospital #: _____   Room #: _____   Age: _____

Diagnosis:

Exhibit 15-2 continued

Operating Room – Maintenance of Sterile Technique/Nurse Interview

	MET-1 N/M-2 N/A-3		COMMENTS
1.		What number of thicknesses for cloth drapes are required to insure sterility (Answer: 4 thicknesses)?	
2.		What number of paper drapes are required to insure sterility (Answer: 2 thicknesses)?	
3.		How many minutes are required to flash sterilize an instrument (Answer: 3 minutes)?	
4.		If a drape falls below waist level, should you reach down and re-arrange it (Answer: No, anything below waist level is not considered sterile any longer)?	
5.		If no sterilometer is found in a pack of towels should they be used (Answer: No)? Observation:	
6.		Do all nurses in the Operating Room have their hair tucked under their caps?	
7.		Do all nurses remove surgical garb (cap, mask, booties) before leaving surgery (Check at door of surgery. Comment when not met)?	
8.		When returning to surgery are new caps, masks, and booties applied?	
9.		Are scrubs thrown in to the laundry basket after each use in the nurse's locker room (Check the locker room, if scrubs are lying around mark not met)?	
10.		Are hats, masks and booties properly thrown away in the garbage after use?	

This method for criteria development assures the presence of professional assessment and judgment in the design and execution of the quality assurance process, thus guaranteeing an effective mechanism for peer review. This same professional presence expands the number of available data sources beyond the traditional review of the record and includes patient observation, as well as patient and staff interviews.

Data Collection

The nursing quality assurance study tool is used for three months. During two of those months, data are collected by the members of the nursing quality assurance committee who separate into teams. The nursing quality assurance representative for the unit is a member of the team and interprets any criteria not understood by the other members. A 20 percent sample is collected on each unit. If the topic selected can be applied to all patients on the unit, a random table is used to select the population. If the topic requires specific patients to be reviewed, an accidental sample is used. During the third month, data are collected by the nursing staff on the unit under the direction of the quality assurance representative. This reinforces the standards of practice being measured and increases objectivity in measurement.

The nursing quality assurance representative presents the collected data to the unit supervisor for examination. The supervisor may challenge the judgments of the reviewers at this time. The quality assurance tools are then collected and submitted to the nursing quality assurance chairman for tabulation. A computerized system tabulates the data, indicating the numbers of met, not met, and nonapplicable items. The computer printout and the review tool are sent to the supervisors for completion of the study process.

Data Analysis

The strengths of the nursing staff in the provision of nursing care, as well as any deficiencies and/or variations from the criteria are identified via the study process. However, the process of review and collection of data is only of merit if corrective action is instituted. This is the responsibility of the unit supervisor, working collaboratively with his or her staff to identify the cause of the variance and to determine the plan for corrective action. The supervisor also has responsibility for determining the plan for reevaluation. There are three methods for reevaluation: subsequent reviews, refined studies, and spot checks by the supervisor.

A summary of the study process is prepared and submitted to the clinical nursing director responsible for the various nursing units. He or she, in turn, reports the scope and results of quality assurance activities in his or her area to the vice president of nursing.

A summary of the quarterly activities of the nursing quality assurance committee is submitted to the hospital quality assurance body. The purpose of this summary is to provide information regarding what topics are being addressed and to assure that this activity is ongoing.

This entire mechanism for developing studies has clearly defined the responsibilities of nurses at all levels in quality assurance activities. By virtue of acquiring the skills involved in the design and implementation of the study process, nursing has developed a model that can be expanded to multidisciplinary and physician-nurse collaborative practice evaluations. The broad review of the many disciplines and medical direction of the Alcoholism Treatment Unit is an example of a study process made easier because of nursing's ability to remain impartial. In addition, the principles related to quality assurance can be adapted to risk management and program evaluation.

RISK MANAGEMENT

The principles identified in the study process are readily adaptable for use in risk management. Nursing, by virtue of its direct access to and responsibility for patient care, becomes directly involved in identifying potential risk factors. Nursing is also involved in determining those real situations that occur that may have had a negative impact on an individual patient.

Recognizing the multiple facets of safety, Mercy Hospital and Medical Center has developed a safety program that includes the following components: safety policies and procedures review; safety education programs; environment surveillance; and incident reviews related to patient and employee safety. Each component of the safety program falls under the supervision of a committee chaired by a designated vice president. The committees are charged with establishing guidelines to survey specific related data and to make recommendations that promote overall hospital safety. The total program is coordinated by the executive safety committee, chaired by the president of Mercy Hospital and Medical Center.

That the president of the organization chairs the overall executive safety program speaks clearly to the fact that safety of patients and staff is a primary concern. At the time this safety program was being developed, the president of the hospital and the executive committee deliberated over the appropriateness of the emphasis being placed on safety as opposed to risk management. The determination at the time was to focus on the positive aspects of safety, with emphasis placed on the dignity and well-being of patients and staff. Risk management is, however, a necessary aspect of all safety committees at Mercy Hospital and Medical Center and is considered a part of all plans that relate to determining the actual assurance of safety. Nursing, by virtue of its relationship to patients and staff, plays an active role on all safety committees. However, the committee specifically governing patient safety was designed as the responsibility of the vice president of nursing and general administration.

The patient safety committee is composed of two physicians, the hospital legal counsel, the director of pharmacy services and a staff pharmacist, the director of the laboratory, a clinical director of nursing, and the director of the outpatient clinic. The relative stability of this membership has been a factor in the rapid advancement of the committee's work.

Two assumptions made at the time this committee was formed have facilitated the process of review and evaluation of patient and visitor incidents. The first assumption is that a systematic review resulting in recommended actions would decrease actual patient safety-related incidents. The second assumption is that a system that encourages people to admit and identify mistakes and possible errors through the use of the incident report sheet provides vital data for an analysis of safety factors. This can have a strong positive impact on the prevention of risk situations.

The objective of the patient safety committee is to review all incident reports generated by hospital personnel that relate to the safety of patients or visitors. These incidents include not only situations that have had a specific negative impact on an individual patient, but also those incidents that identify system deficits that can be seen as potentially hazardous. The effect of including incident reports to demonstrate system problems is a strengthening of the emphasis on the need for appropriate systems to protect the patient. In addition, the opportunity is offered to the departments involved to review the design of their system, based on the additional information obtained from the incident report.

Category Selection

Initially, the committee used a monthly summary sheet to record a detailed description of each incident. The summary sheet was prepared prior to the committee meeting. Through careful analysis of the summary sheet, four major patterns of the types of incidents reported were identified and used to categorize incidents to be reviewed. They included patient falls, loss and theft, medication errors, and system breakdowns as they related to laboratory services.

Once these categories were established, a system of identifying and reviewing each category of incidents was delegated to the appropriate committee member. Since all four major categories are influenced by nursing practice, it was determined that nursing would accept the data generated from a focus review conducted by another department representative.

An example of this type of focus is the analysis of all medication incidents. The pharmacy is responsible for reviewing all medication errors and their potential causes. The findings of this review are reported to the committee. (See Exhibit 15-3.) Appropriate actions are discussed and relegated to the joint action of pharmacy services and nursing management as a whole. Since the hospital employs the unit dose distribution system for medications, the discipline involved in the error is readily identifiable. The consequences of this review have been to involve members of the pharmacy in working jointly with members of the departments of nursing. Together, they assess compliance with procedures as they relate to medication distribution. The effectiveness of the existing distribution system is also determined.

This method of using the study process has been repeated for all categories of incidences. Serious incidents that require individual analysis have been treated specifically by members of the committee in a review mechanism clearly designed to prevent the incident from recurring.

Information generated by other committees, such as infection control and utilization review, that have implications for nursing practice are dealt with in the same manner as described in the safety program. This is also true of information generated by other services that provide direct and indirect patient care.

This comprehensive quality and safety assurance program not only requires practical application of the study process but also communication flow between department and legal counsel.

For nursing at Mercy Hospital and Medical Center, the attorney representative for legal affairs provides insight into situations on a prospective basis. The benefits for nursing include the in-house presence of an attorney, the review of forms for appropriate legality, the validation of specific policies and procedures, and the in-servicing of charting systems from a legal standpoint.

The total scope of risk management within the hospital system is the responsibility of many groups. Clearly, roles of all staff working within the hospital must be defined within the system. The flow and use of information obtained from the various safety committees assures problem identification and relegation, action, and resolution or, at the very least, a mechanism to continue to monitor the status of the identified problem. The study process used in this manner assists staff in providing a safe environment for the patients they serve.

PROGRAM EVALUATION

Some say program evaluation revolves around programs or projects. However, it is our belief that program evaluation encompasses all aspects of managerial functions. This concept provides an effective mechanism for accountability as well as control of these diverse functions.

The framework in which nursing service evaluates its program is dependent upon the environment established by administration and the nurse administrator. Key components of nursing service that should be considered when establishing an evaluation program are the management philosophy of the administrator and that of the nurse administrator, external standards to which nursing service is held accountable, and the role of nursing services within the hospital system.

Exhibit 15-3 Types of Reported Medication Errors

I. Nursing Errors
- a. administered med. to wrong patient. . . . .
- b. administered wrong med. to patient. . . . .
- c. administered wrong dose to patient. . . . .
- d. administered med. to patient in wrong route . . . .
- e. administered med. at wrong time . . . .
- f. administered extra dose(s) . . . .
- g. administered med. that had been D/C . . . .
- h. omitted administering med. to patient . . . .
- i. delayed in noting order(s) . . . .
- j. IV being infused too rapidly. . . . .
- k. IV being infused in wrong tubing . . . .
- l. miscellaneous . . . .

II. Pharmacy Errors
- m. entered order on wrong patient profile . . . .
- n. entered wrong drug (or dose). . . . .
- o. entered wrong instructions on profile . . . .
- p. took order off profile when it should not have been D/C . . . .
- q. left order on profile when it should have been D/C . . . .
- r. allergy not caught. . . . .
- s. med. not sent to unit promptly . . . .
- t. dispensed wrong med. . . . .
- u. dispensed wrong dose . . . .
- v. insufficient quantity of med. dispensed . . . .
- w. miscellaneous . . . .

III. Others (or Unclassified)

At Mercy Hospital and Medical Center, the key components of program evaluation are based upon the hospital administration's philosophy of participative management and management by objectives, nursing administration's promotion of the concept of decentralization through the establishment of supportive activities, and the use of unit committees to promote decentralization. These program aspects must be evaluated, since they combine to form a mechanism for controlling a diversity of activities. Another component to be evaluated is the assurance of adequate cost-effective staffing consistent with the type of the patient population. The following discussion will demonstrate how the evaluation process is used to determine the effectiveness of nursing services.

Management by Objectives

The hospital administration, with input from management staff members, develops annual corporate objectives. The division of nursing in turn develops its objectives with input from the nursing leadership group. Each nursing unit supervisor, with input from her or his staff, develops objectives for her or his respective area. The hospital's and nursing division's objectives are broad, while those of the nursing unit are specific. The objectives of the nursing unit reflect the determined focus as it relates to patient care services unique to its clinical area and delineates its responsibility to carry out the corporate and division objectives. At the end of the year, each unit supervisor writes an annual report that reflects progress toward meeting the specific objectives. This process promotes a system of identifying the accountability for each individual unit. (See Exhibit 15-4.)

Staffing Consistent with the Acuity of the Patient Population

The centralized staffing system that uses a cyclical staffing methodology is evaluated by using the staffing analysis sheet. This sheet reflects both the census of the actual staffing pattern and acuity of patients on a 24-hour basis. The nursing administrator reviews and identifies shifts in patterns, problem areas, and cost effectiveness of staffing. Corrective action can then be taken as needed. (See Exhibit 15-5.)

Supportive Activities

The evaluation process has become an integral part of the management activities of the institution. It is used in projects, programs, or new ideas that are operationalized. By using a broadened dimension of the quality assurance model of the study process, the activities occurring at every level within the nursing organization can be evaluated and/or monitored. Orientation activities, primary nursing, and expansion of the role of the orthopedic nurse epitomize the importance of incorporating the study process into the components of the delivery process.

Although it seems logical to use the study process for evaluating learning experiences, little has been done to expand the scope of measuring the effect of programming on actual practice.

A competency-based orientation program was installed in June of 1982. In an effort to look at the effectiveness of this program, a study was designed to measure the extent to which the eight competencies taught within the program were learned by the new employee. In addition, a tool to measure the degree to which these competencies are applied in actual practice was designed. The study, administered immediately following the six-week orientation program, incor-

Exhibit 15-4 Evaluation through Management by Objectives

EVALUATION THROUGH MANAGEMENT BY OBJECTIVES

OBJECTIVES			EVALUATION
Corporate	Division of Nursing	OB/Gyne Nursing Unit	Annual Report Summary
Facilitate the coordination of patient care activity in an effort to promote dignity and respect for each person.	Facilitate the coordination of patient care activities in an effort to promote dignity and respect for the patient and the nursing staff.	Coordinate and facilitate patients' daily activities providing quality care and promoting dignity and respect for the patient, with the goal to provide family center care.	1. Post partum mothers' classes for all patients were planned and implemented December, 1981.
			2. A system for follow-up phone calls by the primary nurse was instituted December, 1981
			3. Primary care of mother and child was fully implemented on the Unit, January, 1982.
			4. The rooming-in program was expanded to 9 hours per day plus 24 hours upon request, March, 1982.
			5. A policy which allowed surrogate fathers to be present during delivery was established March, 1982.
			6. A policy which allowed significant other to be present during rooming-in periods was established March, 1982.

Exhibit 15-5 Staffing Analysis Sheet

STAFFING ANALYSIS SHEET - Division of Nursing   DATE:

UNIT	CENSUS 7AM	7-3:30 RN	LPN	NA	TOTAL NC HOURS	CENSUS 3PM	3-11:30 RN	LPN	NA	TOTAL NC HOURS	CENSUS 11PM	11-7:30 RN	LPN	NA	TOTAL NC HOURS	CLASS. 1	2	3	4	5	6	24 HOUR TOTALS PC HOURS	NC HOURS	BUDGETED HOURS	AVG. CENSUS	HPS/PT.
OB																										
GYN																										
OBN																								120		
LR																								72		
4E																								64		
4W																								104		
ATU																								40		
5/R																								104		
5/R-O																								104		
PEDS																								176		
PICU																								24		
6S/W																								48		
7																								217		
SCU																								48		
8																								232		
9																								232		
10																								232		
11																								144		
11/CSU																								120		
SICU																								192		
ER																										
OR																										
RR																										
CLERKS																										
SUPERS.																										
TOTALS																										
FLOATS																										
STOCK-OFFS																										
AGENCY																										

porates several modes of information gathering: patient interview, patient observation, documentation, and forms review. It will be readministered in six months to ascertain the long-term effect of the program on clinical practice. The results will be tabulated to identify the strengths and weaknesses in the program and to determine appropriate revisions. This approach provides concrete feedback on which to base future decisions concerning the orientation program.

By expanding on this approach, plans are being made to evaluate continuing education programs based on patient outcome criteria. This can be accomplished through a quality assurance study that measures new learning as it affects nursing care delivery. In addition, the quality assurance model for study of activities is being considered to test the inquiry mode for learning and its impact on patient care delivery.

Another component of program evaluation is the monitoring of primary nursing, the nursing care delivery system. An audit was designed specifically to measure the extent to which nurses accepted the responsibility and accountability for the care of their primary patients. These two characteristics are essential if primary nursing is to be operational. The results of the audit indicated that primary nursing, as previously defined, was not being delivered consistently throughout the hospital. During the data collection process, it was also learned that some major problems and roadblocks prevented the nurses from fully implementing their role. As a result of this study, several steps have been taken to correct problems, thus providing the nurses the support they need to enhance their practice.

Finally, the quality assurance model was used to evaluate a program that expanded the role of the orthopedic nurse. This orthopedic expanded role program was designed through a collaborative effort between physicians, staff nurses, and nursing management and has been in effect over the past four years. The nurse, practicing in his or her expanded role capacity, is able to take specific diagnostic and therapeutic actions that promote patient comfort and safety and prevent real or potential complications from occurring.

To institute this program, nursing protocols were written to integrate the new functions into the routine nursing care delivery process.

An intensive educational program, developed and instituted through the collaborative efforts of physicians and nurses, prepared the nurses for expanded activities. Along with the evaluation of learning, a tool was developed to audit the application of any protocol used. The purpose of this tool was to validate the nursing decisions required to act in an expanded role capacity.

A further evaluation of the expanded role was demonstrated by a length of stay study. The results of this activity indicated the length of stay for orthopedic patients decreased by 1.5 days during the 26 months following the implementation of these expanded role activities. These results have given the impetus to expand the role of the nurse in other specialty areas throughout the Division of Nursing.

From these program evaluation efforts, accomplishments were identified as they relate to the overall functioning of the Division of Nursing. These efforts, along with numerous other evaluation activities, have provided the management review necessary to assess and verify the contributions nursing has made to quality patient care.

This discussion of the study process in the various facets of examining nursing practices demonstrates the diverse methodology used to assess and enhance nursing practice as a major component of the hospital's care delivery system. It is the responsibility of nursing service to influence the organizational focus on patient care and to bring the realities of caring for the sick and injured closer to the ideal. It is recognized that much time and energy is expended in evaluating progress toward this end. However, this effort is justified by the growth nurses have experienced in making patient-centered decisions. Final justification is the product of this growth—the enhancement of patient dignity.

Chapter 16

Quality Assurance and Utilization Review

Patricia M. Kearns, M.S.

Historically, utilization review was considered for inclusion in the appraisal of medical care as early as 1960 when it was approved by the American Hospital Association and the American Medical Association. In mid-1963 it was mentioned in the bulletin of the Joint Commission on Accreditation of Hospitals.[1] However, the most significant impact on utilization review efforts came in 1965 with the passage of the legislation that established the Medicare and Medicaid programs. With this legislation came the requirement for utilization review for all Medicare patients; in 1967 utilization review requirements were extended to Medicaid patients.

Finally, in 1972, as an amendment to the Social Security Act, Public Law 92-603 mandated Professional Services Review Organizations to ensure delivery of health care services in the most effective, efficient, and economical manner possible.

The Joint Commission on Accreditation of Hospitals (JCAH) officially entered the arena of utilization review in 1977 when the *Accreditation Manual for Hospitals*, Standard II—Quality of Professional Services, directed "The hospital shall demonstrate appropriate allocation of its resources through the conduct of an effective utilization review program. The results of the utilization review activity shall be contributory to the quality of patient care and shall be reflected in the other quality-protective functions of the hospital and the medical staff."[2]

Further efforts toward utilization review were beginning to be felt in 1978 with the institution of the Voluntary Cost Containment Program by the American Hospital Association, American Medical Association, and the Federation of American Hospitals. This voluntary effort was aimed at maintaining high-quality health care and equitable distribution of services through the reduction in the rate of increase in health care costs.

Since 1977, the JCAH utilization review standard has been somewhat revised. It is still interpreted, however, as the requirement for assuring appropriate allocation of the hospital's resources in striving to provide high-quality patient care in the most cost-effective manner. It further requires addressing overutilization, underutilization, and inefficient scheduling of resources.

Utilization review is not only review of length of stay; it is review of the necessity of admission, of supportive services, and of continued stays. It is review of practices or monitoring, such as blood utilization review, drug utilization review, relating day of admission to day of surgical procedure, analyzing effect of preadmission workups on length of stay, discharge planning, and more. It is, in effect, peer review. It is also a program designed to ensure cost containment or proper allocation of resources without reducing the quality of patient care.

A utilization review program that would assist in maintaining quality patient care and that would ensure effective utilization of hospital services was implemented in 1978 at a small army hospital under the auspices of a quality assurance committee and was chaired by the Chief of Professional Services. The program was designed to comply with the JCAH standard and encompass all aspects of utilization review, including discharge planning. Flexibility of the program was a major consideration since the ultimate utilization review program would be an elaborate computer program that would hold essential statistics and produce them as needed. Out of necessity, an unsophisticated manually operated program was developed that could be expanded when resources become available.

Specifically included in the utilization review plan was the requirement that the quality assurance committee review and evaluate the minutes of the ambulatory patient care committee, nursing audit, infection control committee, therapeutic agents board, and linen management committee. The inclusion of this requirement in the utilization review program was the initiation of compliance with the yet unpublished Joint Commission on Accreditation of Hospital's quality assurance standard.

Another unrelated decision, the establishment of a monthly marathon-type committee day, impacted on the mushrooming comprehensive quality assurance program. To ensure committee meeting attendance and to ease physician appointment scheduling problems, a compacted schedule was developed and implemented as shown in Exhibit 16-1. This schedule did not affect departmental meetings, which were at the discretion of departmental chiefs but in accordance with pertinent regulations.

Results of the marathon day were outstanding regarding attendance of physicians. The impact on the morale of central appointments personnel was dramatic, and patient satisfaction was greatly enhanced. An unexpected result from the committee meeting day was that in overseeing the hospital committee structure, the administrative assistant, who supervised JCAH activities and preparation, the utilization review program, and attended most of the committee meetings in one capacity or another, was beginning to focus in on identification and integration of all available data on patient care. Coordination of most sources of information about patient care was becoming a reality.

Exhibit 16-1 Schedule for Committee Meetings

1st Friday	Professional Staff Conference	0745–0900 hours
2d Friday	Executive Staff	0800–0830 hours
3d Friday	Executive Staff	0730–0800 hours
	Safety	0800–0900 hours
	Budget Committee	0900–1000 hours
	Quality Assurance Committee	1000–1130 hours
	Oct./Jan./Apr./July—Linen Management	1130–1200 hours
	Nov./Feb./May/Aug.—Library	1130–1200 hours
	Infection Control	1300–1400 hours
	Oct./Jan./Apr./July—Ambulatory Patient Care	1400–1500 hours
	Nov./Feb./May/Aug.—Therapeutic Agents	
	Board	1400–1500 hours
	Dec./Mar./Jan./Sep.—Credentials	1400–1500 hours
	Nov./Feb./May/Aug.—Emergency	
	Preparedness	1500–1600 hours
4th Friday	Executive Staff	0800–0830 hours

When the 1980 JCAH *Accreditation Manual for Hospitals* was published in August 1979, the hospital was well on its way to being in compliance with the quality assurance standard that states: "The hospital shall demonstrate a consistent endeavor to deliver patient care that is optimal within available resources and consistent with achievable goals. A major component in the application of this principle is the operation of a quality assurance program."[3] It was evident that the relationship between quality assurance and utilization review was that of inseparability. Although the quality assurance standard appeared to be an offspring of utilization review, it was definitely not a servant to it.

The attention focused on quality assurance by the JCAH, as reflected in its 1980 *Accreditation Manual,* is reflective of the national emphasis to increase the quantity, improve the quality, and decrease the cost of hospital services provided in this country. Quality assurance was conceived to enhance utilization review, but in reality it envelops utilization review along with program evaluation, auditing, credentialing, continuing medical education, monitoring, and risk management. It envelops and at the same time is composed of the preceding tools, for without them there would be no efficiency no effectiveness, and no quality.

Prior to formalization of the quality assurance program, an analysis of quality assurance functions was required before problem areas were identified and assessments or procedural revisions of the utilization review plan could be accomplished. Through this analysis, line of authority, accountability, and communication were clearly evident, and a flow chart was developed. However, it was also evident there was a real need to develop a cooperative atmosphere in which to foster the growth of quality assurance.

To expand the program into a quality assurance program, it was necessary to specifically include: (a) quality of care (problem solving, credentialing, continuing medical education, monitoring); (b) utilization review; and (c) risk management under a quality assurance umbrella, as illustrated in Figure 16-1. The JCAH requirement for a written utilization review plan can be accomplished by incorporating all utilization review requirements into the written quality assurance plan. In other words, inclusion must be ensured for all mandated requirements, such as delineation of responsibilities and authority of those involved in utilization review activities; a conflict-of-interest policy; a confidentiality policy; a description of the methods for identifying utilization-related problems, including appropriateness and medical necessity of admission, continued stays, and supportive services; procedures for concurrent review, including the period within which review is to be initiated and length of stay norms and percentiles to be used; and a mechanism for discharge planning.

To emphasize JCAH's requirement that the quality assurance program be problem focused, comprehensive, and cost effective, the plan was written to include provisions to hold each discipline responsible for identifying, assessing, and resolving their own problems relating to patient care. The main thrust of the plan was to ensure documentation of the numerous problem-solving efforts that already took place on a day-to-day basis. An annex to the quality assurance

Figure 16-1 Quality Assurance Umbrella

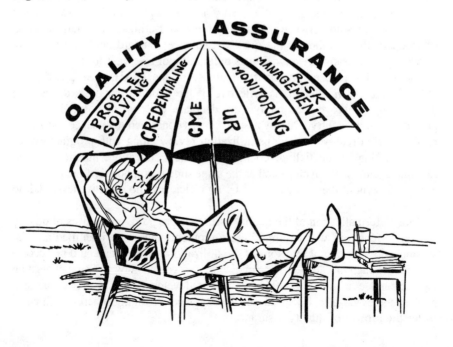

program was developed to ensure that each department or service was aware of their responsibilities and to enhance timely submission of documented problem evaluations. (See Exhibit 16-2.)

The mechanisms for problem identification are numerous and, in addition to medical records, include monitoring activities, morbidity/mortality review, prescription review, incident reports, financial data review, utilization review findings, interviews, observation, and committee minutes review.

It was evident that minutes review was vital to an effective quality assurance program. However, the hospital needed to revise the committee meeting schedule to ensure a better flow of quality assurance activities and to centralize data. As evidenced in the revised schedule (shown in Exhibit 16-3) the time period from marathon day meetings, to funneling into the quality assurance committee for review and comments, to approval by the executive committee and presentation to the professional staff, is one month. The quality assurance committee became capable of identifying and addressing problems in a very systematic and very timely manner.

Problem assessment, including prioritization, can be accomplished prospectively, concurrently, or retrospectively but requires written criteria that, when applied to practice, can result in improved care or performance. When inappropriate patterns of patient care are discovered, remedial action to correct such problems should be implemented. Problems that are department specific can be corrected simply with quality assurance committee notification and concurrence on a standard hospital approved form, such as is reflected in Exhibit 16-4.

On the other hand, if, for example, the emergency room has a problem with documentation that has not been appropriately nor timely filed in patients' medical records, and it is also discovered that STAT results have not been returned promptly, the second problem cannot be corrected by any one department's action. An assessment of both problems by the emergency room should be forwarded to the quality assurance committee. The emergency room's problem or the first problem, the inappropriateness or lateness of documentation, can be corrected within the department. Corrective action should be implemented and a resolution report should be forwarded to the quality assurance committee. The second problem, the delay in receipt of STAT results, should be assessed and recommendations forwarded on another resolution report to the quality assurance committee. The committee should, in turn, review the problem and concur with the recommendations or recommend alternatives and then notify or ''task'' the responsible departments to implement the corrective action.

Corrective action must always be specific to the identified problem and may include continuing medical education or training programs, amended policies or procedures, increased or realigned staffing, provision of new equipment or facilities, or adjustment in staff privileges. Follow-up studies should be conducted in a timely manner and continue until it is demonstrated that the problem has been corrected.[4]

Exhibit 16-2 Quality Assurance Activities

Evaluation by QAC will include consideration of:

1. Prioritization
2. Problem (focused)
3. Assessment
4. Implementation
5. Follow-up

	Frequency	Criteria	Medical Records	Physician Input	Nursing Input
A. Medical Staff Functions					
1. Executive committee	M	X		X	X
2. Surgical case review (Tissue function)	M	X		X	
3. Blood utilization review	Q	X		X	
4. Antibiotic usage review	M	X		X	
5. Pharmacy and therapeutics function	Q	X		X	X
6. Medical records function	Q	X	X	X	X
7. Credentialing	Q	X		X	X
B. Clinic Department Services					
1. Surgical	R	X		X	
2. Medical	R	X		X	
3. Pediatrics	R	X		X	
4. Nursing	Q	X			X
C. Hospital Functions					
1. Infection control	M	X		X	X
2. Safety committee	M	X		X	
3. Preventive maintenance program	R	X			
D. Support Services					
1. Anesthesia (C, surgery)	Q	X		X	X
2. Ambulatory care— hospital (C, PCCM)	Q	X	X	X	X
3. Emergency services (C, PCCM)	M	X	X	X	X
4. Radiology (C, radiology)	Q	X			
5. Pathology (C, pathology)	A	X			
6. Dietetics (C, food service)	A	X	X	X	X

7. Pharmacy (C, pharmacy)	Q	X			
8. Physical therapy (C, PT)	Q	X		X	
9. Social work (C, CMHA)	B	X	X		
10. Special care unit (C, medicine)	Q	X		X	X

Frequency Code

A = annual; B = biannual; Q = quarterly; M = monthly; R = regular and continuous monitoring, report when identified

The quality assurance program was written to assure accountability of the professional staffs for the care they provide. Accountability can be difficult because of its sensitivity, but with experience and teamwork it was evident that accountability could be ascertained through trending results of problem-focused studies. Before trending can be used, however, professionals must establish their own goals or standards to measure performance so that performance-based training or performance-based credentialing can be initiated as needed. Trending, if used properly, can eventually help motivate professionals to make quality assurance work. (See Exhibit 16-5.)

Performance-based credentialing is the ultimate quality control and can be accomplished when a management information system has been developed that receives problem identification data from a variety of sources and when data are not just documented and filed away. When this information has been compiled, analyzed for trends, and directed toward appropriate committees for action,

Exhibit 16-3 Revised Schedule

3rd Friday	Professional Staff Conference	0730–0930 hours
	Safety	0930–1000 hours
	Budget Committee	1030–1100 hours
	Oct./Jan./Apr./July—Health Consumer	1130–1200 hours
	Nov./Feb./May/Aug.—Library	1130–1200 hours
	Infection Control	1300–1400 hours
	Oct./Jan./Apr./July—Ambulatory Patient Care	1400–1500 hours
	Nov./Feb./May/Aug.—Therapeutic Agents Board	1400–1500 hours
	Dec./Mar./Jun./Sep.—Credentials	1400–1500 hours
	Nov./Feb./May/Aug.—Energy Conservation	1500–1600 hours
	Dec./June—Emergency Preparedness	1500–1600 hours
1st Friday	Quality Assurance Committee	1300–1400 hours
2nd Friday	Executive Staff	0800–0830 hours

Exhibit 16-4 Quality Assurance Resolution Report
(Department or Service)

(Date)

Problem no.:	(to be assigned by Quality Assurance Committee)
Problem:	(short statement outlining the problem as perceived or identified)
Problem identified:	(where or how problem was identified)
Criteria:	(Every problem must have at least one criteria on which a judgment or decision may be based—a standard by which to measure.)
Personnel involved in assessment:	(principal participants)
Objective:	(the goal toward which effort is directed)
Corrective action:	(those efforts required to be taken in order to satisfy the objective.)
Follow-up procedures to determine effectiveness:	(outline of planned actions to ensure proper implementation and effectiveness of corrective action.)
Interim report/status:	(may be used to provide information to the Quality Assurance Committee on status of in-progress studies or reviews and provide information on results of follow-up on previously submitted resolution reports.)

_____

Typed Name and Signature

Quality Assurance Committee Review:

_____   _____

Signature of Chairman   Date

---

performance-based training and credentialing can be developed. It is no longer feasible, particularly financially feasible, to have professionals fill out credentialing forms and automatically renew them every year. Health care facilities are responsible to see if those individuals merit recredentialing.

All hospital continuing medical education activities should be coordinated under the auspices of the quality assurance committee, should be based on performance, and should be problem oriented. For example, if it becomes evident through discharge planning of the lack of staff understanding regarding Medicare and Medicaid, the community health nurse could discuss this subject matter at a professional staff conference. Such performance-based training can be initiated

Exhibit 16-5 Sample of Trending

	Physician Assistant	June Monthly Summation Total Charts Reviewed 180 Variation Per Criterion								
		1	2	3	4	5	6	7	8	9	10
1	68201	0	0	4	2	0	0	1	14	0	0
2	68202	0	0	0	0	2	0	0	10	0	1
3	68203	0	1	1	0	0	0	0	8	0	0
4	68204	0	0	0	0	0	0	0	4	0	0
5	68205	0	0	0	0	0	0	1	11	1	0
6	68206	12	14	16	18	17	18	17	23	9	15
	Total	12	15	21	20	19	18	19	70	10	16

Note: The above example represents the summation of chart review for the month of June for six physician's assistants. It was previously recommended by the quality assurance committee that, to ensure an adequate review, at least 10 percent of monthly charts should be reviewed.

when utilization problems, i.e., inappropriate use of disposables, abuse of STATs, misutilization of time, or excessive use of supplies are identified. Sick leave, an important management indicator, should be receiving increasing emphasis and high-level attention, especially during this period of decreasing budgets and reduced manpower levels.

Quality assurance committee monitoring of actions taken to resolve patient care problems includes numerous mechanisms to further emphasize quality care. Monitoring to identify and track specific problems includes blood utilization review (presented by the pathologist to the surgical committee monthly and further presented to quality assurance quarterly); tissue review (minutes review presented by the chief of surgery to committee monthly); antibiotic utilization review (monthly review of infection control committee minutes including in-patient, outpatient, and emergency usage of antibiotics); mortality review (presented to committee as applicable); drug utilization review (quarterly review of therapeutic agent board minutes and studies of usage pattern for drug by department or prescriber); patient survey review (summarized and presented to committee monthly); review of health consumer committee minutes; review of budget committee minutes; and review of internal audits. The importance of minutes review by the quality assurance committee cannot be overemphasized because problems are sometimes more easily identified by an overall hospital committee than by very interested individuals who chair each separate committee.

Since patient surveys are valuable management information tools, they need appropriate design consideration to facilitate completion and return. It is imperative to include location or services on the form to identify either commendable or problem areas. Moreover, employee cooperation in disseminating surveys can be readily obtained when it becomes evident that surveys are useful in identifying employees deserving of praise.

Although not all concerns identified through patient surveys require formal problem solving, many patient concerns do merit consideration, particularly in regard to patient education and staff attitude problems. Surveys can be extremely helpful in identifying potentially compensable events. Common courtesy in the form of a reply should be afforded to patients who complete surveys and who obviously expect to hear from their input to the hospital. If possible, all surveys should be acknowledged.

Patients do, however, need ample time to complete their surveys. It was found that inpatient surveys should be handed out immediately prior to discharge, while outpatient surveys could best be disseminated when patients turned prescriptions in to the pharmacy. The importance of consumer feedback is vital to an effective quality assurance program. Moreover, consumers need to see the end result of consumer-originated quality assurance recommendations and should be invited to participate on a health consumer committee with health care professionals. This committee can be an excellent mechanism for patient education and feedback.

Through review of patient surveys, it could be pointed out, for example, that a number of inpatients are dissatisfied with beverage temperatures. Therefore, criteria could be developed for the surveying of both hot and cold beverages. Random sampling could then be used occasionally to ensure compliance with the criteria. However, in prioritization of problems, it must always be remembered that the more impact a problem has on a patient's life, the sooner it must be resolved. Therefore, a more immediate concern or problem would be a complaint of a severe allergic reaction from a medication that was prescribed in a clinic and filled at the pharmacy after the patient specifically told the clinician of his or her allergies.

When such a problem is identified and forwarded to the quality assurance committee, it could be recommended that a system whereby patients would document known allergies on the reverse side of their prescriptions would serve as a check to preclude future incidents of this nature. The pharmacy could be charged with implementing the recommendation and may order rubber stamps, post signs, and educate patients in an all-out campaign to ensure prescribed medications are compatible to patients. This, of course, would be in addition to the obvious necessary staff training. Using this recommendation, clinicians could be identified who prescribe Cama (buffered aspirin) for patients allergic to aspirin or Keflex for patients allergic to penicillin. It does no good to simply catch the mistake and get the prescription changed; the individual responsible for the mistake must be held accountable through documentation on an incident report form.

To reduce the inefficiency of overlapping functions, surgical case review can be combined with blood utilization review, and infection control review can be combined with antibiotic usage review. However, a surgical monitoring system that could audit all surgical patients continuously could be implemented in any facility and would be a more efficient method.

Surgical case review or tissue review can be used to identify problems in diagnosis (admitting or discharge), deaths, anesthesia time, or surgical procedure. Professional service review organization screening criteria have been developed for specific surgical procedures. These can be helpful but should be revised to be hospital specific.

Incorporated in the monthly departmental surgical case review can be the quarterly requirement for blood utilization review, which should include blood transfusions; use of whole blood versus component blood elements; actual or suspected transfusion reactions; amount of blood requested, used, and wasted; and the number of emergency and ambulatory care patients who receive blood transfusions. It may be beneficial to do a retrospective patient care evaluation using medical records. In a large institution, it is feasible to have a committee or group review blood usage, but in a small facility an individual member of the medical staff can accomplish the review.

The surgical review (including the blood utilization review) should be forwarded through the quality assurance committee for review or recommendations. It is possible the quality assurance committee could determine from trending of the reports of blood usage that, for example, single-unit transfusions have increased significantly. The committee could debate the need for single-unit transfusions and may decide to monitor this trend. If one particular physician is found guilty of continually abusing single-unit transfusions, he or she may need counseling or training. If the problem continues and is significant, documentation may be needed in his or her credentialing files. Surgical case review and blood utilization are important quality assurance and utilization review mechanisms and as such must be fully supported. Therefore, whatever avenue the quality assurance committee chooses, total support is needed from the administrator, the chief of staff, and the board of trustees.

Antibiotic usage review is an ongoing medical staff requirement and includes clinical review of antibiotics for inpatients, ambulatory care patients, and emergency care patients. This review can be accomplished by the medical staff as a whole, the pharmacy and therapeutics committee, or the infection control committee with the quality assurance committee reviewing their minutes and studies. In addition to the clinical review, statistical studies of antibiotics should be conducted, as well as reviews to identify patients who receive large doses of antibiotics when they show no sign of infection or when they show signs of infection and receive no antibiotics. Trending of antibiotics involved in medication errors is imperative. In addition, any clusters of infection must be identified and determination made of antibiotics prescribed for patients involved.

Under the auspices of the overall quality assurance program, a hospital-specific manual for infection control can be developed by the infection control committee as a guide to infection control practices. Although compiling the manual is a time-consuming task, improvement of patient care can be realized and will offset the manpower and dollars expended.

In an effort to contain drug costs, the quality assurance committee could direct the pharmacy to publish a comparative listing of the most widely prescribed drugs, including cost per dose. The listing could be used to help monitor drug utilization by clinician, department, procedure, or diagnosis and should be widely distributed. The effectiveness of a comparative pharmaceutical list can be reflected in a variety of ways. It could be used, for example, if the infection control committee addressed the use of antibiotics for acute minor infections in outpatients and included a reference to utilization of a specific drug of choice in acute urinary tract infections. The committee could reference the pharmaceutical list and designate a drug of choice that could cost substantially less than another widely used drug. Through cooperative effort, effective utilization of resources can become a way of life.

Inflation, labor, and technology are the main causes for the increase in health care cost. However, in determining the country's health cost, physicians have a major role because they initiate expenses of patients. The Government Accounting Office recently stated that about "70 percent of the $278.5 billion expended in 1981 for health care was estimated to be directly influenced, if not controlled by, the decision of the physicians."[5]

Physician-specific productivity figures can be extremely useful in utilization review and can be computed, particularly in a facility where the physicians are employed by the hospital. The U.S. Army has a staffing guide that designates how many outpatients per month each particular specialist should be treating. For example, in accordance with the staffing guide, an internist should see 300 clinic patients per month, a pediatrician 450, an orthopedist 450, a podiatrist 400, etc. Using the guide or a similar tool, it would not be difficult to determine problems in productivity and then evaluate them.

Making physicians aware of how much it costs for services they order for patients is a utilization review responsibility. Discussing costs, productivity, preadmission screening, necessity for services, and so on at professional conferences is imperative since staff involvement is vital. Moreover, for physicians to be motivated in regard to utilization review, the review must be relevant on a local level. The goal of any utilization review program is a melding of quality with cost containment.

Patterns of utilization must be identified and trended to afford benefit to the quality assurance committee. To ensure that services are necessary, appropriate, and cost effective, utilization by physician or department should be compiled to identify problem areas and to enhance practitioner reappraisals. As discussed previously, it is necessary to determine whether a particular individual merits recredentialing.

Problems identified through any utilization review activity should be forwarded by the quality assurance committee to the appropriate department or service to be corrected per recommendations of the committee. Corrections should comply with the hospital's approved problem-solving technique, with follow-up as required.

The aim of discharge planning is to discharge as soon as an acute level of care is no longer required. Discharge should be initiated as soon as practical. To facilitate this vital aspect of utilization review, a discharge planning coordinator, preferably a social worker, is necessary and should be included in the quality assurance committee to provide feedback on the extent of discharge planning efforts.

Many mechanisms, such as coordination between nursing and medical staff, patient instruction, family involvement, and early identification of patients who may require posthospitalization care, can enhance appropriate discharge planning. All this can be accomplished through a team effort: a team of social workers, nurses, and physicians who, through written delineation of their authority and responsibilities, can facilitate discharge planning. A dietician, physical therapist, community health nurse, and chaplain can be included effectively on the team. Further, authority should be delegated to nonphysician health care professionals to initiate preparations for discharge planning, utilizing team-developed criteria and identifying patients whose diagnoses, problems, or social circumstances require discharge planning.

Day-to-day ward contact is a prerequisite to an effective discharge planning program. In a small facility, this contact can be initiated by a social work technician with a good clinical background who is able to recognize the interrelationships of a patient's psychological, emotional, and physical needs. He or she should review daily admissions, using team-developed criteria, to determine patients considered high risk or high priority for discharge planning.

Based on discharge planning statistics, it was apparent in military facilities that retirees and dependents have a much greater need for assistance with discharge planning than active duty patients. Many of these patients require assistance in obtaining information regarding nursing homes, home care, Medicare, Medicaid, or any service that may be required to improve or maintain the patient's health status.

The quality assurance committee must ensure through concurrent utilization review that inpatient services are necessary and appropriate and could not have been provided effectively on an outpatient basis. It must be remembered, however, that concurrent utilization review is a type of peer review to determine whether a patient requires a particular health service, such as admission, a period of hospital stay, or a specific diagnostic or therapeutic procedure. It is a peer review because the criteria for reviewing appropriateness of admission, certification of admission, and assignment of length of stay must be developed by physicians. The criteria must be used as screens to differentiate those cases that require further review because the criteria are not met.

In regard to length of stay review, the initial length of stay does not necessarily mean that the patient must be discharged in that many days. If there is documentation in the patient's chart for the medical necessity of an extension, an extension should be granted in accordance with the facility's quality assurance committee approved guidelines. If there is no documentation in the chart, the attending physician must write a justification in the chart before an additional length of stay is granted. To keep a patient in the hospital the least amount of days as possible, but as long as medically necessary, is the purpose of length of stay review.

Further utilization review can be accomplished by periodically reviewing specific practices, i.e., relating day of admission and diagnostic tests, determining the effect of preadmission workups on length of stay, and analyzing patterns of postoperative stays. If poor utilization is uncovered, studies should be performed focusing on diagnoses or practitioners with identified or suspected utilization-related problems. Documentation and trending of results is necessary to ensure accountability.

Risk management, which should be included under the quality assurance umbrella, provides for a program to prevent hazardous injuries and risk of financial loss. Risk includes falls, medication errors, medical incidents, or therapeutic misadventures. The importance of incident reports must be stressed to the entire activity so that the system functions and evaluates any unusual incident. Historically, nursing service has been faithful in completing and forwarding incident reports, but anyone who is aware of an unusual incident, or any incident out of the ordinary, should complete a report.

It is obvious that the pharmacy can identify problems in the distribution and administration of drugs on both an inpatient and outpatient basis and should be using incident reports to appraise the quality assurance committee of such. Errors can stem from a variety of problems, such as illegible handwriting, incompatibility, and omission. Many medication errors are of no consequence, but some, however, are deadly.

Moreover, even in an ambulatory care setting, medication errors can become potentially compensable events. If a clinician forgets to explain discoloration of urine when prescribing Pyridium, he or she can forget to explain an effect on driving, such as drowsiness. Or, he or she can forget to tell a patient to take the medication with food or milk, which can produce some discomfort and perhaps noncompliance.

The antibiotic review required by the JCAH must be performed on outpatients and emergency patients, as well as on inpatients. Although this review is vital, it is only an antibiotic review. Consider all the other prescriptions that are written daily and never reviewed. A controlled drug problem may be evaluated on occasion, but the other prescriptions are generally not reviewed except by the pharmacist. A pharmacist is a good ally in the search for, or lack of, quality in the distribution or administration of drugs; he or she should be using incident reports to document identified problems. Accurate incident reporting has several potential benefits, including prevention of future incidents and improvements in patient care, as well as accountability.

The combination of various health workers or professionals in a hospital allows ongoing peer review that can help to achieve quality of performance, but this is not guaranteed. If poor quality work is uncovered, the quality assurance committee must be apprised through use of a resolution report or whatever mechanisms so designated. The objective is to develop a management information system that receives and analyzes problems so that performance-based credentialing can become an actuality.

With the inclusion of risk management under quality assurance, monthly minutes of the safety committee should be reviewed and evaluated by the quality assurance committee, as well as monthly summations of incident reports. Trending of reports can provide valuable information in addressing potentially compensable events. A patient safety audit, with criteria tailored specifically to the hospital, can be conducted to assist in the identification of possible problems and, for example, could identify that a helicopter safety education class should be conducted for personnel who assist in transferring medical evacuation patients. The committee could recommend a class designed to educate personnel to the hazards of approaching and disembarking from aircraft and to familiarize personnel with the complexities involved in an actual flight.

To complete the quality assurance umbrella, a top-level administrator is absolutely necessary for assuming responsibility of the overall management of quality assurance activities. The administrator must ensure the umbrella does not collapse. Administrators should have sufficient personnel to enable them to perform their mission and that of the health center, and administrators should also have the authority to do so. The administrator should encourage teamwork and be able to preclude fragmentation of effort and inefficient use of personnel, to coordinate activities and integrate and utilize data, to initiate remedial action in the alleviation of problems, and to ensure resolution of all such problems. The umbrella of quality assurance must be broad and all-encompassing if it is expected to contribute to an improved staff attitude toward patient data systems and if it is expected to contribute to quality care. However, no umbrella will be able to protect or shield patients from the destructive rays of potentially compensable events without the support of the ribs of administration.

As reflected in JCAH's directives, management and control of any quality assurance/utilization review program requires continual coordination, evaluation, and education. Moreover, compliance with the JCAH's annual review and revision requirements ensures addressing the constantly changing problems in today's health care system. Quality health services rely on teamwork and motivation brought about when the work environment builds a sense of trust and cooperation and when the psychological needs of employees are meshed with the needs of the organization. How well the utilization of resources is combined with the people element, i.e., trust, respect, integrity, self-reliance, cooperation, and pride, will determine the success of quality assurance efforts.

NOTES

1. American Medical Association, *Utilization Review* (Chicago, 1968), p. 1.

2. Joint Commission on Accreditation of Hospitals, *Accreditation Manual of Hospitals*, 1977 ed. (Chicago, 1977).

3. Joint Commission on Accreditation of Hospitals, *Accreditation Manual of Hospitals*, 1980 ed. (Chicago, 1980), p. 151.

4. P.M. Kearns, "Utilization Review Expanded Into Quality Assurance," *Hospitals* 54 (1980):62.

5. American Hospital Association, *Hospital Week* 18, no. 4 (1982):2.

Chapter 17

Combining Risk Management and Quality Assurance

Jesus J. Peña, M.P.A., J.D.; Beatriz M. Peña, M.P.H.;
and Bernard Rosen, Ph.D.

As hospital staff become more aware of the alarming number of incidents happening daily at their facilities and the costly implications of some incidents, more institutions across the country are working toward the creation of programs on loss prevention and examination of problem areas. The same situation has been a source of concern to the Joint Commission on Accreditation of Hospitals, insurance companies, and unions. As a result, a great number of hospitals have developed combined risk management and quality assurance programs that focus on this new dimension of the health care industry.

There is no doubt that quality assurance and risk management share: (1) the commitment to eliminate or reduce problems in patient areas; (2) in efforts aimed at loss prevention; and (3) in analyses of related data.

The four most common reasons for the creation of the combined programs have been:

1. The new quality assurance standard passed by the Joint Commission on Accreditation of Hospitals (JCAH), which went into effect January 1, 1980, set new requirements for risk management and quality assurance programs and, furthermore, required their integration.
2. High insurance premiums or the move to self-insurance programs have transferred the problem of risk management from the insurance company to the hospital itself.
3. A more militant attitude on the part of many unions has led to a new awareness of occupational hazards and their implications to employees and patients.
4. The integration of risk management and quality assurance made good business sense as a means to improve patient care, reduce liability, and maintain harmony in the union force.

In support of this theory, the American Hospital Association has suggested that, with the integration of quality assurance and risk management programs, duplication of efforts will be eliminated, total program cost will be reduced, the risk of malpractice loss will be lessened, and hospitals will have in place systematic, effective methods to improve the quality of care.[1]

The roots of risk management are traceable to the malpractice insurance crisis of 1974 to 1976. At that time, those hospitals that sought favored status with commercial insurance carriers established risk management programs. The promise of reduced premiums based on in-house risk identification, evaluation, reduction, or elimination and consequential favorable claims history may have provided the initial motivation of boards of trustees and administrators. Hospitals that self-insured all or part of their potential liabilities and those that participated in captive arrangements were required by federal regulations to initiate risk management programs.[2]

Central Islip Psychiatric Center started to integrate their quality assurance and risk management efforts in 1978 with the reevaluation of the incident review committee. During 1978, a total of 3,293 incidents were reviewed. Accidental injuries represented approximately one-third of all reported incidents. The other major categories were leave without consent, patient fights, and assaults. The manual process caused an apparent similarity of incidents, difficulties in recalling particular details, and a need to establish a systematic way of reporting. The manual count of all incidents for the first time included their analysis and the examination of possible trends. It resulted in the creation of educational programs aimed at reducing risk and upgrading quality of care. This convinced the members of the committee in 1979 to devise a computerized incident report system to provide the administration with detailed information as to the types of incidents, nature, frequency, number and type of witnesses, sex and age of the patient, most common days and hours of occurrence, and other characteristics that could provide indications of trends. The program was aimed in two directions: (1) to improve patient care by minimizing any risk to patient and staff; and (2) to save moneys paid in insurance claims by having an investigation immediately ready to shield the institution against unfounded claims.

By having all incident data available in easy-to-read summary form, it is easy to spot certain trends. Educational programs could be developed to reduce a particular risk. Also, some of the insurance claims could be avoided as a result of the educational programs.

Before the actual computerization of the incidents, it was realized that a clear definition of *incident* was needed and, due to the magnitude of the program, an extensive training phase was necessary to familiarize all members of the staff with the new reporting mechanism, as well as with the new definition.

Instead of narrowing the definition, it was decided to use the broadest concept in order not to miss any incident. *Incident reporting* (instead of *incident*) was defined as "a mechanism for informing the administration of the occurrence of, and circumstances surrounding, individual problematic events (incidents) in a given setting.'' Although the specific criteria for determining whether or not a given event should be considered an incident may vary, incidents are

1. events contrary to plans for, or implementation of, best quality patient care
2. events that inappropriately place some patient or staff member at risk
3. events that put a program or facility in a tenuous legal or political position that may be costly
4. events to be avoided to the greatest extent possible.

INCIDENT REVIEW COMMITTEE

Prior to the establishment of the program, it was debated whether a risk management coordinator or committee was needed to carry out the program and its integration to quality assurance. It was concluded that, from the point of view of risk management, the first step was risk identification, and the oldest method of accomplishing this was the incident reporting system. Once risks were identified, the next step was to analyze, or measure, the risks. Risks can be separated into two classes. The first class includes those risks that require some immediate action to deal with a specific patient, employee, or visitor involved in a specific incident leading to a potential malpractice, Worker's Compensation, or general liability claim. Because patients represent the highest risk group in most hospitals, they deserve the most attention, even though the areas of Worker's Compensation, general liability, and directors' and officers' liability claims are increasing. The first concern is how to deal with the patient involved in a particular incident. The second concern, from a loss prevention or quality assurance standpoint, is how to deal with the circumstances that allowed the incident to occur. The second class consists of potential risks.

The decision was a revamping of the old incident review committee to bring different areas of expertise to the committee to identify problems and provide areas of experience on educational programs aimed at improving quality assurance. It was recognized that utilization review coordinators could assist by pointing out potential problems. The infection control coordinator must work closely with the committee. The entire nursing department is invaluable to this committee since they often have the most direct, immediate contact with the patient. The safety committee must help in identifying and reducing risk. The program evaluation department analyzes patterns and trends. Working with all these groups in a coordinated fashion, in a result-oriented system of problem identification, investigation, evaluation, and development of proper educational programs, was the first step toward a good risk management program.

Educating staff members to understand their responsibility for providing high-quality care in a safe environment from the outset has been accepted as a major element in the risk management program. Because incidents are more often the result of people failures than equipment failures, a well-trained and highly motivated staff is a hospital's best resource for reducing the potential for patient injury.[3]

Prior to the establishment of the program, educational sessions were held to instruct all personnel in the new reporting procedures, with heavy emphasis on the physicians. To analyze the incidents and coordinate the work related to it, clinical and support personnel, a representative from the union, and a representative from the Mental Health Information Service (the branch of the court that protects the patients' interests) were included in the committee. The committee meets every second Thursday afternoon to evaluate the incidents according to their severity. The committee sorts the incidents in descending order as A, B, or C. At the same time, the committee orders investigations when the information is contradictory or when the severity of the incident requires more detailed information. The committee recommends personnel action or the establishment of specific educational programs to prevent the recurrence of similar incidents.

After this process, all incidents are coded and fed into the computer. The committee constantly stresses the importance of prompt reporting, and a deadline of 24 hours after the incident is set for completing all parts of the incident report. Initially, it was debated whether to rename the committee, but it was decided to continue calling it the incident review committee until the total integration of risk management and quality assurance was accomplished.

COMPUTERIZED INCIDENT REPORTING SYSTEM

In 1979 after a full year of operation, the committee decided to institute a fully computerized incident reporting system in order to more easily identify the trends and make the program more viable.

Computer capability was secured on a rental basis. A total of 29 pieces of information were to be coded for each incident, including data identifying the patient; the specific place, date and time of the incident; how many people (patients and/or staff) were involved and what their roles were (aggressor, victim, etc.); the general cause of the incident; and so on. The 29 variables are presented in Exhibit 17-1. Over 30 types of incidents, ranging from animal bites or stings to incorrect medication, assaults, and suicides, were categorized. Exhibit 17-2 lists the incident categories.

Once coded, the information is keyed into the computer and is then available in a flexible form to answer a variety of questions.

An initial report on incidents for a given period of time will generally include a breakdown of types of incidents by service unit. Comparing a series of these types of figures can give an accurate indication of trends in various types of incidents over time. Such reports have to focus attention on relevant questions

Exhibit 17-1 Incident Report Variables

Variable	Columns
Patient #	1–6
Age	8–9
Sex	10
Date of incident	11–16
Time of incident	17–20
Unit (bldg.)	21–22
Ward	23–25
Ward census	26–28
# Employees	29–30
Location of incident	32
Specific location	33–34
Witness present	35
Who involved	36
# of patients involved	37
Type of injury	38–39
Disposition	40–41
Incident class	42
Incident type	43–44
Cause of incident	45–46
Patient's role	47
Action(s) by unit	48–49
Other patient(s)'s #	50–55
Other patient(s)'s role	56
Date report received	58–63
*Date committee signed	65–70
*Committee role	71
*Status after LWOC (Escape)	73
Case coded in incident	76
Incident #	77–80

*Information no longer coded as of January 1981.

and, once problem areas have been identified, more detailed reports can easily be generated that focus on specific types of incidents.

RESULTS

In 1979, the incident review committee analyzed and coded a total of 2,856 incidents. At the time, the average population of the hospital was 2,049 patients. See Table 17-1.

The initial aim was to analyze incidents in relation to the type of unit that housed the patients. Units 1 to 3 housed short-term, young, active patients. They accounted for 28.4 percent of all incidents reported in 1979. Units 4, 5, 6, 7,

Exhibit 17-2 Incident Codes
(Numerically ordered)

1. Suicide death	21. Intentional fire
2. Suicide attempt	22. Theft (alleged theft)
3. Sudden death	23. Sexual abuse (forced)
4. Accidental death	25. Verbal abuse
5. Homicide	26. Physical health episode (fainting,
6. Assault	seizures, etc.)
7. Patient fight	27. Injury found by employee (of un-
8. Accidental injury	known origin)
10. Serious drug reaction	28. Animal bite or sting
11. Medication error	29. Choking
12. Patient abuse—(pending)	30. Drinking
13. Escape	31. Destructive behavior
14. Self-inflicted injury	32. Attempted LWOC (Escape)
15. Property damage	33. Leave without consent
16. Sexual act between consenting	34. Abuse confirmed
adults	35. Abuse dismissed
17. Property damage *plus* injury	40. Other
18. Drug abuse (pot smoking)	
19. Drug overdose	
20. Accidental fire	

8, and 9 housed geriatric patients. They accounted for 48.3 percent of all incidents, but they amount to 77.9 percent of all patients at Central Islip Psychiatric Center. Unit 10 housed 210 very ill patients, combining long-term patients, patients committed under court order, and a security ward for aggressive and crisis patients. It accounted for 17.3 percent of all incidents reported. Unit 11 housed a 99-bed, medical/surgical unit that provided medical and surgical services to the inpatient population of three large psychiatric hospitals in the area (approximately 8,000 patients in the three hospitals). Unit 11 was staffed following general hospital guidelines and with the same standards for utilization review. The number of incidents reported represented 2.6 percent of all reported. Unit 12 housed a 56-bed Community Preparation Program aimed at preparing long-term patients for community placement. It accounted for 3.3 percent of all incidents.

After the review of incidents by buildings, the incident review committee decided to look into the types of incidents by shifts. See Table 17-2.

The findings were that 43.4 percent of all incidents happened during the daytime; 42.1 percent took place during the evening; and 14.5 percent during the night shift.

The analysis of Table 17-2 provided the hospital with an insight on the most common types of incidents that happened during the day—accidental injury,

Table 17-1 Total Incidents during 1979

UNIT #

	1	2	3	4	5	6	7	8	9	10	11	12	Total
No.	498	152	162	328	480	52	80	186	256	494	74	94	2,856
%	17.4	5.3	5.7	11.5	16.8	1.8	2.8	6.5	8.9	17.3	2.6	3.3	100.0
Adj.	92.22	36.19	31.39	10.09	14.13	1.48	3.88	3.54	15.02	19.60	7.71	20.08	12.15
Avg. 1st of month census for period	45	35	43	271	282	292	172	438	142	210	80	39	2049

No. = Actual number incidents during period for unit.

% = Unit's percentage of all incidents occurring in the hospital.

Adj. = # of incidents per month per 100 patients in daily census for that unit. Adjusts incidents for census differences to facilitate comparison across units. Adjustments based on average first of month census for period.

Table 17-2 Most Common Incidents by Shifts (1979)

Type of Incident	Shift			Total
	Night	Day	Evening	
Accidental Injury	194 (17.8)	523 (47.9)	375 (34.3)	1,092
Patient Fight	64 (19.9)	128 (39.7)	130 (40.4)	322
Assault	44 (15)	137 (46.6)	113 (38.4)	294
Self-Inflicted Injury	7 (7.3)	47 (48.9)	42 (43.8)	96
Destructive Behavior	5 (7.6)	34 (51.5)	27 (40.9)	66
Suicide Attempt	3 (5.6)	22 (40.7)	29 (53.7)	54
Leave without Consent	14 (3)	127 (27)	328 (70)	469
Medication Error	5 (20)	15 (60)	5 (20)	25
Health Episode	10 (18.2)	37 (68.2)	7 (13.6)	54
Others	68	170	146	384
	414 (14.5%)	1,240 (43.4%)	1,202 (42.1%)	2,856

assault, self-inflicted injury, and destructive behavior—indicating that the most aggressive types of incidents happened during the day, which has led to the training of staff to cope with this behavior. As a contrast, during the evening, the categories of incidents tend to be more toward self-destruction than aggressiveness, such as suicide attempts.

Assuming that most patients' activities are conducted during the day, it was logical to expect a high number of incidents during this period; but to have almost the same number during the evening was attributed to previous understaffing situations during the evening shift. The committee recommended a redistribution of staff to increase the number assigned to the evening shift. As a result, the number of incidents decreased by 24.9 percent, and the severity of the incidents was also minimized.

It was also observed that a disproportionate number of incidents occurred during hours when shifts were changing. When provided with this information, the administration was able to analyze the specific procedures that were used in various units for patient coverage during the change of shift, and plans were drawn for a more proper distribution of staff according to number of incidents per shift. In some units, it was necessary to start a system of staggering shifts. As a result of this system, the situation was completely eliminated, and the following year not only was there a reduction in the number of incidents, but there was also no discernible pattern of time of occurrence.

The committee instituted a report consisting of a breakdown in the number of incidents in the different categories according to the sex of the patient. See Table 17-3. It was observed that incidents in male wards outnumber incidents in the female wards with the exception of accidental injury, self-inflicted injury, destructive behavior, and medication errors. The "Others" category includes the 31 remaining categories in Exhibit 17-2.

As a result, specific education programs based on behavior modification were developed for the female population to try to change their self-destructive behavior. After a year of evaluation, a decrease was shown in self-inflicted injuries in the female population mainly due to the awareness developed in the staff by the educational programs, which led to an earlier identification of patients with the propensity for self-destruction.

Although the committee discovered that sex was not an important factor in the breakdown of incidents, the opposite situation was evident when the committee analyzed the incidents according to the patients' ages. See Table 17-4. Although patients over 65 comprised 62 percent of the hospital population, they accounted for only 29.4 percent of all incidents.

Table 17-3 Incidents by Sex (1979)

Type of Incident	Sex		Total
	Male	Female	
Accidental Injury	523(47.9%)	569(52.1%)	1,092
Patient Fight	180(55.9%)	142(44.1%)	322
Assault	182(61.9%)	112(38.1%)	294
Self-Inflicted Injury	30(31.2%)	66(68.8%)	96
Destructive Behavior	32(48.5%)	34(51.5%)	66
Suicide Attempt	32(59.3%)	22(40.7%)	54
Leave Without Consent	319(68.0%)	150(32.0%)	469
Medication Error	8(32%)	17(68%)	25
Health Episode	39(72.2%)	15(27.8%)	54
Others	280(72.9%)	104(27.1%)	384
	1,625(56.9%)	1,231(43.1%)	2,856

Table 17-4 Incidents by Age (1979)

Type of Incident	Age Group			Total
	18 to 29	30 to 64	65 to 97	
Accidental Injury	123(11.3%)	360(33.0%)	609(55.7%)	1,092
Patient Fight	96(29.8%)	186(57.8%)	40(12.4%)	322
Assault	97(33.0%)	160(54.4%)	37(12.6%)	294
Self-Inflicted Injury	45(46.9%)	45(46.9%)	6(6.2%)	96
Destructive Behavior	34(51.5%)	26(39.4%)	6(9.1%)	66
Suicide Attempt	28(51.9%)	23(42.6%)	3(5.5%)	54
Leave Without Consent	246(52.4%)	210(44.8%)	13(2.8%)	469
Medication Error	4(16.0%)	7(28.0%)	14(56.0%)	25
Health Episode	11(20.4%)	30(55.6%)	13(24.0%)	54
Others	114(29.7%)	172(44.8%)	98(25.5%)	384
	798(27.9%)	1,219(42.7%)	839(29.4%)	2,856

The committee suggested a series of conferences to increase the awareness and knowledge of the staff regarding suicidal attempts. It was noticed that the population aged 18 to 29, even if they only comprised a small percentage of the patient population, accounted for 51.9 percent of all suicidal attempts, followed by the 30 to 64 age group with 42.6 percent. The over-65 population only accounted for 5.5 percent of all suicide attempts. During 1980, the number of incidents declined by 24.9 percent. This decline was attributed to the success of the computerized risk management program and its educational component.

Starting in 1980, the committee decided to focus more attention on the number of accidents as opposed to the total number of incidents. It was concluded that accidents represent the largest single type of incident reported in the hospital (1,113 were reported for 1980, which was 51.9 percent of the 2,145 incidents reported during the year). The committee examined these 1,113 accidents in an initial attempt to isolate possible patterns that might have provided clues for reducing the center's accident rate.

Table 17-5 presents the number of accidents reported by each unit during 1980 and also indicates the number of patients who were reported to have one or more, two or more, or three or more accidents in each unit. For the center as a whole, 745 individual patients were involved in the 1,113 accidents, with 223 patients being involved in two or more, and 87 being involved in three or more accidents during the reporting period. The number of accidents for individual patients ranged from one to ten. The number of patients in each unit remained fixed during 1980 for comparison purposes. (See Table 17-1.)

Table 17-5 Number of Accidents and Number of Patients Having at Least One, Two, and Three Accidents by Unit (1980)

Unit	Number of Accidents	Number of Patients Having 1 or More Accidents	Number of Patients Having 2 or More Accidents	Number of Patients Having 3 or More Accidents
Unit 1	38	32	6	0
Unit 2	36	29	5	2
Unit 3	41	35	5	1
Unit 4	72	53	14	5
Unit 5	48	42	6	0
Unit 6	198	129	46	14
Unit 7	248	152	55	22
Unit 8	172	120	35	11
Unit 9	142	82	32	15
Unit 10	36	30	4	2
Unit 11	53	48	5	0
Unit 12	4	3	1	0
Unit 13*	25	21	3	1
Tot. Hospital**	1113	745	223	87

*New Unit added to the Hospital 12/30/79

**Total figures (except for Number of Accidents column) are different than the totals of the Unit figures because some patients occupied more than one Unit during the course of the year.

Table 17-6 presents, for each unit, the average first of the month census and the number of accidents reported for the period. The percentage each of these figures represents of the hospital totals is also given in the last two columns. These figures can be used to determine which units seem to have a disproportionate number of accidents as related to their census. The units with the highest proportion of multiple accident patients were Unit 6 (36 percent), Unit 7 (36 percent), and Unit 9 (39 percent). Table 17-7 summarizes this type of comparison into a single index. It shows number of incidents reported per patient in the average daily census.

For the most part, the relationships shown in these tables are expected. The acute admission units have a high and fairly even rate per patient. The chronic units, which include the geriatric admission wards, have noticeably high rates, followed by the Medical/Surgical Unit. These units would be expected to rank high in accidents given the nature of the patients they serve.

Table 17-6 Comparison of Census (Number and Proportion of CIPC Total) and Reported Number of Accidents (Number and Proportion of CIPC Total) by Unit—1980

Unit	Average 1st of Month Census 7/1/79 - 6/1/80	Number of Accidents Reported	% of Total Hospital Patients in Unit	% of Total Hospital Accidents Occurring in Unit
Unit 1	44	38	2.2	3.4
Unit 2	42	36	2.1	3.2
Unit 3	45	41	2.3	3.7
Unit 4	171	72	8.7	6.5
Unit 5	171	48	8.7	4.3
Unit 6	284	198	14.5	17.8
Unit 7	292	248	14.9	22.3
Unit 8	419	172	21.4	15.5
Unit 9	137	142	7.0	12.8
Unit 10	197	36	10.1	3.2
Unit 11	78	53	4.0	4.8
Unit 12	29	4	1.5	0.4
Unit 13	51	25	2.6	*
Total Hospital	1960	1113	100.0%	100.0%

*New Unit

Note: Table 17-7 summarizes this type of comparison into a single index, the number of incidents reported per patient in average daily census.

Table 17-8 presents the number of accidents reported for each unit by shift. In all cases but two (Medical/Surgical and Unit 2), the highest proportion of accidents were reported to have occurred during the day shift. For the facility as a whole, 48.2 percent of all accidents occurred during this shift. In general, the second highest proportion of accidents occurred during the evening shift with the exception of Medical/Surgical and Unit 2 for which the most accidents were reported for this shift.

These patterns seem reasonable given the amount of activity present during the day and evening shifts. What may be surprising is the proportion of accidents that occur during the night shift (19.5 percent in 1980 and 24.5 percent in 1979) when activity should be at a minimum. This may be partly explained by the fact that of the 213 accidents that occurred during the night shift, 149 (70 percent) occurred between the hours of 6 a.m. and 8 a.m. when ward activity is resuming. These 149 accidents represent 13.4 percent of all accidents reported, which may indicate that the early morning hours (when staffing is still low) represents a

Table 17-7 Number of Accidents per Patient in Average Daily Census—1980*

Unit	Accidents per Patient*
Unit 1	7.2
Unit 2	7.1
Unit 3	7.6
Unit 4	3.5
Unit 5	2.4
Unit 6	5.8
Unit 7	7.1
Unit 8	3.4
Unit 9	8.6
Unit 10	1.5
Unit 11	5.7
Unit 12	1.1
Unit 13	6.1
Total	4.7

*Figures are number of accidents reported during the year per patient in average first of month census.

high-risk period. In fact, 30 percent of all accidents occurred from 6 a.m. through 10 a.m.

During 1980, the committee also concentrated on the location of the accidents. In general, the largest proportion of accidents occurred in the patients' sleeping areas and in the dayrooms. This is particularly true of the chronic units. Hall and bathroom areas also account for a large proportion of accidents, with shower and dining areas accounting for the fewest accidents of those areas specifically identified. A large number of accidents also occurred in the "other" category which includes recreation and program areas, staircases, areas outside of buildings and/or off-facility property, and general "other."

The emphasis in this chapter has been on the role of the incident review committee in upgrading the quality of care. How does that role affect the risk management programs?

The incident review committee plays a key role in risk management if it is true that the solution to malpractice problems is the implementation of programs of prevention that will reduce risk to patients. Such programs should be related to general incidents in hospitals, such as falls and medication errors, and to specifically medical incidents, such as events that occur during surgery. Since

Table 17-8 Number of Accidents by Shift by Unit—1980

	Day		Evening		Night		Total**	
	N	%	N	%	N	%	N	
Unit 1	20	(54.1)	10	(27.0)	7	(18.9)	37	(100)
Unit 2	11	(30.6)	17	(47.2)	8	(22.2)	36	
Unit 3	23	(57.5)	17	(42.5)	0	(0.0)	40	
Unit 4	34	(50.0)	24	(35.3)	10	(14.7)	68	
Unit 5	28	(59.6)	9	(19.1)	10	(21.3)	617	
Unit 6	103	(52.6)	48	(24.5)	45	(22.9)	196	
Unit 7	115	(47.3)	74	(30.3)	55	(22.5)	244	
Unit 8	83	(48.8)	47	(27.6)	40	(23.5)	170	
Unit 9	64	(45.7)	56	(40.0)	20	(14.3)	140	
Unit 10	14	(41.2)	13	(38.2)	7	(20.6)	34	
Unit 11	18	(34.0)	27	(50.9)	8	(15.1)	53	
Unit 12	2	(50.0)	2	(50.0)	0	(0.0)	4	
Unit 13	12	(48.0)	10	(40.0)	3	(12.0)	25	
Total	527	(48.2)	354	(32.4)	213	(19.5)	1094	

**Time of incident was not reported in 19 cases. Percentages are based upon totals of available data.

recent court decisions increasingly have held hospitals liable for everything that occurs within them, it is essential that hospitals take appropriate steps to implement programs of prevention that cover the spectrum from identification of risk, to patient grievance mechanisms, to appropriate feedback and intervention.

The absolute commitment and involvement of a hospital's board of trustees and management is crucial to any risk management program. The board has the ultimate responsibility for what happens to patients, from medical care to environmental safety.

A system for regular and prompt reporting of all incidents of patient injury is integral to an effective program of prevention. Staff members must be trained to understand that early reporting of incidents allows early identification of problems, including human error and system problems, and allows for corrective intervention. Of course, staff reporting must be followed by immediate action by department heads. Supervisors' and managers' responses must encourage and support the incident reporting system. An environment in which reprisals are allowed for reporting errors is counterproductive.

The most sensitive aspect of such a system is reporting physician-related incidents. Physicians traditionally have been reluctant to report incidents involving themselves or their colleagues, preferring instead to handle the situations informally. Nurses and certain other personnel traditionally have done the same. For example, the wall of silence that traditionally has surrounded the operating room must be breached.

Once chosen, the risk manager should be invested with enough authority to feel secure that his or her recommendations and those of the risk management committee will be heeded. At the earliest opportunity, the risk manager should make the rounds of the department heads in the institution, spell out his or her responsibilities to them, and request their cooperation in meeting those responsibilities. This task will not always be an easy one because some managers do not appreciate other managers looking over their shoulders. Since this will be a necessary part of the job, the risk manager should try to identify and alleviate potential difficulties at the outset.

The composition of the risk management committee will, of course, be determined by the size and makeup of the hospital, but in all cases those actually delivering the care—physicians and nurses—must be represented. Preferably, the hospital's legal counsel will also sit on the committee. This committee will assist the risk manager in initiating and following through a step-by-step program designed to ensure that the hospital is doing all it can in the area of risk management.

Obviously, a hospital cannot eliminate all of the dangerous medical procedures performed within its walls. An element of risk has always accompanied the practice of medicine and seemingly always will. But the risk manager and the committee should, nonetheless, be attentive to the possibility that certain needlessly dangerous procedures are being performed on the premises. Perhaps a particular medication is still being prescribed through habit even though a safer substitute has been found. It generally will be a simple matter to eliminate this avoidable risk. On the other hand, there may be a physician who is particularly recalcitrant about his or her medication preferences. Then steps should be taken to absolve the hospital of any culpability for the use of a dangerous drug. It may be necessary, in this instance, to have the physician sign a release form removing the hospital from any liability for the drug's use.

In some cases, the hospital that is not able to eliminate a high-risk procedure may be able to limit its use. Certain once-marginal techniques may have proliferated into a routine simply through lack of oversight. The risk manager should work closely with representatives of the nursing and medical staffs on the risk management committee to explore areas in which cutbacks might be made. Decisions regarding changes in the way in which care is delivered should be approached cautiously. Of course, nothing should be done to compromise the quality of care, but there still may be ways of broadening the margin of safety in delivering that care. If the level of risk can be reduced sufficiently, the hospital may more confidently consider assuming that risk itself through an internally funded and operated insurance mechanism. In almost every instance, this self-insurance will prove to be less expensive than that provided by an outside insurer.

Liability was long ago acknowledged by those in industry as a necessary part of the cost of doing business, and so they had to develop means to deal with it. One handy tool they came up with was the "hold-harmless" agreement. These agreements are now commonplace among wholesale and retail suppliers in the business sector, but they are only beginning to be seen in hospitals. A hold-harmless agreement does not pass off legitimate responsibility to another; it merely ensures that the hospital is liable only for that which is of its own doing. Hospitals would do well to enter into such agreements, whenever possible, with the numerous drug and equipment manufacturers to whom they give their business. The manufacturer, for example, not the hospital, should bear the responsibility for the damage caused by a malfunctioning dialysis machine. These agreements will help see to it that the responsibility for negligence always falls in the right place.

A hospital's malpractice premiums of self-insurance reserves are costs that must be passed on to the patient or to a third party payer or be absorbed. The recent sharp increase in malpractice premiums has occurred at a time when government leaders, employers, union officials, and others are becoming seriously concerned about hospital costs. Several states have restricted Medicaid reimbursements; some health insurers are requiring second opinions before surgery; two states have established a broad prospective budget review system; and the new federal administration has proposed a far-ranging cost-containment program. These programs point toward a financial structure that will reward those hospitals that can control liability risks in a cost-effective manner.

CONCLUSIONS

The first step in any risk management operation is risk identification. At Central Islip Psychiatric Center, one of the oldest methods of risk identification, the incident reporting system, was used.

The program was started in 1978. During the first year, the committee reviewed 3,293 incident reports. During the second year of operation, the committee reviewed 2,856, a decrease of 13.3 percent. During the third year, 2,145 incidents were reviewed, a decrease of 24.9 percent from the 1979 figure.

At present, the committee has representation from the medical staff, nursing, administration, legal counsel, program evaluation department, and other committees of the hospital and the unions. Occasionally, it requires the expertise of members of the infection control committee, safety committee, and other committees. This multidisciplinary approach has allowed good and objective evaluation of the different problems. In addition, the multidisciplinary approach has facilitated the creation of educational programs and has helped to develop a constant awareness of potential risks.

Before the committee suggests any training, it helps to identify the need and the objective for the training. Strong preventive measures have been part of the suggestions developed by the committee. A clear interaction has been established between quality assurance, risk management, and other hospital functions as they relate to quality patient care.

The rental of the computer time to implement the system during the first year amounted to $1,000, but that time was also used to experiment with programming of medication to notify the staff when medication hadn't been changed for a long time, if no progress notes had been made, if symptoms had changed, or if there was inadequate response to treatment.

At the end of the third year of the program, the committee is now considering computerizing all safety and fire reports to integrate them with the incident reports and, in conjunction with the quality assurance program, to create a liability control program aimed at reducing the number of incidents, safety violations, fire hazards, potentials for accidents, etc. The new program will be coordinated through an umbrella risk management program that will involve all segments of the facility. The aim is that the combined risk management and quality assurance program will help the administration to make rational decisions regarding utilization of resources in the delivery of cost-effective patient care.

The interdisciplinary nature of the committee facilitated the evaluation of its function. As goals are established to identify, reduce, or eliminate risk, quantifiable criteria are established against which performance can be measured. This technique is explained to personnel in staff training sessions and becomes part of the crucial monitoring for effective action of the risk management function with the understanding that, with the reduction of risk, the quality of patient care will improve and patients and employees will benefit.

Effective steps to minimize losses from incidents that have occurred should receive as much attention as efforts to prevent compensable incidents from occurring.

A risk management program should involve persons who are responsible for the insurance function. Whether the hospital insures fully or retains all or a part of the risk, it should involve persons with insurance experience and expertise in planning and implementation. Not only is it important to achieve an appropriate balance between retention and transfer of risk, but also insurance representatives must be involved in loss control activities and in feeding back claims information so that more refined prevention strategies can be worked out.

NOTES

1. J.E. Orlikoff and G.B. Lanham, "Quality Assurance and Risk Management: Learning to Live Together," *Journal of Quality Assurance* 2 (Fall 1980):8–12.

2. T.A. Dunn, "Self-Insurance Treatment for the Hospital Malpractice Coverage Crisis," *Risk Management* 24 (1978):10–14.

3. M. Jones and D. Dodge, "Training Model Helps Staff Eliminate Risk," *Hospitals* 54 (1980):40–42.

Part V

Conclusion

Chapter 18

The Future of Health Care

Robert M. Refowitz, M.D., Ph.D.

INTRODUCTION

Prediction of the future characteristics of health care is at once a challenging and essentially impossible endeavor. It is safe to state that the delivery system will continue to have three primary components: the institutions, the providers, and the technological and scientific base. In the coming years, each of these will be reshaped by combinations of complex and basically unpredictable social, economic, and political forces. However, given our country's long tradition of political compromises, it is unlikely that there will be any radical departure from the basic fabric of existing resources and institutions.

The major issue in the delivery of health care for the immediate future is cost containment. On the basis of history, adjustments in entitlements and experimentation with financial incentives to the major institutions and/or practitioners should be expected. The current political climate augers for fiscal solutions to what are seen as solely fiscal problems. The results of today's efforts may only be predicted with temerity. This chapter will offer insights into possible significant developments in the future. Its principal focus will be that of the interdigitation of activities of quality assurance and utilization review with the more traditional mainstream of health care.

THE INSTITUTIONS

The term *medical institution* conjures up visions of vast complexes of solid, ultramodern hospital buildings. In addition, there are essential social and economic infrastructures: the insurance system(s), the legal framework for professional practice, the burgeoning malpractice issues, and the basic ethical trust of medicine itself.

The watchwords for the future include cost effectiveness, cost containment, and the quality of care.[1] The adaptability of many of the established institutions will be sorely tested. Hospitals will be forced into competition both with each other and with the ever-widening array of stand-alone facilities (prepaid clinics, emergicenters, etc.). At the same time, hospitals will have to endure the pressures of less liberal reimbursement incomes.[2] For-profit institutions will continue their expansion, and money will become the central issue for much of the health care system. Not only will money become relevant for total operational costs but also for its relationship with the ethics and behavior of health care providers. A primary profit maximizer (i.e., businessman) and the public's expectations for a physician are simply not the same.[3,4]

The advent of reimbursement by diagnosis (DRG) makes the hospital responsible for the excesses and inefficiencies of its attending and full-time staffs. The challenge is clear; the institutions must assume control over expenditures. While that would seem straightforward in other settings, the unusual nature of the hospital as the doctor's workshop makes cost containment a complex task. Furthermore, public charity no longer cushions hospitals against their deficits. It is likely that hospital administrators will be caught between the Scylla of capped reimbursements and the Charybdis of the need for tight monitoring of physician-generated expenditures and the competition among local institutions in bed surplus areas for doctors and their patients.

A major force reshaping medical care will be the malpractice problem. Ever-escalating insurance premiums may succeed in driving practitioners (particularly new ones in the high-risk areas of medicine) into institutional (i.e., paid malpractice insurance) settings, while the direct and indirect costs will clearly be passed along to the purchasers of care. Unresolved is the potential limit, if any, to the events and outcomes that will be alleged to be malpractice. Will the solution(s) to the inevitable future crises be some form of no-fault? And will the legal profession allow a lucrative aspect of its endeavor to be summarily ended?

Clearcut malpractice rarely has been the problem for the system; usually these cases are readily settled. The dilemma is where to draw the line(s) between the unsatisfactory results of a case or the social welfare needs of an individual patient and the definitions of malpractice. Up to this point, malpractice has not been intended to be the cornucopia for the disabled or needy in whom some relationship, however tenuous, can be shown between their infirmities and the receipt of medical care. This social decision is, of course, always subject to change. The case of retrolental fibroplasia rings all too loudly—yesterday's cure is today's "malpractice."

Analyses of malpractice cases reveal that proper documentation and a standard of care compatible with that held nationwide are crucial. With the evolution of increased institutional responsibility, there will be more substantive review of practices and practitioners. While this will incense the "rugged individualist" physicians, it will be a matter of necessity for the institution. The more compliant practitioners will chafe but adapt. It is unfortunate that with regard to malpractice many practitioners feel rather like the main character in Kafka's *The Castle*[5] (the basis for the familiar television show of a few years ago, *The Prisoner*). Practitioners never can quite find out the ever-changing rules, and they never can find out what they've done wrong.

THE TECHNOLOGY

The past decade or so has been one of incredible change in the technology of medicine. So much has happened in recent years that it is difficult for those under 35 or 40 years of age to understand the state of medicine in the first half of this century. Penicillin was first introduced into clinical practice in about 1946. Prior to that, the only antibiotic was sulfa, which had been available only since 1937. Fewer and fewer modern clinicians remember the great scourges of public health—smallpox, yellow fever, cholera, diphtheria, polio—and many might not recognize them today as isolated cases.

Sputnik was launched in 1959, and a scant dozen years later men were walking on the moon. Similar progress has been made in the technology of medical care. Computerized Tomography (CT) scanners are rapidly moving through their fourth generation; computers are creating digitally enhanced angiograms, radioimmunoassay (RIA) techniques are permitting the measurement of minute quantities of biological materials; and monoclonal antibodies have been used experimentally to eliminate the excess digoxin in life-threatening overdose situations. The future is clearly technological; invasive and noninvasive techniques are rapidly providing quantification of heretofore undreamed specificity and precision. Some have said that the danger is, in fact, the increased ability to quantify without a commensurate ability to act. Clearly a balance needs to be struck, although if tradition is maintained, scientific explorations will continue all but unabated.

What will the substance of medical practice be once much of the new technology is incorporated? Will a physical exam be replaced by the handheld scanner used by Dr. McCoy ("Bones" of *Star Trek*)? It is hard to believe that not so very long ago Buck Rogers serials were the Saturday afternoon fare at the movies, and people marveled at the wrist-radio-television, the space travel, and the laserlike weaponry. Will the physician become obsolete?

Artificial intelligence, once the realm of computer theorists, is now rapidly approaching practical application to medical care. Initially, computers provided simple data acquisition and recordkeeping. The next advances were made into real-time monitoring. Critical care units and operating suites are now all laden with sophisticated electronics. The next generation of developments will probably be quite profound. The lines of division between machines and humans will become blurred as interactive decision-making functions become computer based. Such changes will be met with intense opposition from many physicians. Their lack of familiarity with computers and the quantification implicit in computing will be hard to overcome. Such resistance will impede the day-to-day application of this technology and may also serve as a wedge between the "sophisticated" newcomers (often institutionally based) and the "old timers" in the community.

Important new areas of medical computing are differential diagnosis and patient care management. Internist-I, a recently heralded general internal medicine "diagnostic consultant" program models over 500 individual diseases and their 3,500 associated manifestations. It forms differential diagnoses from the relative importance, frequencies, and specific diagnostic values of the several manifestations. It models human procedures by formulating alternative hypotheses and through heuristic algorithms provides what are said to be excellent results in complex cases (e.g., the clinical pathology cases (CPCs) of the *New England Journal of Medicine*).[6]

Computers are quite adept at managing the volume of information that constitutes the basis of medical practice. With reasonable development efforts, microcomputers or time-shared mainframe systems can be created to do much of the recordkeeping and simple patient management. This will go far beyond today's familiar computer-based patient appointment and accounting systems.[7,8,9,10] It is quite practical to put a clinical data base into memory and to use this and well-accepted differential diagnosis decision trees to monitor care. Patient care plans will have to reflect specific goals. To these ends, the computer will act to focus the management to the deliberate pursuit of the stated goals. Testing will be performed in a set sequence and will reflect the constraints of efficiency and cost effectiveness. It will become far more difficult to admit patients to "find out what's wrong with them."

From a utilization review and quality assurance perspective, computer assistance will measurably impact on day-to-day care. Concurrent reviews will be facilitated and, more significantly, will incorporate a requirement for a clear plan based on the history, a physical exam, and reasonable initial lab or X-ray studies. In essence, it will be possible to monitor the efficacy of the several facets of care based on solid expectations for the studies or procedures undertaken.[11,12]

PHYSICIANS

Will patients be dealing just with doctors in the future? Given the groundswell of activity around the fringes of medicine, this is a very germane question. The past decade has seen the revision of nursing practice acts to accommodate nurse practitioners and, in some cases, independent nursing practitioners. In a parallel situation, psychologists, social workers, and many others are staking claims to parts of mental health care. Chiropractic is not dampening its drive for privileges in traditional hospital settings, and the power of a determined group of lobbyists (practitioners and true-believer patients) should not be underestimated. Optometry has gained the use of drugs for diagnosis in many states and the use of therapeutic pharmaceuticals in a smaller but significant number of states. California's Board of Medical Quality Assurance is seriously looking into the evidence that the existing Medical Practice Act unreasonably (unfairly?) excludes approaches that have proven to be effective. To some this is open season on medicine as they know it, but to others it is a long due reform lifting the tyranny of the medical monopoly over disease. Regardless of the current arguments and their validity, this is an idea whose time appears to have come.[13]

The medical education process is far from static. Now that the perceived manpower shortages of the past are all but resolved, the content of the education merits reconsideration. The major issue is the proper preparation of medical personnel to meet the unpredictable challenges of the real world of tomorrow. The interests of the private practitioners and the academics are often different. The uncertainties of the future make it mandatory that appropriate skills be imparted. Openmindedness about computerization must be commonplace, and the whole process of practicing medicine must be available for scrutiny and adaptation. Students should be selected for their adaptability, maturity, and interpersonal skills. It may not be long before the role of rote memory is all but eliminated in routine medicine. The more openly discussed cheating by students must also be actively explored. Perhaps it is a real clue that the actual (rather than the stated) goals of the educational process need change. Why reward the best recall of simple facts when they are readily available to all? Appropriate role models for the future must be identified and nourished. Most medical practice is relatively isolated despite the trappings of professional cross-fertilization. An unimpeachable intellectual honesty is a worthy goal for selection and training. That would be the best equipment for an otherwise qualified aspiring physician.

Subspecialization, while the brunt of many well-deserved jokes, is a rather serious issue for the future. The trend to subspecialization has been seen as a way of dealing with the uncertainty of medicine (i.e., a better chance of mastering at least one small field); as a prestige item or status; and as a straightforward means of increasing professional earnings. All are correct to some extent. The emergence of a revitalized primary care focus (family and primary care) among physicians is welcomed as it meets the needs of the vast majority of medical problems that are either self-limited or relatively straightforward. The dilemma is how to maintain a proper balance between these generalists and the increasing sub- and subsubspecialists. It is further exacerbated by the economic realities of supply and demand. Subspecialists are now diffusing into all but the smallest communities, and the prevalence of diseases dictates that they must practice general medicine or surgery. What is the proper balance of generalists and specialists? How will the public's interests best be served?

A related development in medical "turf allocation" is so-called "specialty licensing." In essence, this limits the professional's scope of practice by criteria as yet unestablished. Although this idea properly reflects the realities of modern medicine, it further fragments the unity of its authority and, in a way, invites the proliferation of alternative providers. With the possible exception of some generalists, it would seem that the threat of malpractice action would serve to keep this quiescent. However, with the increased competition for patients in the future among the greatly increased number of physicians, some abuses are quite inevitable.

A totally different perspective on medicine will be introduced with the growth in the numbers of administratively oriented physicians. Whether they bear the label of preventive medicine, public health, occupational medicine, or quality assurance, the impact will be the same. The performance of physicians will be subject to both scrutiny and disapproval. Physicians, perhaps the last of the rugged individualist professionals, just simply will no longer escape outside accountability.

Despite any coverage in the press, to this point in time little serious quality of care enforcement has occurred outside of the controlled substance area. Some efforts to contain costs have been undertaken, and with them have come some enforcement on overt fraud. Overutilization is often discussed as an area ripe for enforcement, but little if anything has actually been done.

The impending switch of financial reimbursement schemes for hospitals from cost (or cost-plus) reimbursement to either prospective total cost or diagnostic group reimbursement will precipitate major changes in utilization review. The physician, as the *identified* originator of many of the incremental costs of hospitalization, will become a target for cost-containment activities. Initially, these might involve those cases with excessive lengths of stay or totally inappropriate admissions. No financial sanctions would probably be imposed on the physician at first. Once the hospital becomes comfortable with the reimbursement methods, penalties of some type might be inevitable. This would be a complete turnaround from the current situation where extra days of hospitalization are desirable since those days generate a relative "profit" for the hospital. (The average per-day reimbursement exceeds the real daily costs at the end of acute illness stays.) The newly created Professional Review Organizations (PRO) have a more formal cost-containment mandate than their predecessors, the PSROs. It may be anticipated that the PROs will expand on the well-entrenched notion of norms for the treatment of specific (common) diseases. The penalty they might exact for deviation could be substantial and could affect either the institution or the practitioner. If the practitioners are subject to direct penalties, it is likely that their activities can be more markedly influenced. However, as this represents a dramatic change from the present system, it is not likely to evolve quickly.

Another tack in cost containment is provided by the fact that the physician is acting as the patient's agent in expending moneys to secure the patient's treatment. At present, the patient is fully responsible for the hospital charges he or she incurs. Medicare even requires the patient to sign a notice to that effect in the context of PSRO-conducted reviews. If the physician, in his or her actions as the patient's agent, does not exercise his or her responsibility for cost containment properly, shouldn't the patient have recourse? Since the parallel to attorneys and other similar professionals is apparent, it is not surprising that this area has received scant attention in the state legislatures. Nevertheless, the legal doctrines are well established, and under more difficult circumstances they might be applied. It should not be forgotten that ours is not the only possible means of reimbursing physicians. The health maintenance organization (HMO) movement, the British system of capitation and panels, and the traditional Chinese system where the doctor was paid only while the patient was healthy—not during any illness—all offer potential alternatives. Change may be coming to the American medical system.

QUALITY OF CARE

Utilization review and quality assurance are now both formally included in medical practice. This legitimacy does not, however, imply any significant influence. Most of the power of utilization review and quality assurance stems directly from the efforts of the U.S. government in its role as the payer for Medicare enrollees. The overwhelming emphasis has been on cost containment, with quality of care issues taking a secondary role.

Utilization review and quality assurance activities are mandated by the Joint Commission on Accreditation of Hospitals (JCAH). Each institution is, in principle, required to have a vigorous program in these areas. The reality is usually rather different. Utilization review and quality assurance are perfunctory in the eyes of most physicians, and these committees rarely exceed pro forma activity status.

The initial thrust of PSRO was intended to be quality of care. While this never came to pass, societal pressures are mounting for activities of this type. Hospitals, in particular, are under special pressures to ensure quality care. First, they will soon have new financial obligations for cost (and quality) control. Second, malpractice litigation is seemingly ever expanding. And third, the increasing numbers of full-time hospital employees (especially physicians) raises the institution's exposure to lawsuits. Taken as a group, these factors should pressure hospitals to adopt more substantial quality of care efforts.

Public discussion of the existence of impaired physicians has long been overdue. With these admissions, it is now possible to deal with this heretofore "nonproblem." It is probable that real improvements can be effected for some of the impaired practitioners, as well as major changes made in the beliefs of physicians in general. With the acceptance of the concept of impairment, there is the implicit acceptance that there are detectable variations and gradations in the quality of care. There will now be a greater peer awareness of the entire issue and some obligation (as yet unframed) to identify problems for remedial action. Taken as a totality, all of these changes will lead to better care.

The days of the individualist who might say, "I have colleagues but no peers" are ending. The rise of institutionalized medical practice with its large cadres of well-trained practitioners who are not pressured to maintain a practice in the community constitutes a pool of reviewers. This trend in reviewing will increase as full-timers replace or supplement those whose incomes as consultants are derived from direct referrals by community-based doctors. In fact, the recent success of organized medicine in defeating PSROs may backfire. The functions of the PSRO—utilization review and quality assurance—will not be abandoned. Rather, they will be taken up by the providers of payment (e.g., the insurance companies), and the doctors will no longer have the unappreciated luxury of peer reviews.

Other ongoing trends portend equally significant consequences. First, the growing numbers of "closed staffs" at hospitals (in fact or in practice) will heighten the economic turf battles. Second, the tacit supposition that a minimum number of continuing medical education (CME) credits annually equates with continued competence will be questioned. Most practitioners will readily admit that CME can frequently be "time in a chair, awake or otherwise," a signature on the attendance list at an approved conference, or even moneys paid and a certificate picked up at the end of a course. Unless the program is well done and the doctor puts himself or herself on the line in some way (e.g., a test), the value may be very limited. Specialty board recertification will be the way of the future. It might be edged along by a differential reimbursement of some type, the universal American free-market carrot-and-stick approach. Finally, how can medical practice management courses conducted on cruises credibly convince anyone of renewed medical competence?

Another major issue for the future will be medical teaching. Currently, time spent as a teacher brings prestige and often is needed to maintain appointments to medical staffs. Teaching may also meet the personal needs of doctors to further their own educations or those of future physicians. Teaching is a modest surrogate for some minimum standard of quality; however, it may not always be more than that. Titles and appointments are often poorly correlated to abilities and are rarely relinquished or revoked. Teaching is an art, and the need for best teacher awards at most medical schools underscores this.

Last, within the existing framework for medical care reimbursement, the Blue Cross and Blue Shield plans (the "Blues") are perhaps best described as "cost-plus" operations. Their utilization review and quality assurance activities exist in all locations but it is the author's belief that they are far from vigorously pursued. Many younger and healthier people are hospitalized for far more tenuous reasons if they have Blue Cross-Blue Shield than if they are under Medicare's stricter (but far from strict) scrutiny. This may, however, eventually change. The spiraling costs of medical care and the growing awareness on the part of large scale purchasers of care (e.g., the government, unions, and large employers) of the need for and benefits of utilization review and quality assurance will lead to enhancement of these activities.

Quality assurance and utilization review in the future will scarcely resemble the efforts seen today. A combination of greatly improved technology—both in computers and software—and the increase in the numbers of professional quality assurance personnel will facilitate the changes. Record linking between various institutions and practitioners is really not far off; it needs only hardware and moneys. (The IRS computer system is a good example.) Physicians forget that their Medicare and Blue Shield provider profiles are the stuff from which quality assurance activities can readily develop.

The literature is replete with first- and second-generation computer programs for the diagnostic evaluation of patients.[13,14,15,16] They take various probabilities of disease based on symptom complexes and make statistical inferences (often using Bayes' Theorem).[17] At this point in time, the physician plays a crucial role in the decision analysis feedback loop. The future may bring far more sophisticated, stand-alone systems needing much less human interaction.

Computer algorithms for quality assurance and utilization review would be somewhat different than those for diagnosis and far simpler to create. They would be structured around consensus decisions as to the differential diagnosis or workup of major problems and conditions. Both the sequence of evaluation/ testing and the actual content of this process could be readily monitored, with atypical or nonconforming cases singled out for physician review.

Computerization and the centralization of reimbursement data will jointly facilitate better utilization review and quality assurance. According to Donabedian's framework for the quality of care, evaluations can be performed on one of three bases: (1) structure; (2) process; or (3) outcome.[18] Using this framework, quality assurance and utilization review will be propelled from the use of retrospective reviews and structural criteria to a more complete use of concurrent reviews and process criteria. Structure refers to the possession of the so-called proper personnel and facilities by an institution. Process standards measure the ways in which care is delivered—the testing, treatments, and even the formulation of the differential diagnosis. Outcome, the last of the types of criteria, refers to the notion that good care gives a satisfactory outcome. As this is far from certain in current medical care, it is not likely to be applied except in terms of populations. Individual variability still reigns supreme in the determination of the outcome of a specific disease in a particular person.

Cost effectiveness is a natural concomitant of any routine review process. Unneeded lab tests, extra diagnostic studies, or even unnecessary hospital days could be identified. The "therapeutic trial of barium" so irreverently cited in *The House of God*[19] might finally be abandoned. In addition, minimum standards could be set for the case management of certain conditions, the use of radiology and nuclear medicine scans, and other facets of medical evaluation. For example, should all proven myocardial infarctions (MIs) have a predischarge graded exercise evaluation? Should all cholecystectomies (excision of the gallbladder) have intraoperative T-tube cholangiograms? Should all suspected acute cholecystitis patients have a hepatobiliary iminodiacetic acid/diethyl paraisopropyl-iminodiacetic acid scan as their first major test? Shouldn't all permanent cardiac pacemakers be implanted for specific, documented criteria? The possibilities are limited only by the willingness of those in control to declare standards and sustain their power to do so.

Another benefit of increased computerization might be the reduction of the delay time encountered in obtaining most in-hospital test results. In most institutions, the actual result is not on the chart for some time, often days in all but the most common tests. Unless the practitioner is specifically notified of the result(s) or inquires, it is not incorporated into the therapeutic program for the patient until sometimes much later. The often cited response to quality of care initiated inquiries in hospital that arise from unattended problems is "it was ordered" or "requested" or "the slip was sent" or even "it was done." That, in effect, is treating the chart mainly for the benefit of any possible retrospective review, not the patient.

The ritual of daily hospital rounds may be in for serious reevaluation. It is apparent that such a practice is often highly inefficient. It often prolongs hospitalization and potentially places the patient at risk should results reported (to the chart) not be seen as significant for a particular case. The traditional excuse of "it wasn't on the chart yet" was supposed to vanish with the electronic (i.e., paperless) chart. Experience to date with these systems has not shown them to meet their highly touted expectations. That is not to say that such a system is unattainable. Furthermore, as the turnaround time between writing an order for a test in the chart and actually acting on the result may often approach 72 hours in the traditional methods, it may become advantageous (or necessary) for the physician to hook up a personal, portable computer to that of the hospital by telephone. This is already quite commonplace in science and business. With proper and readily available password safeguards and existing technology, this could be implemented today.

If all these potential advances are implemented, there may be some question as to the role(s) the physician would play. Clearly, some activities would not be needed. Autoregulation of blood glucose by sophisticated (implanted or portable) units would obviate much dose setting and even careful dietary controls. Computers might easily monitor every patient in the CCU, step-down/observation units, and paramedic ambulances and perhaps automatically medicate or even defibrillate. The computer is far more attentive to monitoring than any human could ever be, particularly in a routine situation. However, given the complexity of the human condition and biological diversity, physicians or their futuristic counterparts will always be needed. Nonetheless, a caveat is in order.

Natural selection may very well apply to professions. Fortunately, Lamarckian inheritance of acquired characteristics does too.

NOTES

1. J. Hadley et al., "Special Report—The Financially Distressed Hospital," *New England Journal of Medicine* 307 (1982):1283–1287.

2. J. Iglehart, "Health Policy Report—The New Era of Prospective Payment for Hospitals," *New England Journal of Medicine* 307 (1982):1288–1293.

3. R. Cunningham, "Sounding Board—Changing Philosophies in Medical Care and the Rise of the Investor-Owned Hospital," *New England Journal of Medicine* 307 (1982):817–819.

4. "Money and Medical Ethics: Will Patients Stop Trusting Doctors?" *Observer* (American College of Physicians) 2 (1982):2, 15.

5. F. Kafka, *The Castle,* translated by E. Willa Muir (N.Y.: Borzoi Books, 1948).

6. R. Miller et al., "An Experimental Computer-Based Diagnostic Consultant for General Internal Medicine," *New England Journal of Medicine* 307 (1982):468–476.

7. J. Cottrell et al., "Critical Care Computing," *Journal of American Medical Association* 248 (1982):2289–2291.

8. T. Ziporyn, "Computer-Assisted Medical Decision Making: Interest Growing," *Journal of American Medical Association* 248 (1982):913–918.

9. "Medical Data Bank Is Just a Phone Call Away," *Medical World News* 23 (1982):28–30.

10. R. Ball, "Computerized Medical Records: An Idea Whose Price Has Come," *Medical World News* 23 (1982):121, 123.

11. P. Griner et al., "Selection and Interpretation of Diagnostic Tests and Procedures: Principles and Applications," *Annals of Internal Medicine* 99 (1981):453–600.

12. R. Galen and S. Gambino, *Beyond Normality: The Predictive Value and Efficiency of Medical Diagnosis* (New York: John Wiley & Sons, Inc., 1975).

13. J. Carlova, "Will Low-Cost Healers Replace MD's?" *Medical Economics,* August 8, 1974, pp. 84–90.

14. L. Goldman et al., "A Computer-Derived Protocol to Aid in the Diagnosis of Emergency Room Patients with Acute Chest Pain," *New England Journal of Medicine* 307 (1982):588–596.

15. D. Eddy, "Clinical Policies and the Quality of Clinical Practice," *New England Journal of Medicine* 307 (1982):342–347.

16. J. Kassirer et al., "Toward a Theory of Clinical Expertise,' *American Journal of Medicine* 73 (1982):342–347.

17. T. Colton, *Statistics In Medicine* (Boston: Little, Brown & Co., 1974), pp. 71–74, 91–94.

18. A. Donabedian, *A Guide to Medical Care Administration: Vol. II: Medical Care Appraisal—Quality and Utilization* (New York: American Public Health Association, 1969), p. 9.

19. S. Shem, *The House of God* (N.Y.: Dell Publishing Co., 1978).

Index

285